This book is dedicated to the two "sweeties" in my life: Lorin & Alexandra. Thanks for understanding my personal need to write this book.

Many thanks also to my parents, Dr. Mary Ann and Richard Valinski, who spent countless days reading my book and offering suggestions.

HOW TO USE THIS RESTAURANT GUIDE

Many people are under the assumption that it is nearly impossible to "eat right" while "dining out." This book demonstrates that it just isn't so! Many restaurants offer menu items that are low in both calories and fat. In addition, just about every restaurant has menu items that can be modified to meet your healthy eating program.

The information in this book was up-to-date at the time of the printing. All nutritional information from the restaurants was obtained from and reviewed by their corporate headquarters prior to printing.

Before you order foods at these restaurants based on the information in this book, consider the following. Restaurants frequently change menus, recipes, and chefs. In addition, there may be errors in the contents of this book due to typographical mistakes or misunderstandings between myself and my sources. So always verify the information in this book before ordering.

Dining Lean is a guide book that lists menu items including the lowest fat and calorie menu items available at each restaurant. These are not exact prescriptions of what *you* should be eating. As with any book that suggests foods for better health, it is impossible to generalize to the entire population. Always consult with a Registered Dietitian or Medical doctor regarding how to tailor this restaurant guide to your particular health needs. Bon Appetit!

Dr. Joanne Lichten

Dining Lean

How to Eat Healthy in your Favorite Restaurants

Joanne V. Lichten, RD, PhD

Nutrifit Publishing

Dining Lean

How to Eat Healthy in Your Favorite Restaurants

Joanne V. Lichten, RD, PhD

Published by:
Nutrifit Publishing
PO Box 690452
Houston, TX 77269-0452
(281) 955-LEAN
(888) 431-LEAN

Printed in Canada

Publisher's Cataloging In Publication data:
Lichten, Joanne V.
Dining Lean: How to eat healthy in your favorite restaurants/ Joanne V. Lichten.
288p. 22cm. Includes index.
ISBN: 1-880347-90-3: $16.95
1. Nutrition - Handbooks, manuals, etc. 2. Restaurants - United States - Guidebooks. 3. Low-fat diet.

TX907.2   1998
613.2-dc20

Cover design by Pat Packard, Houston

Table of Contents

PART

1

The Beginning

Introduction

Nearly half of all Americans eat out on a typical day.

Eating out used to be a rare social event. Now, as a result of dual career families, business meetings planned around meals, hectic schedules, and fatigue, we eat out more frequently. According to the National Restaurant Association, nearly half of all adults eat out on a typical day. Of the meals we eat out, half of these meals are takeout or delivered food. And...

Many Americans want to eat healthier.

The average American gains a pound a year after they reach the age of 25, contributing to nearly half of all adults being overweight. Studies reveal that Americans are constantly trying to lose weight. Since heart disease is the number one killer in the United States, many of us are also concerned with our serum cholesterol. For those reasons, about 40% of all restaurant customers are trying to eat healthier food items not only at home, but also when eating out. Dining out can no longer be used as an excuse for unhealthy eating habits. Because...

Restaurants are responding with healthy foods.

A recent survey of table service restaurants confirmed that 40% currently feature healthful menu items. Results from another study indicated that nearly half of the restaurants plan to add more nutritious menu items in the future. Even fast food restaurants (representing one third of all restaurant visits) are serving new, good-tasting, healthy foods. And...

DINING LEAN has made it easier than ever to select the healthiest food at every restaurant.

This book provides you with the following information:

■ Your daily recommendation of calories, fat, and sodium.

■ How much calories, fat, and sodium you actually *consume* each day.

■ Calorie, fat, and sodium content of thousands of restaurant food items.

■ "Calorimeter" charts and portion size depictions for estimating the calories and fat grams of *any* food when nutritional information is not available.

■ Exchanges for people with diabetes or on a weight management program.

■ Lists of recommended preparation and serving modifications to request.

Why does DINING LEAN stress low fat menu selections?

In the second chapter, you will discover that it is the excess fat in our diet that is increasing our serum cholesterol and keeping us fatter than we would want to be. Most people don't realize that:

■ Fats have twice as many calories as equal weights of carbohydrates or protein.

■ Fats in the foods we eat are very close in composition to the fat on our body. Whenever we eat more fat than we need - they are just "sucked up" by our fat cells.

■ All fats, whether "healthy" fats (such as margarine or vegetable oil) or "unhealthy" fats (like butter or lard), have the same number of calories and make us *equally* fat.

■ "Cholesterol Free" *does not* mean the product is calorie-free, lower in calories, fat-free, or lower in fat.

■ Simply cutting back on dietary cholesterol is not enough to lower your blood cholesterol; cutting back on your fat intake will.

Therefore, the bottom line is: if you want to lower your serum cholesterol or lose weight decrease your *fat* intake!

How this Book is Organized

The next two chapters in **Dining Lean** include a discussion of nutritional needs and general guidelines for eating out healthy at *any* restaurant. The remainder of the book is organized into separate chapters based on the type of food served. Each chapter, illustrated with easy-to-read comparison charts and lists, contains recommendations on how to reduce your intake of both calories and fat. Nutritional information (calories, fats, and sodium) is provided for all commonly served foods including specific items found at your favorite restaurants. Exchanges are also listed for persons following a diet for diabetes or for weight loss and maintenance. There is no implied comparison of one restaurant against another.

Other Important Information

The calories, grams of fat, and sodium listed in the introductory sections of the chapters were obtained from USDA food composition tables, averages from restaurant's nutritional information, food manufacturers, and scientific literature. The nutritional information listed under each restaurant was obtained directly from that restaurant. Prior to publication, each restaurant reviewed the written text. Calories were listed exactly as the numbers were provided; fat grams larger than one, were often rounded to the nearest whole number for simplicity. Some exchanges were provided by the restaurant but most were calculated by the author using the restaurant-provided nutritional information.

No Nutritional Information Available? No Problem!

Most restaurants do not provide nutritional information. Even if you could find the food in a calorie book, it is still difficult to know how many calories were in *your* food since portion sizes will vary greatly.

For example, if the calorie book lists an *average* roll as having 150 calories, you still don't know how many calories are in *your* roll. What is an *average* size roll look like anyway?

If your calorie guide book states there are 600 calories in a 10 oz serving of lasagna, are you any closer to knowing how many calories you consumed? Is a 10 oz serving of lasagna a small portion or a large one?

It doesn't have to be confusing to accurately calculate the calories in your favorite meals. We just need two pieces of information: ❶ the weight, measurement, or size of the food and ❷ the number of calories per ounce or per a specific measurement of that food. **Dining Lean** provides you with the information you need.

❶   Weight or size of the food. Throughout the book you will find size descriptions of many food items (such as the *"the size of a deck of cards"*). There will also be measurements and drawings depicting portion sizes of many types of foods. These measurements, descriptors, and pictures make it easy to determine the specific measurement or portion size of the foods you selected.

❷   Calories per ounce for specific food items. In **Dining Lean** you will use what the author has termed *Calorimeters* to assist you in calculating the number of calories *at a glance*. All foods have roughly between zero and 200 calories per ounce. Pure fat, such as butter or oil, has 200 calories per ounce. Water, at the other extreme, has zero. All other foods fall somewhere in between these two numbers.

What is a Calorimeter?

The calorimeter is an easy to use chart that illustrates calories in a specific portion. Food items are logically grouped for comparative purposes. The calorimeter, at a glance, will enable you to compare food choices by the ounce and by the serving size. This simple tool enables you to make well-informed food selections. Let's take a look at a calorimeter of *all* foods.

Calorimeter: Calories per ounce

200	Pure Fats
180	Nuts
150	Chocolate Candy
140	Brownie
130	Cookies, Plain Croissants, Cake Doughnuts
120	Chocolate Cream Filled Doughnuts
110	Danish, Cheesecake, Plain & Frosted Cakes, Pasta (plain)
100	Muffins, Coffee Cake, Yeast Doughnuts, Sausage, Fried Meats
80	Bagel, Custard Pies
75	Thin Crust Cheese Pizza, Steaks
70	Bread, Lowfat Muffins, Fruit Pies
60	Ice Cream
50	Fruit Cobbler, Chicken
40	Soft Serve, Ice Milk
30	Fish
0	Water

As you can see, all foods have between zero and 200 calories per ounce. To find out how many ounces are in each food, each calorimeter is accompanied by pictures depicting the most common portion sizes. For example, knowing that a 3 oz portion of meat is the size of a deck of cards, you can easily estimate the calories and fat grams of your meat portion.

Do you want to Lose Weight?

In the next chapter you will learn that by eating 100 fewer calories each day, you can lose a pound a month, effortlessly! To help you lose weight, there are numerous suggestions preceded by a check (✓). Frequently, these suggestions are combined with an example of the calorie and fat savings.

Dining Lean Basics:
Facts about Calories, Fat, & Sodium

Did you know that you can begin losing weight or prevent the typical trend of gaining weight as you age by making *very small* changes in how you eat? This chapter explains how to maintain a healthy weight *and* keep your cholesterol level normal while you enjoy eating out!

$E=MC^2$

There is only one reason why we gain excess weight. It is simply because we **E**at **M**ore **C**alories than our bodies need. There are two general solutions to treat and prevent excess weight gain: ❶ eat fewer calories and ❷ exercise more to burn more calories.

Some diets promote a specific pattern of foods to eat, when to eat it, and exactly how much to eat of it. These programs often state or imply a mindset of the presence of good and bad foods. **Dining Lean**, instead, suggests that each of us determine how many calories we need in a day so we can decide how to best *spend* our calories. Think of the number of calories we need in a day as a budget. When you eat more calories than you need, you will gain weight. When you eat fewer calories than you need each day, you will lose weight. It really is that simple.

The options on how to spend your calories are nearly limitless, but no single food is "off" the program. Certainly, eating all fried foods or high sugar foods on a daily basis would not be healthy. But eating these foods on an infrequent basis is still acceptable. According to research conducted by the author, people who have been successful at losing weight are the ones who have made *slow*, healthy changes in their lifestyle and didn't give up all the foods they love. Typically, when you cut out all the foods you love, it becomes difficult to "stick with the program." Have some flexibility - it's a lot more fun and gives you the greatest chance of success in the long run.

How Many Calories Should I Be Eating?

The number of calories we need every day to maintain our present weight can be calculated using the simple formula below.

Estimating Daily Calorie Needs

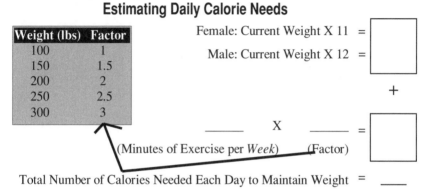

Weight (lbs)	Factor
100	1
150	1.5
200	2
250	2.5
300	3

Female: Current Weight X 11 = ☐

Male: Current Weight X 12 = ☐

+

_____ X _____ = ☐
(Minutes of Exercise per *Week*)   (Factor)

Total Number of Calories Needed Each Day to Maintain Weight = ____

If you want to lose weight, you will have to either ❶ eat fewer calories or ❷ exercise more to burn more calories. Read on to find out how you can eat fewer calories.

A Calorie is a Calorie is a Calorie - Or is it?

Calories come from three basic nutrients: carbohydrates, proteins, and fats. Vitamins, minerals, and water (the other three nutrients) have no calories.

CALORIES

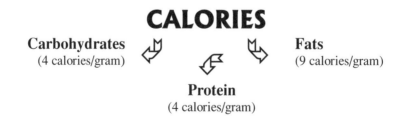

Carbohydrates
(4 calories/gram)

Fats
(9 calories/gram)

Protein
(4 calories/gram)

FACT: Fats are more than twice as caloric (or fattening) as carbohydrates and proteins. While carbohydrates and proteins have only 4 calories per gram, fats have a whopping 9 calories per gram. That translates to approximately 112 calories per ounce of protein or carbohydrates. One ounce of fat has over 250 calories!

That's why you can eat a greater *quantity* of foods that are low in fat than of those that are high in fat. For example, a medium sized apple (high in carbohydrates) has no more calories than two tiny pats of margarine (pure fat).

To illustrate the point further, a cup of white flour has 400 calories and a cup of sugar has 800 calories. In contrast, a cup of oil (pure fat) has 2000 calories!

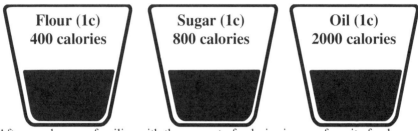

| Flour (1c) | Sugar (1c) | Oil (1c) |
| 400 calories | 800 calories | 2000 calories |

After you become familiar with the amount of calories in your favorite foods, you can decide how to spend your calories so that you are eating fewer calories than you currently eat. The choices can be individualized. For example, if you look forward to dessert you may consider saving calories in your dinner. Check out the difference illustrated in this next example.

A Typical Dinner	Calories	Fat (g)	More Food/Less Calories	Calories	Fat (g)
4 oz. Margarita	240	0	Glass of Wine	100	0
1 sl Bread w/1 t. Butter	125	5	1 sl Plain Bread	80	0
Salad w/ 3T. Dressing	250	24	Salad w/ 1T. Dressing	105	8
Loaded Baked Potato	400	25	Dry Baked Potato	160	1
8 oz. Fried Fish	600	32	8 oz. Broiled Fish w/	250	5
¼ c. Tartar Sauce	320	36	lemon		
Broccoli/Cheese Sauce	125	12	Steamed Broccoli	25	0
			Cheesecake (big 6 oz)	600	35
TOTAL:	2060	134	TOTAL:	1320	49

Both meals represent the same quantity of food prepared in a different manner. The meal on the right side has added dessert (cheesecake!) and still has fewer calories than the meal on the left.

FACT: There are 3500 calories in each pound of body fat. Eating just 10 calories extra every day could contribute to one pound gained each year.

10 calories/day X 365 days = 3650 extra calories a year

That's just 1 hard candy, 1 nibble of a cookie, a sip of soda, *or* a thin smear of butter. Just one of these ten additional calories every day could account for the average one pound many Americans gain each year.

An extra 100 calories consumed each day adds up to nearly a pound a month.

100 calories X 30 days = 3000 extra calories a month

That extra pound each month could come from eating just a third of a doughnut, 8 oz of beer, 8 oz of soda, an extra tablespoon of salad dressing, ²/₃ oz of chips, *or* just 10 French fries extra each day.

Conversely, if you eat just 100 calories *less* each day, you can lose almost a pound a month or 10 pounds a year with very little effort. This book is loaded with numerous small changes you can undertake to make a *major* impact upon your weight.

FACT: The more fat you eat, the fatter you become. Excess fat consumption works against weight control and weight loss efforts in two ways. The first, and more obvious, is the calories per gram as compared to the other two nutrients. The second, and more insidious, is the way our bodies process the fats we eat.

Our bodies change all of the three calorie-containing nutrients (carbohydrates, proteins, and fats) into fuel that our body runs on. Whenever we eat more calories (from any source) than we need each day, our body stores the extra calories as *body fat*.

Eating an extra 100 calories of carbohydrates or an extra 100 calories of protein does not build as much body fat as eating an extra 100 calories of fat. A recent study at the Stanford Center for Research in Disease Prevention demonstrated that dietary fat might be even more caloric than the 4/4/9 ratio indicated.

When we eat more carbohydrates or proteins than we need, twenty three percent (23%) of all the calories are lost in switching the carbohydrates chemically to stored fat. Because the fat that we eat is very much like the fat that we store on our body, very few calories (3%) are needed to convert it. So, nearly all of the fat calories become excess fat on our body. Therefore, fats are probably *three* times more fattening than carbohydrates and proteins.

Simple mathematics makes a demonstrable case for controlling fat consumption. By cutting back on the fats we eat, we can enjoy more real food and lose weight painlessly.

Cut Back on Fats to Decrease Your Cholesterol

FACT: Heart disease is the #1 killer in the United States. Half of all Americans die of heart disease. That's why so many people are concerned about their serum cholesterol level. Levels over 200 mg/dl are considered high for most adults. Research demonstrates that lowering your serum cholesterol level can reduce your risk of developing heart disease.

FACT: Simply cutting back on your dietary cholesterol intake will not lower your serum cholesterol level! Many people think that simply cutting back on the cholesterol content of their food will reduce their serum cholesterol level. While this may have an effect, it is *far more important* to lower your total intake of fat. When you eat *excess fat* your liver simply responds by making *more serum cholesterol*. Cutting back on your cholesterol intake will not necessarily lower your fat intake. Lowering your fat intake usually lowers your cholesterol intake as well.

FACT: There are two types of fats. The fats we eat can be categorized into either HEALTHY fats or UNHEALTHY fats. Decades ago, we were told to simply replace the UNHEALTHY fats with the HEALTHY fats. The HEALTHY fats tend to lower the serum cholesterol while the UNHEALTHY fats tend to raise the serum cholesterol.

HEALTHY FATS (*lowers* cholesterol)	UNHEALTHY FATS (*raises* cholesterol)
Monounsaturated Fats: Avocado Cannola Oil Olive Oil Peanut Oil	**Saturated Fats:** (*Animal*) Bacon Lard Sausage
Polyunsaturated Fats: Corn Oil Cottonseed Oil Soybean Oil Sunflower Oil Safflower Oil	(*Vegetable*) Coconut Oil Palm Oil Palm Kernel Oil **Hydrogenated Fats:** Hydrogenated Vegetable Shortening

Unfortunately, many people believe that HEALTHY fats can be eaten in unlimited quantity. It is not that simple. The *total* fat content of our diets must be lowered. That's why the American Heart Association has been saying for years that we need to reduce our fat intake to less than 30% of our total calories.

FACT: All fats have the same number of calories per gram. Fats all have 9 calories per gram or about 250 calories per ounce. One level tablespoon of butter and margarine both have 100 calories. Oil and lard each have 120 calories per level tablespoon. Although the HEALTHY fats may be a bit better for your heart - healthy and unhealthy fats are both equally fattening!

FACT: Only animals have livers so only animals can produce cholesterol. Cholesterol is manufactured in the liver. Since only animals have livers, only animal products contain cholesterol. That is why cholesterol can be found in animal products such as butter, lard, meat, cheese, and eggs.

FACT: *NO* vegetable products have cholesterol. Vegetables do not have livers so vegetables cannot produce cholesterol. Non-animal products such as wheat, vegetables, fruits, olive oil, margarine, vegetable oils, and tofu (soy bean curd) do not have any cholesterol. A vegetable oil that claims to have "No Cholesterol" may be misleading if you were to conclude that the product has been modified. Vegetables don't have livers; therefore, vegetable oils never had cholesterol and never will.

FACT: Cholesterol Free *does not mean* it is calorie-free or fat-free. "No or low cholesterol" products result from either food that is *naturally* low in cholesterol or from food in which some of the cholesterol has been removed. You can remove the majority of cholesterol from animal products by removing the fat. There is very little cholesterol in skim milk and cheeses made with skim milk. Egg substitutes are made of egg white; the high cholesterol egg yolk has been mostly or completely removed. Unfortunately, some egg substitutes have added vegetable oil, which increases the fat content.

Manufacturers of many "no or low cholesterol" foods have just simply changed the type of fat used in a food product. They may have replaced some or all of the animal fat with a vegetable fat in products such as imitation cheese, crackers, or French fries.

In many cases, a "cholesterol-free" product has just as much fat as the original - and therefore, just as many calories. A vegetable oil is pure fat. Lard (animal fat) is pure fat. Vegetable oil may be a little healthier for your heart, but it is just as caloric as lard. Advertising campaigns have successfully misled many consumers.

FACT: There is no such thing as a no-cholesterol, no-fat oil. You can't remove the fat from oil because vegetable oil is 100% fat - removing the oil would leave you with an empty bottle. Diet margarine has less calories only because some of the fat has been replaced with water and then whipped together. You can't cook well with diet margarine for that reason; the water simply evaporates. Because water has no calories, 100% of all the calories in diet margarine are *still* coming from fat.

Don't believe it if someone tells you that they are frying with a no-cholesterol, *no-fat* oil. There simply is not such a product. There are sprays that have 0 calories per spray (or less than 0.⁵ mg by labeling law) but are still made up of fat. These still need to be used with caution; over spraying can still add on calories.

FACT: Fat-free salad dressings may not really be fat-free. It's true. The Food and Drug Administration allows manufacturers to label foods fat-free if one serving contains less than 0.[5] gram of fat. But one serving is just two level tablespoons. If you eat salads with a large serving of salad dressing, that fat-free dressing could still add up to a significant number of calories and grams of fat. Comparing the same serving sizes, the fat-free salad dressing is still a better choice over regular salad dressing.

FACT: The American Heart Association recommends that Americans eat no more than 30% of their total calories from fat. Simply cutting back on your dietary cholesterol intake *will not* lower your serum cholesterol. That's why the American Heart Association has been recommending for years that we eat less than 30% of all our calories in the form of fat. Simply replacing butter with margarine and frying with vegetable oil instead of lard will not significantly lower your cholesterol. You need to cut back on the total amount of fat.

What Foods Are High in Fat?

Most of the fat we eat is not from visible fat such as butter on bread or on a potato. It is hidden from us in the form of egg yolks, meat, cheese, whole milk, fried foods, foods prepared with fat, salad dressing, margarine on vegetables, or sauces.

FACT: Many foods in their natural state are low in fat and calories.

LOWER FAT FOODS	HIGHER FAT FOODS
Most fruits and fruit juices	Avocados, coconuts, olives, nuts, seeds, and peanut butter
Vegetable juices, vegetables prepared with little or no added fats, starchy vegetables (corn, potatoes) made with little or no added fats	Fried vegetables such as fried mushrooms, onions, okra, zucchini or French fries; vegetables with added fats such as broccoli with cream sauce or greens prepared with bacon drippings; loaded baked potatoes; potato skins
Legumes (beans, peas) prepared with little or no fats	Refried beans
Pasta, plain or with tomato sauce, rice or couscous with little added fats	Pasta with butter or a cream sauce, pasta with a meat sauce, fried rice, "dirty" rice prepared with sausage

LOWER FAT FOODS	HIGHER FAT FOODS
Bread and flour products with little added fats: tortillas, yeast rolls, bagels, pancakes	Cornbread, fried tortillas, biscuits, garlic bread, buttered bread, croissants, waffles, chips, nachos
Most cereals	Granola, cereal with nuts, grits with butter and/or cheese
Desserts such as sorbet, ice milk, lower fat frozen yogurts, low-fat and fat free muffins	Cake, cookies, pies, danish, doughnuts, muffins, ice cream
Skim, nonfat or 1% low fat milk Yogurt, cottage cheese, and aged cheeses made with skim or 1% low fat milk	2% milk, whole milk, yogurt made with whole milk, most cheeses, coffee creamer, non-dairy coffee creamer, sour cream, cream cheese
Egg whites or low fat egg substitute	Egg yolks
Baked or grilled lean protein sources such as fish or shellfish, chicken or turkey without skin, lean beef round, trimmed pork tenderloin, or wild game without skin	Fried shrimp, fried oysters, fried catfish, fried chicken pieces or nuggets, poultry with skin, heavily marbled beef, pork chops, Chicken fried steak, hot dogs, prime rib, hamburger, sausage, bacon
Broth-based soups	Cream based soups
Fat free salad dressing, flavored vinegar, picante sauce	Regular salad dressings
Cooking with herbs, broth or water	Butter, margarine, oil, bacon drippings, lard, hydrogenated vegetable shortening

How much Fat Could I Possibly be Eating?

Picture yourself placing an entire stick of butter on a slice of bread. Roll up that slice of bread and take a bite. Do you think that is disgusting? Well, many Americans eat more fat than the equivalent of a stick of butter each day!

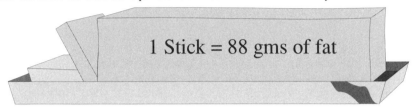

1 Stick = 88 gms of fat

Considering that each stick of butter (or margarine) has 88 gram of fat, let's look at a few typical meals eaten out:

Breakfast	Fat (g)	Italian Lunch	Fat (g)	Mexican Dinner	Fat (g)
2 Scrambled Eggs	15	Salad w/3T. Italian Dressing	26	18 Tortilla Chips	18
3 Slices Bacon	12	Minestrone Soup	5	Mexican Rice	10
1 Spoonful Fried Potatoes	10	2 Buttered Breadsticks	12	3 Cheese Enchiladas	50
Plain Biscuit, 1	8			Refried Beans	10
TOTALS:	**45g**		**43g**		**88g**

These three meals add up to a total of 176 grams of fat or 2 sticks of butter. How much fat do you eat each day? Are you feeling queasy yet?

Calculating the Percentage of Fats in Foods

FACT: The average American eats 35 - 40 percent of all their calories in the form of fat. How do you know if you are hitting the target of "less than 30%?"

Dietary fats such as margarine, butter, oil, or shortening get nearly 100% of all their calories from fat. On the other hand, most of the fruits, vegetables, and starches in their unadulterated state derive less than 10% of all their calories from fat.

FACT: Calculating the percentage of fat in an individual food is easy. To calculate the percentage of fat in a food, use this simple formula:

Calculating the Percentage of Fat in a Food

Step 1→	Grams of Fat X 9	= Calories from Fat
Step 2→	$\dfrac{\text{Calories from Fat}}{\text{Total Calories}}$ X 100 = % Fat	

FACT: Food labels that claim the "percentage *fat-free*" are misleading. Fats have more than twice as many calories as the same amount of carbohydrates or proteins. Therefore, the percentage of calories coming from fat will also be disproportionately higher than it would appear from the numbers on a food label. This is illustrated in the following example.

	½% Milk, 1 c.	Whole Milk, 1 c.
Calories:	90 calories	150 calories
Fat (g):	1 gram fat	8 gram fat
Step 1→	1 X 9 = 9	8 X 9 = 72
Step 2→	9/90= .10	72/150 = .48
	.10 X 100 = **10% FAT**	.48 X 100 = **48% FAT**

Even lean meats can get a large percentage of calories from fat. As you can see, the labeling of a certain percent fat-free (such as 95% fat-free luncheon meats) has *nothing* to do with the American Heart Association's recommendation of 30% fat. The manufacturer is referring to the percentage of *the weight of the product* that is fat-free and not the percentage of *calories*.

	95% Fat-free Meats, 1 oz	Bologna, 1 oz
Calories:	35	72
Fat (g):	2	7
Step 1→	2 X 9 = 18	7 X 9 = 63
Step 2→	18/35= .51	63/72 = .88
	.51 X 100 = **51% FAT**	.88 X 100 = **88% FAT**

FACT: Eating just a "dab" of margarine, oil, or dressing can really add up over time. Even though vegetables and starches, as they are found in nature, are fairly low fat, adding fats can make a BIG difference. All you need for sustained health is "a dab" of fat a day, but instead most of us add "just a dab" to everything we eat. And that adds up quickly as you can see in the next two examples.

Vegetable Salad, without Dressing	Vegetable Salad with 2T. Dressing
Calories: 30	190
Fat (g): 0.2	16

Step 1→ $0.2 \times 9 = 1.^8$	$16 \times 9 = 144$
Step 2→ $1.^8/35 = .05$ $.05 \times 100 = $ **5% FAT**	$144/190 = .76$ $.76 \times 100 = $ **76% FAT**

Yeast Roll, no butter or margarine	Yeast Roll with 1 teaspoon margarine
Calories: 110	145
Fat (g): 1	5

Step 1→ $1 \times 9 = 9$	$5 \times 9 = 45$
Step 2→ $9/110 = .08$ $.08 \times 100 = $ **8% FAT**	$45/145 = .31$ $.31 \times 100 = $ **31% FAT**

These illustrations were to demonstrate that many foods are more than 30% fat. This does not mean that you should not be eating them. There is a far simpler way to decrease our fat intake than calculating the fat percentage in each and every food. A easier way involves three steps:

❶ Determine how many total *grams* of fat you need each day (see the chart on the next page),

❷ Examine the fat grams in each food (using the Calorimeters and nutritional information throughout this book), and

❸ Keep your fat gram intake within the level noted in step 1.

How Much Fat Should I Be Eating?

Fats contribute to the texture and taste of foods, and our satiety level (feeling of fullness) but cutting our fat intake back to 30% is a sensible and achievable level. To calculate 30% of your total calories you eat in a day, use this simple formula:

Calculating 30% of your Total Calories

Step 1→	Number of Calories You Eat X .30 = Calories Coming from Fat
Step 2→	$\dfrac{\text{Calories Coming from Fat}}{9}$ = Recommended *Maximum* Grams of Fat

For example, a person eating 2000 calorie diet each day should keep their fat intake to *less than* 67 grams of fat (2000 calories X .30 = 600 calories from fat; 600/9 = 67 grams of fat). For simplification, use this next chart.

What are the *Maximum* Grams of Fat I Should Eat?

Calories	30% Fat (g)	20% Fat (g)	10% Fat (g)
1000	33	22	11
1200	40	27	13
1500	50	33	17
1800	60	40	20
2000	67	44	22
2500	83	56	28
3000	100	67	33

As referenced earlier, 30% fat level is the *maximum* number of fat grams to be consumed each day, according the American Heart Association. The 20% fat level was included in the previous chart for those people interested in maintaining a lower fat intake.

Some weight loss programs encourage us to decrease our fat intake to less than 10% of our total calories. For most of us, this lower level is not realistic or practical. Because Mother Nature provides a small amount of fat in just about every food item (in it's natural state) you can keep your fat intake to 10% of total calories only if you exclude nearly all meat, chicken, fish, eggs, cheese, salad dressing, oil, margarine, avocados, and nuts. This level of strictness greatly restricts food choices.

Should I Restrict my Sodium Intake?

High blood pressure increases your risk of strokes, heart attacks, and other forms of heart disease. For that reason, the Joint National Committee on Detection, Evaluation, and Treatment of High Blood Pressure recommends that persons with high blood pressure should take off excess weight, cut back on alcohol, increase their physical activity, eat more foods high in potassium, and eat less sodium. Notice that to decrease high blood pressure, reducing sodium is not the *only* recommendation - often losing excess weight brings about more dramatic results.

The typical American eats 4000 milligrams (mg) of sodium eat day while the National Academy of Sciences recommends that healthy individuals consume no more than 2400 mg of sodium per day. A teaspoon of salt contains 2100 mg of sodium. However, very little comes directly from the salt shaker on the table; 80% comes from processed foods.

What Foods are High in Sodium?

LOW SODIUM FOODS	HIGHER SODIUM FOODS
Fresh and frozen fruits and vegetables	Canned vegetables, canned tomato sauce, sauerkraut, soups, broth, canned vegetable juices, processed potato products, olives
Fresh & dried herbs and spices such as basil, cinnamon, curry powder, paprika, and sage; vanilla & almond extracts, lemon juice, vinegar	Table salt, cocktail sauce, soy sauce, most gravies, steak sauce, catsup, tartar sauce, teriyaki sauce, meat tenderizer, garlic salt and other herbs & spices made with salt such as garlic salt, MSG, chili con queso
Chicken, beef, turkey, veal, fish (fresh water & salt water), fresh roast beef or sliced turkey	Bacon, ham, bologna, salami, sausage, pastrami, corned beef, hot dogs, pepperoni, canned tuna & other canned fish, pickled herring, anchovies, prepared meat salads such as tuna salad, casseroles
Pasta, rice, fresh beans	Pasta with sauce, rice prepared with sausage or broth, canned beans
Low sodium cheeses	American and aged cheeses, cottage cheese
Unsalted nuts, unsalted chips, puddings made from scratch	Pickles, salted nuts, potato chips, instant pudding
Oil, unsalted butter *or* margarine	Salted butter & margarine, prepared salad dressings
Fresh fruit, gelatin, frozen yogurt	Baked desserts

General Recommendations to Decrease Sodium

■ Request grilled or baked foods rather than fried foods.

■ Choose fresh meats rather cold cuts or sausage. Avoid smoked or pickled foods.

■ Order salads, burgers, tacos, omelets, and other foods without cheese.

■ Ask that your food be prepared without salt, MSG (monosodium glutamate), or soy sauce.

■ Request unsalted butter or margarine. Ask to have all sauces served on the side.

■ Have salad with minimal dressing instead of soup.

■ Order your sandwich without the pickle.

■ Use lemon or oil & vinegar instead of bottled salad dressings.

■ Ask for fresh fruit instead of chips with your sandwich.

■ Enjoy yeast breads rather than biscuits, cornbreads, or other quick breads prepared with baking soda or baking powder.

■ Order fruit, low fat ice cream, frozen yogurt, or gelatin instead of baked desserts.

Now that you have mastered a basic understanding of your calorie, fat, and sodium needs, the nutritional information in the balance of the book will be more valuable. As an additional reference, read the next chapter on *General Guidelines for Dining Lean*. These are suggestions you can use in any restaurant.

General Guidelines for Dining Lean

If you think you lack the willpower it takes to dine out low fat, read on. There really is no such thing as willpower. What you need to prevent overeating is pre-planning skills. This chapter includes some of the skills that will help you eat right when you are dining out. Each change will deliver significant savings of calories and grams of fat.

Speak to the Manager

It may be difficult to know what to order just by looking at the menu. The staff may also be too busy (or may not know enough about the food) to really help you with your decisions. Instead, contact the restaurant ahead of time and ask the manager specific questions about serving sizes and preparation methods. Tell the manager about your nutritional concerns and ask what they may be able to prepare for you. The best time to call the manager is between the hours of 9 and 11 in the morning and between 2 and 5 in the afternoon.

Be Assertive

At the restaurant, be assertive about what changes you want. If it seems that the server did not understand your request - repeat it and emphasize the words such as "without butter." Send it back if it doesn't come the way you requested it. Remember that *you* are paying for it!

Did Mother say "Never Play with your Food"?

If the food delivered to your table does not comply with your special request and you do not want to wait for another dish to be prepared, feel free to play with your food. Using your knife, wipe off the extra sauce, trim away the fat, or remove the skin off your chicken. Pour the sauce off your dinner plate and onto an empty bread plate. Use a paper napkin to blot away the extra fat on your slice of pizza.

Get the "Doggie Bag" with Dinner

Since most restaurants serve twice as much food as you really need, ask for a doggie bag as soon as you get your dinner. Put half of the dinner in the doggie bag for tomorrow's lunch. Remember that the starving children in Africa will not benefit from your overeating. If you do not carry the extra food in a doggie bag, you will carry it out on your "waist" (*read* "waste") line.

Don't Feel Guilty About Eating

Eating is necessary for sustaining life; eating should be pleasurable. There's no need to feel guilty about enjoying the foods you love. This book was written to educate you on the nutritional value of specific foods available in restaurants. Use this information as a tool to help you decide exactly how you are going to *spend* your calories and grams of fat. A frequent question you should be asking yourself is: "Considering the calories and fat grams in this food, is it worth it?"

This book is not written as a prescription; set your own priorities. One person may order salad *with* dressing and *fried* fish. Another person may eat both the salad and the potato dry and order the fish baked, just so they can "splurge" on a rich, creamy dessert. This book is about making informed decisions.

Eating low fat may require some time to get used to - don't make all of the recommended changes at the same time or you might find the food unpalatable. Make these changes slowly and your taste buds will adapt.

Eat Slowly and Taste Every Bite

Some people eat more than they need simply because they are speed eaters. They are focused on the physical process of eating as opposed to savoring the food. If you don't swallow until all the flavor of the food is gone, you will enjoy the food so much more and you will end up eating less. Logically, this suggestion is more significant when the food contains a lot of calories. If you have decided to spend the extra calories on a dessert, for example, take thin slivers and savor every bite!

Eat Till you "Feel Fine" - Not Stuffed!

Special occasions, in the past, were celebrated by dining out. The infrequency often led to overindulgence. Today, due to the frequency of dining out, the quantity consumed needs to be moderated. Start listening to your body. Remember that it takes 20 minutes for the full stomach to tell the brain that it is full. So eat slowly! Give the brain time to do its job. Stop when you feel comfortable. Don't feel compelled to clean your plate - the restaurant staff will do that for you.

Concentrate on the Atmosphere

Focus on people you are with and the conversation that is going on around you. Then you can concentrate less on the food.

Proximity can be a Problem

Does just seeing certain foods prompt you to eat? If so, keep food reminders to a minimum. That may sound difficult in a restaurant, but here are some ideas:

- Stay away from all-you-can-eat buffets or at least don't sit next to the buffet.

- Ask for a table away from the steady traffic coming from the kitchen.

- Have the bread, chips, and butter removed from the table or at least moved outside your reach.

- Be assertive with your requests regarding serving sizes; ask for just one piece of bread or just a half serving of a meal or dessert. That's easier than having a full serving and telling yourself to eat just half. Remember you can't eat what isn't there!

- Hand the dessert and liquor menus back to the server.

- Ask the server not to bring the dessert cart to the table.

Have Closure to the Meal

Most of us need a signal that the meal is over. For many of us, it is when the food is gone and the plate is empty. But since restaurants serve more than most of us need to eat using that signal is a prescription for weight gain. Other suggestions for signals include:

- When you've eaten enough and feel *comfortable*, not stuffed, ask for the doggie bag.

- If you will not be taking the leftovers home, ask your server to clear off your plate so you won't have to look at the temptation.

- If the server is nowhere around, make your food unpalatable so you won't continue to nibble. Try salting your food excessively or pouring on the hot sauce. Another method is to get the food out of sight by placing your napkin over the plate.

- Sip coffee or hot tea; use this activity as your signal that the meal is over.

Order the "Luncheon" or "Appetizer" Portion

Some restaurants will allow you to order the "luncheon" portion at dinner for a discounted price. The luncheon portions are generally half of the dinner portions. These restaurants generally do not mention this on the menu - you need to ask.

Studies conducted by University of Pennsylvania marketing professor Brian Wansink, PhD proved that consumers tend to use more of a food product if it comes in a larger package. Is that also true for *you* in restaurants?

Know the Menu Terminology

Knowing how to read and interpret the menu can help you to make wiser decisions. If you don't understand a menu item or the description, *ask* your server.

■ Leaner ways to cook meats and vegetables include broiling, roasting, char-grilling, grilling, poaching, stir-frying, boiling, and steaming.

■ Restaurants may still brush or baste the meats with fats during or after the cooking process.

■ Some meat may be marinated in oil or a high fat substance, which can add both calories and fat.

■ The term "Prime" often refers to meat that is very high in fat.

■ Many restaurants add margarine, butter, oil, or other sauces before serving boiled or steamed vegetables. Ask that it be left off.

■ Terms that indicate a high fat food:

Fried	Pan-fried	Hollandaise
Crispy	Escalloped	Creamed
Creamy	Stewed	In its own Gravy
Buttery	Casserole	Au Gratin
In a Butter Sauce	Hash	Parmesan
In a Cream Sauce	Pot Pie	In a Cheese Sauce

Don't Drink Your Calories!

Always have a calorie-free beverage such as water, mineral water, club soda, unsweetened iced tea, black tea or a diet soda nearby so you can quench your thirst. These fluids also help to fill you up. Watch out for the latest fruit juice sparklers - most have over 100 calories per 10 oz serving. Nearly all restaurants in this book offer some non-caloric options other than water, coffee, and tea.

Look at the measuring cups in your kitchen to become familiar with fluid ounces. Eight fluid ounces is equivalent to a one cup measuring cup. This is about the size of a small Styrofoam coffee cup. Keep in mind that most of us drink these beverages in portions larger than 8 oz.

Most people don't realize how many calories there are in the beverages they drink. Look at the comparisons in the *Beverage* chapter.

Make Appetizers the Meal

Many appetizers are fried; just eating one choice could easily blow your fat allotment for the whole day! But if you are going to eat something fried - at least eat it in an appetizer portion instead of the entree portion.

If you find some leaner appetizers such as shrimp cocktail or beef strips on a skewer - consider making that your entree. Appetizer meat portions are often only 2 to 4 ounces, rather than the 8-10 oz entrée size.

Pasta, in Italian restaurants, is often offered in both the entree and the appetizer portion. Having two or three appetizers for a meal can be a viable option or an appetizer, salad, and some bread.

Breads Aren't Fattening

Plain bread or yeast rolls are relatively low in fat and calories. It's the butter and oil that is added that does the damage. Most plain, unbuttered breads have only about 70 - 80 calories per ounce (the size of an average slice of bread). Garlic bread can often have twice as many calories!

Cornbread, croissants, buttered breadsticks, and muffins can add on substantially more calories than the plain yeast rolls. These are often 100-125 calories per ounce even before you butter them. For more details, see the discussion in the chapter entitled *Breads & Spreads.*

Salads Aren't Always Low Calorie Fare

Raw vegetables are low in fat. But, the dressing and the mayonnaise-laden salads can really add up the fat and calories.

Salad dressings have about 80 calories per level tablespoon and most restaurants are generous! They usually put on 3 or 4 tablespoons (that's about 200 calories of pure fat) on a *small* garden salad. Oil and vinegar isn't much better - remember oil has 125 calories per tablespoon. Read the *Salads* chapter to discover why a salad can sometimes have more calories and fat than a hamburger and fries.

Beware of "Reduced Calorie" Salad Dressings

Don't rely on restaurants to carry very low-calorie dressings. Even if they do have lower calorie dressings, they may not be as low as you had hoped. While regular salad dressings have about 80 calories and 9 grams of fat per tablespoon, lower calorie salad dressings may range anywhere from 6-50 calories and 0-5 grams fat. Generally, salad bars have the lower calorie dressings while the more upscale restaurants select those in the higher calorie range.

Always Ask for Your Dressing on the Side

Don't let the person in the kitchen determine how much salad dressing you like and how many calories you need. Always ask for your salad dressing on the side so *you* can control how much to add. A good way to get a taste with every bite is to dip your fork into the salad dressing and then into your salad.

There are other Low Calorie Dressings Available

Vinegar is almost always available although rarely mentioned as a dressing option. Many of them are flavorful such as red wine vinegar, balsamic vinegar, and tarragon vinegar. A squirt of lemon on your salad may satisfy your palate. Picante sauce (at 10 calories per tablespoon) also makes a great low calorie dressing or a topping for your baked potato.

Bring Your Own Dressing

Some food companies such as Estee, Dieter's Gourmet, Weight Watchers, Skinny Havens, and Pritikin sell dressings in individual, one-serving packets. If you are going to a restaurant that doesn't serve a lower calorie dressing, bring your own!

Stay Away from Fried Foods

Frying generally doubles in the calories in a given food. Appetizers are notoriously the worst because almost everything is fried. Reviewing the examples below, you may begin to realize that fried foods just may not be worth it!

Order Baked or Grilled rather than Fried:		Calories	Fat (g)
Fried Fish, 8 oz		550	25
Baked Fish, 8 oz		240	3
	Savings:	310	22
French Fries, 10		160	8
Plain Potato, ½ c		100	<1
	Savings:	60	8

If it says "Low Fat" is it Really?

Some restaurants use small red hearts or the terms "heart healthy," "low fat," or "light" to designate menu items that are lower in cholesterol and/or fat. According to new regulations by the Food and Drug Administration, the restaurant must now be able to back up the claim. Typically, that information is not on the menu but can be requested from the server. But keep in mind that there is still the possibility that the cook may not follow the preparation instructions exactly.

Request Healthier Fats

Even if butter is served at the table or used in the cooking, margarine or vegetable oil is almost always available. Request this when ordering. Margarine and oil still has the same number of calories, but it's healthier!

Limit the Animal Protein Portions

Beef, chicken, and turkey are good sources of protein but, unfortunately, they also contain fat - especially saturated fats. Chicken, turkey, and fish are generally leaner than beef but the American Heart Association recommends that we eat no more than 6-8 ounces of animal protein *each day*. That's comparable to eating a piece of meat the size and thickness of a deck of cards for lunch and another piece the same size for dinner.

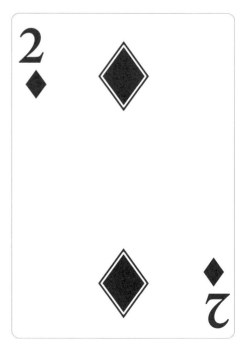

Unfortunately, meat portions served in restaurants are often 6-8 oz at lunch and 8-10 oz at dinner. Occasionally, you will find luncheon portions closer to 3-4 ounces. Ordering appetizers that have 2 or 3 ounces of meat instead of an entree is an excellent way to keep your meat protein to a minimum.

Split an Entree and have an Extra Salad

Again, since entrees are much larger than most people should be eating, consider splitting an entree. Then order an extra salad, a plate of steamed vegetables, or a baked potato.

Simplicity is Best in Entrees

Simply prepared foods are usually the lowest in fats and calories. Butter or oil is often added while cooking the individual servings and can often be omitted if you request. Ask that the vegetables, potatoes, and meats be prepared without added fats.

Broiled foods can be prepared with wine or lemon juice instead of butter. Fish, even with the added fats used when broiling, is usually a better choice than beef. Grilled chicken is almost always offered as well.

Those Little Extras can Really Add Up

Always ask what is added to the menu items that you want to order. Review the chapter on *Salads* to find out how many calories and grams of fat are in salad dressings, croutons, and sunflower seeds. Dozens of sauces are listed in the *Entrees & Sauces* chapter. The chapter on *Mexican Restaurants* discusses the calories in avocados, sour cream, and shredded cheese.

Just a few croutons and a sprinkle of cheese can add an extra hundred calories. Is that how you want to spend your calories and fat? Or would you rather have some dessert? It's up to you!

Order all Sauces on the Side

Most sauces are very high in fat. Unless you know that they are lowfat, it is best to order *all* sauces on the side. That way you can control how much you really want. Dip your fork into the sauce and then into the food for a taste with every bite. This is true for the lemon butter sauce that comes on the fish, the gravy added to the chicken fried steak, the dressing on the salad, and the Alfredo sauce on the fettuccine.

Fill up on Fat-Free Fare

Pure unadulterated starches, vegetables, and fruit are often very low in fat. Plain bread, noodles, potatoes, beans, corn, broccoli, strawberries and melons are all low in fat. It's the toppings that add up the calories and fat grams. A healthy meal includes a small portion of meat and larger amounts of these fat-free fare.

Split Dessert, if You Must

Fruit makes a low calorie and sweet ending to a meal. Even if fresh fruit is not listed on the menu, it is often available. Make sure it is not covered with cream or liquor or served with cheese.

Calories for most other desserts are in the range of 400 to 1000 calories per portion. So if you must, split one with another person or with the whole table. Our taste buds are mostly sensitized to those first few bites anyway. So take small bites and really enjoy it.

Know the Abbreviations and Measurements

Throughout this book, calories and grams of fat are given for a specific measure of a food item. Measurements such as teaspoon or tablespoon refer to level portions not *heaping* spoons!

Take out the measuring spoons and cups out of your kitchen cupboard and use them when serving yourself at home so you can become familiar with how much is served in a restaurant. Use a postage scale to weigh your food portions at home so you can easily estimate the portions served at the restaurants.

Common Measurements:

3 t (teaspoon) = 1 T (Tablespoon)
4 T   = ¼ c (cup)
8 T   = ½ c
16 T   = 1 c

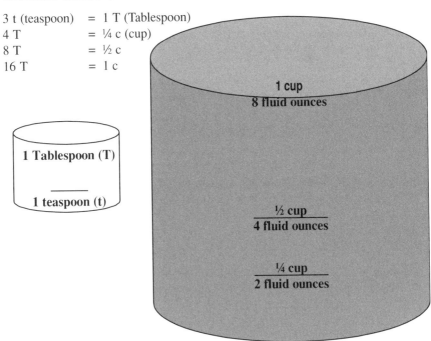

1 cup
8 fluid ounces

1 Tablespoon (T)

1 teaspoon (t)

½ cup
4 fluid ounces

¼ cup
2 fluid ounces

Abbreviations:

c	= cup		med	= medium
cal	= calories		mg	= milligrams
CB	= cheeseburger		na	= not available
ch	= cheese		oz	= ounce (s)
choc	= chocolate		pkg	= package
chol	= cholesterol		pkt	= packet
ea	= each		sl	= slice
fl oz	= fluid oz		sm	= small
gm	= gram(s)		SW	= sandwich
HB	= hamburger		t	= teaspoon
lg	= large		T	= tablespoon
lb	= pound		w/	= with
mayo	= mayonnaise		w/out	= without
			<1	= less than 1

Exchange Abbreviations

Persons with diabetes and people on weight loss programs often use exchanges as simplified way of keeping track of what to eat and how much. Exchanges are lists of foods that are grouped together because they share similar amounts of calories, carbohydrates, proteins, and fats.

Exchanges were provided by some of the restaurants. Whenever possible, exchanges were calculated for the remaining foods listed in this book according to the 1995 edition of Exchange Lists for Meal Planning (American Diabetes Association & American Dietetic Association). For more information or to locate a Registered Dietitian to plan an exchange program for you, call the American Dietetic Association/National Center for Nutrition and Dietetics Hot Line at (800) 366-1655.

Carbohydrate Group:

ST	= Starch
FR	= Fruit
SkMk	= Skim Milk
LfMk	= Low Fat Milk
WMk	= Whole Milk
CHO	= Other Carbohydrates
V	= Vegetables

Meat and Meat Substitute Group:

VLM	= Very Lean Meat
LM	= Lean Meat
MFM	= Medium Fat Meat
HFM	= High Fat Meat

Fat Group:

FAT	= Fat

PART

2

Breakfast, Lunch, & Snacks

Breakfast

Chapter Contents:

- Fresh Fruits, Dried Fruits, & Fruit Juices
- Cereal & Milk
- Eggs & Egg Substitutes
- Breakfast Meats & Potatoes
- Pancakes, Waffles, & French Toast
- Your Favorite Breakfast Restaurants

Most of us are off and running in the morning. Often that means no time for breakfast. No problem, you say, "If I don't eat in the morning I'll have more calories to *spend* later in the day, right"?

WRONG! Research evidence indicates that people, who skip breakfast, eat larger meals later in the day when their bodies are the least active. Breakfast skippers tend to be more overweight than those that eat breakfast.

When you skip breakfast, you are telling your body that you are still fasting from the night before. That signals a lowering of your metabolism throughout the day. Breakfast literally means "**Break Fast**"- the meal that breaks your fast.

Our weekends can be equally disastrous if we sit down to a more leisurely BIG breakfast or brunch. Often these meals are loaded in both fat and calories. This might be all right if we were to "eat breakfast like a king, lunch like a prince, and dinner like a pauper." But how many of us eat dinner like a pauper? Most of us do not!

Even if eaten just once a week, the traditional bacon, eggs, and biscuit meal can put on excessive unwanted pounds. Check out the calories and fat grams!

A High Fat Breakfast:

	Calories	Fat (g)
Orange Juice, 1c	110	0
Bacon & Cheese Omelet	512	42
Hashbrowns, ¾ c	250	15
Biscuit, 3 oz	375	22
Margarine, 2t	70	8
TOTAL:	1317	87

What should you eat? If you like a big breakfast, consider making some of the changes noted in this example.

A Large Healthy Breakfast:

	Calories	Fat (g)
Fresh Orange, 1	65	0
Vegetable Omelet made with Egg Beaters	100	5
Grits, ¾ c unbuttered	110	1
Bagel, 3 oz	240	3
Margarine, 1t	35	4
Jam, 1T	54	0
TOTAL:	604	13

The healthiest breakfast is a low fat, high fiber, high carbohydrate meal. This would consist of fresh fruits and juices, low fat cereals and skim milk, low fat breads, and spreads within your fat limit.

A Smaller Healthy Breakfast:

	Calories	Fat (g)
Fresh Orange	65	0
Wheat Flake Cereal & Skim Milk, 1 c each	190	1
English Muffin, 2 oz	130	1
Jam, 1T	54	0
TOTAL:	439	2

Next time you think you have no time for breakfast - grab a piece of fruit and a toasted bagel or English muffin with minimal margarine. It's not only fast, it's a healthy choice!

One question to ask yourself is "How do I want to spend my calories"? Secondly, and perhaps more importantly, "What breakfast provides me with the energy that I need for my busy day ahead?"

Fresh Fruits, Dried Fruits, & Fruit Juices

✔ **Fresh fruits, dried fruits, and fruit juices are high in vitamins and minerals and have virtually no fat**; they're great ideas for breakfast. Fresh fruits are also high in fiber and will fill you up quickly. Fresh fruit also makes an excellent topping for pancakes, instead of the usual butter and syrup.

✔ **Dried fruits are considered high in calories** even though they are just as caloric as the fresh fruit they are derived from. A raisin has just as many calories as the grape from which it came from. Only the water was removed. Unfortunately, many people have a tendency to eat far more raisins than they would of the fresh grape.

Select Fresh Fruit Instead of Dried Fruit:

	Calories	Fat (g)
36 Raisins or 2T	60	0
36 Small Grapes or 1c	60	0
Savings:	**0**	**0**

✔ **Fruit juices are concentrated in calories**. Ounce for ounce fruit juice has approximately the same calories as most sugar-sweetened sodas. If you are watching your weight, you may want to order the *small* glass of juice. Or better yet, enjoy the high fiber benefits of fresh fruit instead.

Select Fresh Fruit Instead of Fruit Juice:

	Calories	Fat (g)
½ c Orange Juice	54	0
½ c Diced Cantaloupe	28	0
Savings:	**26**	**0**

Fruits, Fruit Juices, & Dried Fruit

	Calories	Fat (g)	Sodium (mg)	Exchanges
Fresh Fruit:				
Apple Ring, ea	15	0	3	¼FR
Apple, whole medium	80	0.5	1	1½FR
Apple, 1/6 slice	15	0	0	¼=1FR
Applesauce, 2T	25	0	1	½FR, ¼c=1FR
Applesauce, ½ c	100	0	4	1½FR
Banana, 1	110	0	0	1½FR
Banana/Strawberry Medley	108	1	6	1½FR
Blueberries, ¼ c	20	0	2	¾c=1FR
Cantaloupe, diced, ½ c	30	0	7	½FR
Cantaloupe, slice	10	0	2	3=½FR
Fig, 1 raw	40	0	1	½FR
Figs canned in heavy syrup, 3	80	0	1	1½FR
Fresh Fruit Chunks, ½ c	60	0	2	1FR

Fruits, Fruit Juices, & Dried Fruit (continued)

	Calories	Fat (g)	Sodium (mg)	Exchanges
Glacéd Fruit, ¼c	50	0	5	1FR
Grapes, 25	60	0.^{5}	2	1FR
Grapefruit, ½	60	0	0	1FR
Grapefruit, canned, ¼ c	25	0	5	½FR
Honeydew, slice	15	0	4	¼FR
Kiwi, slice	10	0	1	6 slices=1FR
Orange, whole medium, ea	65	0	2	1FR
Orange Sections, slice	7	0	0	2 sl=¼FR
Peaches, sliced & drained, 1 pc	20	0	0	3 pc=1FR
Pears, ea	100	0.^{7}	1	1½FR
Pineapple, slice	20	0	1	3 sl=1FR
Pineapple, chunked, 4 pc	20	0	0	12 pc=1FR
Pineapple Bits, 1T	10	0	2	3T=½FR
Prunes, canned, 1	20	0	0	3=1FR
Strawberries, 1 ea	10	0	0	6=1FR
Tangerine, ea	40	0	1	½FR
Watermelon, diced, 1c	50	0.^{7}	3	¾c=1FR
Watermelon, sliced, ea	10	0	1	3=½FR
Dried Fruit:				
Apricots, dried, 7	60	0	1	1FR
Dates, dried, 3	68	0	0	1FR
Figs, dried, 2	95	0.^{4}	4	1½FR
Peaches, dried, 2	62	0.^{2}	2	1FR
Pears, dried,	92	0	2	1½FR
Prunes, dried, 3	60	0	0	1FR
Raisins, 2T	60	0	0	1FR
Fruit Juice:				
Tomato Juice, 6 oz	40	0	0	1FR
Apple Juice, 6 oz	85	0	13	1½FR
Cranberry Juice, 6 oz	110	0	8	2FR
Grape Juice, 6 oz	120	0	5	2FR
Grapefruit Juice, 6 oz	70	0	2	1FR
Orange Juice, 6 oz	85	0	1	1½FR
Prune Juice, 6 oz	130	0	8	2FR

Cereal & Milk

✔ **Select skim or low fat milk** instead of whole milk at breakfast. This substitution will save you a substantial amount of calories and fat.

✔ **Most cold cereals are low in fat** provided you select skim milk to go with it. Granola-type cereals or those with added nuts will have substantially more calories and fat.

Avoid Granola Cereals:

	Calories	Fat (g)
1 c Granola	490	20
1 c Wheat Flakes	100	1
Savings:	**390**	**19**

✔ **Birchermuesli, is a cold cereal consisting of a blend of oats, fruits, and nuts**. Some restaurants use only nonfat plain yogurt in its preparation so it is fairly healthy (the nuts will contain both fat and calories). Most restaurants still prepare it in the traditional high fat Swiss manner using heavy cream or half & half. Ask before ordering this item.

✔ **Grits and oatmeal, prepared plain, are very low in fat,** but the calories go up when fats are added. Ask if the grits can be prepared without butter or margarine. Oatmeal usually is served with milk on the side. Request skim or low fat milk to save calories.

✔ **Sugar has 16 calories per teaspoon**. Doesn't sound like too much you say? One teaspoon a day translates to extra pound and a half of fat each year! Try artificial sweeteners on your cereal or eat it plain. Your taste buds will adjust to the taste difference within a couple of weeks.

16 calories X 365 days in a year = 5,840 calories

5840 calories / 3500 calories = **1.^{7} pounds of fat on your body!**

Cereal & Milk

	Calories	Fat (g)	Sodium (mg)	Exchanges
Cold Cereals:				
Flake Cereal, ½ c	75	1	200	1ST
Granola, ½ c	245	10	45	1ST+1CHO+2FAT
High Fiber Cereal, ½ c	105	0	470	1½ST
Raisin Bran Cereal, 1 c	170	1	370	1¾ST+½FR
Shredded Wheat, 1 c	170	1	0	2ST
Sweet Puff Cereal, 1 c	120	1	200	1½CHO
Wheat or Corn Flakes, 1 c	100	1	290	1½ST
Hot Cereals:				
Oatmeal, ½ c	75	1	300	1ST
Grits, unbuttered, ½ c	75	0.^{5}	300	1ST
Grits, ½ c w/ 1 t margarine	120	6	420	1ST+1FAT
Milk (1c):				
Whole Milk	150	8	120	1SkMk
2% Low Fat Milk	120	5	120	1LfMk
Skim Milk	90	0	120	1WhMk

Eggs & Egg Substitutes

✓ **Eggs are a good source of protein**; one egg has as much protein as an ounce of meat. Egg whites have no fat or cholesterol, but one egg *yolk* contains 5 grams of fat and 270 mg cholesterol. For this reason, the American Heart Association recommends no more than 3 egg yolks per week.

✓ **Order egg substitutes** instead of eggs. Egg substitutes are basically colored and flavored egg whites. Their taste has greatly improved over the years.

Request Egg Substitutes Instead of Eggs:	Calories	Fat (g)
Two eggs scrambled in 1 t margarine	200	15
Egg substitutes scrambled in 1 t margarine	60	4
Savings:	**140**	**11**

✓ **Many restaurants will prepare your order with "egg whites only" or with egg substitutes, even if it is not on the menu!** This includes omelets, frittatas, and even French toast.

✓ **Request that your eggs or egg substitutes be prepared with a non-stick spray.** Otherwise, cooks will use generous amounts of butter or oil to prepare these products.

Eggs	Calories	Fat (g)	Sodium (mg)	Exchanges
Egg, poached or boiled, 1	75	5	70	1MFM
Egg, scrambled or fried, 1	100	8	150	1MFM+½FAT
Egg whites, 2	32	0	100	1VLM
Scrambled Eggs, ¼ c	100	8	150	1MFM+½FAT
Egg substitutes, ¼ c	25	0	80	1VLM
Egg Dishes:				
Eggs Benedict w/ ½ muffin	480	36	1280	½ST+3MFM+4FAT
Vegetable Frittata w/2 eggs	230	15	250	2MFM+1V+1FAT
Meat Frittata w/2 eggs	320	23	600	2MFM+1HFM+1FAT
Quiche Lorraine, 1/6 pie	500	37	460	2ST+2HFM+4FAT
Quiche Florentine, 1/6 pie	410	25	650	2ST+3MFM+1FAT
Quiche, w/ham & cheese, 1/6 pie	460	27	500	2ST+3MFM+2FAT
Omelets:				
Plain, 3 egg	325	26	520	3MFM+2FAT
Cheese, 3 egg	440	36	695	4MFM+3FAT
Ham & Cheese, 3 egg	470	37	850	4MFM+3½FAT
Mushroom, 3 egg	435	37	615	3MFM+1V+4FAT
Mushroom & Cheese, 3 egg	550	47	790	4MFM+1V+5FAT

Breakfast Meats & Potatoes

✔ **Order ham or Canadian bacon instead of bacon or sausage.** Ounce for ounce ham and Canadian bacon is higher in protein and lower in fat. Some people add bacon and sausage to their breakfast thinking they are high in protein. Yet more than 70% of their calories comes from *fat!*

	Bacon, 1 slice	Sausage, 1 oz patty
Calories:	36	100
Fat (g):	3	8
Step 1➜	3 X 9 = 27	8 X 9 = 72
Step 2➜	27/36 = .75	72/100 = .72
	.75 X 100 = **75% FAT**	.72 X 100 = **72% FAT**

✔ **All we need is just six ounces of protein a day** or meat the size of two decks of playing cards. Each egg or serving of egg substitutes counts as an ounce of meat. What meal and source of protein would best satisfy your needs? It's up to you.

✔ **Bacon, ham, sausage, and smoked salmon are all high in sodium** that is added during the processing.

✔ For breakfast steaks and other meats, see the *Entrée & Sauces* chapter.

✔ **Hash browns, home fries, or any other fried potato products are high in fat.** Most have more than 50% of their calories coming from fat.

✔ **Ask for a substitute of tomato slices, fresh fruit, or unbuttered grits instead.** Most restaurants will comply.

Accompaniments

	Calories	Fat (g)	Sodium (mg)	Exchanges
Breakfast Meats:				
Bacon, 1 slice	36	3	101	1FAT
Breakfast Ham, 1 slice	25	1	295	½LM
Canadian-style Bacon, 1 slice	42	2	360	¾LM
Country Ham, 1 oz	60	4	400	1MFM
Smoked Salmon, 1 oz	35	1.[2]	333	1LM
Sausage, 1 oz patty	100	8	350	1HFM
Sausage, link	52	5	105	1MFM
Breakfast Potatoes:				
Hashbrowns & Home Fries, ½ c	165	10	50	1ST+2FAT
Potato Puffs, ½ c	140	7	460	1ST+1½FAT

Pancakes, Waffles, & French Toast

✓ **Buttermilk pancakes have just 55 calories per ounce**. These shadings demonstrate the size of 1 and 2 ounce pancakes that are ½" thick. If your plate contains pancakes that are 6½" across (an inch wider than this book), you can safely estimate that they are at least 4 ounces or 220 calories each! Whole grain pancakes typically have a bit more calories and fat. They are also heavier so pancakes of the same size as discussed earlier will actually have more calories.

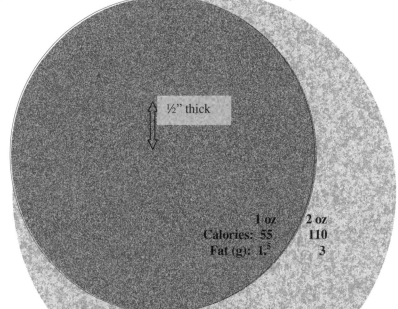

½" thick

	1 oz	2 oz
Calories:	55	110
Fat (g):	1.5	3

✓ **Waffles are higher in fat and calories than pancakes.** Think about sharing the Belgium waffle with a friend.

✓ **Ask for the non-stick spray**. Waffles are usually prepared with a non-stick spray. Request the spray for the pancakes and French toast as well.

✓ **Ask for French toast to be prepared with egg substitute**. This substitution is not available for pancakes since the batter is usually prepared in advance.

✓ **Stay away from deep-fried French toast** unless you can afford the calories.

✓ **Use a minimal amount of syrup**. At approximately 50 calories a tablespoon, the calories in the syrup can be damaging to your waistline. Most restaurants have *diet* syrup (about 10 calories/tablespoon). If your taste buds are not yet ready for the diet syrup, try mixing the regular and the diet together in a small bowl.

✓ **Applesauce, sprinkled cinnamon, and fresh fruit also make delicious, lower calorie toppings.**

✓ Specify "**no butter, powdered sugar, fruit toppings, whipped cream, or other toppings on top.**" Request for these toppings on the side; these additions are what converts pancakes and waffles into nutritional disasters.

Order the Pancakes, Waffles, and French Toast Served Plain:	Calories	Fat (g)
Three 2 oz pancakes, plain	330	9
Plus 1T whipped butter & 1T powdered sugar	110	9
Total:	**440**	**18**

✓ **Order a short stack of pancakes.**

✓ **Order pancakes, waffles, and French toast without meat.**

Pancakes, Waffles, & French Toast

	Calories	Fat g	Sodium mg	Exchanges
Pancakes:				
Buttermilk Pancakes, 2 oz	110	3	460	1ST+1FAT
Buckwheat Pancakes, 2½ oz	135	5	370	1ST+1FAT
Wholegrain Nut Pancake, 2½ oz	160	6	390	1ST+1½FAT
Waffles:				
Small Waffle, 4" X 4" X ½"	100	3	230	1ST+½FAT
Regular Waffle, 4 oz	300	15	460	2ST+3FAT
Belgian Waffle, 6 oz (7" round)	420	20	880	3ST+4FAT
Wholegrain Nut Belgium Waffle, 6 oz (7" round)	450	28	880	2½ST+5½FAT
French Toast:				
Regular-sized Bread, 1 slice	90	2	210	1ST+½FAT
Thick-sized Bread, 1 slice	135	3	315	1½ST+½FAT
Deep-fried toast sticks, order	450	24	475	3ST+5FAT
Sauces & Toppings (1T unless noted):				
Applesauce, ¼ c	50	0	2	1FR
Butter	108	12	123	2½FAT
Diet Syrup	9	0	6	FREE
Fruit Flavored Syrup	55	0	0	1CHO
Fruit Topping	24	0	3	½FR
Fruit Topping, ¼ c	100	0	11	1CHO+½FR
Jelly, Jam, or Marmalade	50	0	3	1CHO
Maple Syrup	50	0	20	1CHO
Margarine	100	11	100	2½FAT
Powdered Sugar	29	0	0	½CHO
Whipped Butter	81	9	80	2FAT
Whipped Margarine	70	7	70	1½FAT
Whipped Topping	12	1	2	¼FAT

Your Favorite Breakfast Restaurants

ARBY'S®

Breakfast Items:	Calories	Fat (g)	Sodium (mg)	Exchanges
Bacon, 2 strips	90	7	220	1HFM
Biscuit, plain	280	15	730	2ST+3FAT
Blueberry Muffin	230	9	290	1ST+1½CHO+2FAT
Cinnamon Nut Danish	360	11	105	4CHO+2FAT
Croissant, plain	220	12	230	1½ST+2½FAT
Egg, portion	95	8	54	1MFM+½FAT
French-Toastix, 6 pieces w/out pow'd sugar	430	21	550	2ST+1½CHO+4FAT
Ham	45	1	405	1LM
Sausage	163	15	321	1HFM+1½FAT
Swiss	45	3	175	½HFM
Table Syrup, 1oz	100	0	30	1½CHO

AU BON PAIN®

	Calories	Fat (g)	Sodium (mg)	Exchanges
Hot Croissants:				
Ham & Cheese	380	20	690	2ST+1½LM+3FAT
Spinach & Cheese	270	16	330	1½ST+½MFM+½V+ 2½FAT
Dessert Croissants:				
Plain	270	15	240	2ST+3FAT
Almond	560	37	260	3CHO+7½FAT
Apple	280	10	180	3CHO+2FAT
Chocolate	440	23	230	3CHO+4½FAT
Cinnamon Raisin	380	13	290	1FR+3CHO+2½FAT
Raspberry Cheese	380	19	300	3CHO+4FAT
Sweet Cheese	390	22	330	3ST+4½FAT
Low Fat Muffins:				
Triple Berry	270	3	560	3CHO+1FR+½FAT
Chocolate Cake	290	3	630	4CHO+½FAT
Gourmet Muffins:				
Pumpkin with Streusel Topping (seasonal)	470	18	550	1FR+3½CHO+ 3½FAT
Raisin Bran	390	11	1030	1FR+3CHO+2FAT
Blueberry	410	15	380	1FR+3CHO+ 3FAT
Carrot Nut	480	23	650	3CHO+1V+4½FAT
Chocolate Chip	490	20	560	4½CHO+4FAT
Corn	470	18	570	4½CHO+3½FAT

AU BON PAIN® (continued)

	Calories	Fat (g)	Sodium (mg)	Exchanges
Danish:				
Danish with Lemon Filling	450	24	410	3½CHO+5FAT
Danish with Sweet Cheese Filling	420	26	380	2½CHO+5FAT
Scones & Other Specialties:				
Cinnamon Scone	520	28	230	4CHO+5½FAT
Orange Scone	440	23	240	3½CHO+4½FAT
Pecan Roll	900	48	480	7CHO+9½FAT

BOB EVANS®

Breakfast: Egg Beaters® can be substituted for eggs in the scrambled eggs or omelets. Request that non-stick spray be used in the preparation of the eggs instead of the liquid margarine. Choose dry toast, English muffin, or bagel with jelly or jam for the leanest bread choice. Request the home fries to be left off.

When ordering Traditional Buttermilk pancakes, margarine is served on the side. Sugar free syrup is available upon request. Other leaner choices include Oatmeal, a Fruit Plate, or Lite Sausage Breakfast (Bob Evans Farms Country Lite™ Sausage Link, Egg Beaters® [prepared with non-stick spray], fresh fruit, and a bagel with Philadelphia Brand Light™ Cream Cheese.

BURGER KING®

Breakfast:	Calories	Fat (g)	Sodium (mg)	Exchanges
Croissan'wich® w/Sausage, Egg & Cheese	550	42	1110	1½ST+2½HFM+4½FAT
Croissan'wich® w/Sausage & Cheese	450	35	940	1½ST+1½HFM+4½FAT
Biscuit	330	18	950	2½ST+3½FAT
Biscuit with Egg	420	24	1110	2½ST+1HFM+3FAT
Biscuit with Sausage	530	36	1350	2½ST+1HFM+5½FAT
Biscuit with Bacon, Egg, & Cheese	510	31	1530	2½ST+2HFM+3FAT
French Toast Sticks	500	27	490	2ST+2CHO+5½FAT
Hash Browns, sm	240	15	440	1½ST+3FAT
A.M. EXPRESS® Grape Jam	30	0	0	½CHO
A.M. EXPRESS® Strawberry Jam	30	0	0	½CHO
A.M. EXPRESS® Dip	80	0	20	1½CHO

CARL'S JR.®

Breakfast:	Calories	Fat (g)	Sodium (mg)	Exchanges
French Toast Dips® w/out syrup	410	25	380	2½ST+5FAT
Sunrise Sandwich®, bacon/sausage not included	370	21	710	2ST+1½HFM+1½FAT
Breakfast Burrito	430	26	810	2ST+2HFM+1½FAT
Scrambled Eggs	160	11	125	2MFM
English Muffin w/ Margarine	230	10	330	2ST+2FAT
Breakfast Quesadilla	300	14	750	2ST+1½HFM+1FAT
Bacon, 2 strips	40	3.^{5}	125	½HFM
Sausage, 1 patty	200	18	530	1HFM+2FAT
Bakery Products:				
Blueberry Muffin	340	14	340	2ST+1FR+3FAT
Bran Muffin	370	13	410	3½ST+2½FAT
Cinnamon Roll	420	13	570	4CHO+2½FAT
Spreads & Syrups:				
Grape Jelly	35	0	0	½CHO
Strawberry Jam	35	0	0	½CHO
Table Syrup	90	0	5	1½CHO
Milk/Juice:				
Orange Juice, 6 fl oz	90	0	0	1½FR
Milk 1% Fat, 10 fl oz	150	3	180	1½SkMk

COUNTRY KITCHEN®

Right Choice™ Menu Items:	Calories	Fat (g)	Sodium (mg)	Exchanges
Pancake Breakfasts (request fresh fruit instead of breakfast meats):				
Blueberry Pancakes	355	12	na	na
Best Cakes in Town, full stack	430	12	na	na
Short Stack of Pancakes	370	10	na	na
Other Breakfasts:				
Garden Omelette (request fresh fruit instead of hashbrowns; dry toast with jelly only)	365	6	na	na
Healthy Egg Breakfast (cholesterol-free eggs, fruit, dry toast & jelly)	310	5	na	na
Hot or Cold Cereal, fruit, 2% milk, dry toast, & jelly	465	6	na	na

DENNY'S®

	Calories	Fat (g)	Sodium (mg)	Exchanges
Fit Fare™ Breakfast:				
Slim Slam w/syrup	638	12	1772	3ST+3½CHO+3LM
Blueberry Topping	106	0	15	2FR
Strawberry Topping	115	1	12	2FR
Cherry Topping	86	0	5	1½FAT
Cereal Combo:				
Choice: Toast, dry, 1 sl	92	1	166	1ST
English Muffin, dry, whole	125	1	198	1½ST
Bagel, dry, whole	235	1	495	3ST
Choice: Oatmeal	100	2	175	1ST
Grits	80	0	520	1ST
Cereal (average)	100	0	276	1ST
2% milk	87	5	70	½SkMk+1FAT
Choice: Applesauce	60	0	13	1FR
Cantaloupe	32	0	16	½FR
Grapefruit, ½	60	0	0	1FR
Grapes	55	1	0	1FR
Honeydew	31	0	22	½FR
Banana, 1	110	0	0	2FR
Banana/Strawberries	108	1	6	1½FR
Choice: Apple Juice	126	0	24	2FR
Grapefruit Juice	115	0	0	2FR
Orange Juice	126	0	31	2FR
Tomato Juice	56	0	921	2V

Breakfast (nutritional information *doesn't* include syrup or margarine):

	Calories	Fat (g)	Sodium (mg)	Exchanges
Original Grand Slam	795	50	2237	4ST+3HFM+5½FAT
French Slam	1029	71	1428	4ST+3½HFM+9FAT
Super/Play It Again Sam	1192	75	3555	6ST+4½HFM+8FAT

Breakfast (nutritional information *doesn't* include bacon or sausage):

	Calories	Fat (g)	Sodium (mg)	Exchanges
Belgian Waffle Supreme	433	23	218	1ST+2½CHO+4FAT

Breakfast (nutritional information *doesn't* include bread choice):

	Calories	Fat (g)	Sodium (mg)	Exchanges
Scram Slam	974	80	1750	2ST+5HFM+8FAT
All American Slam	1028	87	1924	1½ST+6HFM+8FAT
Ultimate Omelette	780	62	1360	2ST+3½HFM+7FAT
Veggie-Cheese Omelette	714	53	955	2ST+3HFM+6FAT
Ham'n'Cheddar Omelette	743	55	1518	1½ST+5HFM+4FAT
Farmer's Omelette®	912	69	1816	2ST+4HFM+1V
Sausage Cheddar Omelette	1036	86	1841	1½ST+6HFM+7½FAT
Eggs Benedict	860	56	1943	3½ST+4MFM+7FAT
Chicken Fried Steak & Eggs	723	56	1505	2ST+3HFM+6FAT
Porterhouse Steak & Eggs	1223	95	1369	1ST+10HFM+3FAT
T-bone Steak & Eggs	1045	82	1191	1ST+8HFM+4FAT
Sirloin Steak & Eggs	808	64	952	1ST+5HFM+5FAT

DENNY'S® (continued)

Other Breakfasts:

	Calories	Fat (g)	Sodium (mg)	Exchanges
Pork Chops & Eggs	555	36	968	1½ST+4MFM+3FAT
Southern Slam	1065	84	2449	3ST+4HFM+10FAT
Moons Over My Hammy (no potato)	807	48	2247	3ST+5MFM+4½FAT
Waffle, plain	304	21	200	1ST+½CHO+4FAT
French Toast, 2 plain	510	25	413	3½ST+5FAT
Pancakes, 3 plain	491	7	1818	4ST+2CHO+1FAT
One Egg	134	12	61	1MFM+1FAT
Sunny Fresh Egg Substitute	94	7	91	1MFM
Ham	94	3	761	2VLM
Bacon, 4 slices	162	18	640	1½HFM+1FAT
Sausage, 4 links	354	32	944	2HFM+3FAT
Hashed Browns	218	14	424	1½ST+2½FAT
Covered	318	23	604	1½ST+1HFM+2½FAT
covered & smothered	359	26	790	1½ST+1HFM+3FAT
Blueberry Muffin	309	14	190	3ST+½CHO+3FAT
Biscuit, plain	375	22	750	2½ST+4FAT
Biscuit & Sausage Gravy	570	38	1475	3ST+7FAT

Other tips: Egg substitutes may be requested instead of eggs in any of the egg dishes. You may substitute fresh fruit or tomato slices for either the breakfast meats or hash browns.

HARDEE'S®

Breakfast Menu:

	Calories	Fat (g)	Sodium (mg)	Exchanges
Rise 'N' Shine™ Biscuit	390	21	1000	3ST+4FAT
Jelly Biscuit	440	21	1000	3ST+2½FR+4FAT
Apple Cinnamon 'N' Raisin™ Biscuit	200	8	350	1ST+1FR+1½FAT
Sausage Biscuit	510	31	1360	3ST+1HFM+4½FAT
Sausage & Egg Biscuit	630	40	1480	3ST+2HFM+5FAT
Bacon & Egg Biscuit	570	33	1400	3ST+2HFM+3FAT
Bacon, Egg & Cheese Biscuit	610	37	1630	3ST+2HFM+4FAT
Ham Biscuit	400	20	1340	3ST+1MFM+3FAT
Ham, Egg & Cheese Biscuit	540	30	1660	3ST+2MFM+2HFM+3FAT
Country Ham Biscuit	430	22	1930	3ST+1HFM+3FAT
Big Country Breakfast®, Sausage	1000	66	2310	4ST+5HFM+5FAT
Big Country Breakfast®, Bacon	820	49	1870	4ST+3½HFM+4FAT
Frisco™ Breakfast Sandwich, Ham	500	25	1370	3ST+2½MFM+2½FAT
Regular Hash Rounds™	230	14	560	1½ST+3FAT
Biscuit 'N' Gravy™	510	28	1500	3½ST+6FAT
Three Pancakes	280	2	890	3½ST+½FAT
Ultimate Omelet™ Biscuit	570	33	1370	3ST+2MFM+3FAT
Orange Juice, 12 oz	140	<1	5	2FR

JACK IN THE BOX®

Breakfast:	Calories	Fat (g)	Sodium (mg)	Exchanges
Breakfast Jack®	300	12	890	2ST+2MFM
Pancakes with Bacon	400	12	980	3¾ST+2½FAT
Sausage Croissant	670	48	940	2½ST+2MFM+7FAT
Sourdough Breakfast Sandwich	380	24	1120	2ST+2HFM+1½FAT
Supreme Croissant	570	32	1240	2½ST+2MFM+4½FAT
Ultimate Breakfast Sandwich	620	36	1800	2½ST+4MFM+3FAT
Hash Browns	160	11	310	¾ST+2FAT
Country Crock Spread®	25	3	40	½FAT
Grape Jelly	40	0	5	¾CHO
Pancake Syrup	120	0	5	2CHO

KRYSTAL®

Breakfast Items:	Calories	Fat (g)	Sodium (mg)	Exchanges
Plain Donut	150	9	135	1ST+2FAT
Donut w/Chocolate Icing	212	11	165	1ST+1CHO+2FAT
Donut w/Vanilla Icing	198	9	135	1ST+1CHO+2FAT
Sunriser	259	17	544	1ST+1½HFM+1FAT
Biscuit	244	12	437	2ST+2½FAT
Bacon Biscuit	308	17	726	2ST+3½FAT
Country Ham Biscuit	334	17	1147	2ST+1½HFM+1FAT
Egg Biscuit	327	19	481	2ST+1MFM+3FAT
Gravy Biscuit	419	26	980	2½ST+5FAT
Sausage Biscuit	437	30	668	2ST+1HFM+4FAT
Bacon, Egg, Cheese Biscuit	421	26	899	2ST+1HFM+3½FAT

McDONALD'S® (Nov 1997)

Breakfast:	Calories	Fat (g)	Sodium (mg)	Exchanges
Egg McMuffin®	290	12	710	2ST+2MFM
Sausage McMuffin®	360	23	740	2ST+1MFM+3FAT
Sausage McMuffin® w/Egg	440	28	810	2ST+2MFM+3FAT
English Muffin	140	2	210	2ST
Sausage Biscuit	470	31	1080	2ST+1HFM+4½FAT
Sausage Biscuit w/Egg	550	37	1160	2ST+2HFM+4FAT
Bacon, Egg & Cheese Biscuit	470	28	1250	2ST+2HFM+2½FAT
Biscuit	290	15	780	2ST+3FAT
Sausage	170	16	290	1HFM+1½FAT
Scrambled Eggs, 2	160	11	170	2MFM
Hashbrowns	130	8	330	1ST+1FAT
Hotcakes, plain	310	7	610	3½ST+1FAT
Hotcakes, w/2 pats margarine & syrup	570	16	750	3½ST+3CHO+3FAT
Breakfast Burrito	320	19	600	1½ST+1½MFM+2FAT

McDONALD'S® (Nov 1997) (continued)

Breakfast:	Calories	Fat (g)	Sodium (mg)	Exchanges
Muffins/Danish:				
Low Fat Apple Bran Muffin	300	3	380	4CHO
Apple Danish	360	16	290	3CHO+3FAT
Cheese Danish	410	22	340	3CHO+4FAT
Cinnamon Roll	400	20	340	3CHO+4FAT

PERKINS® FAMILY RESTAURANT

Breakfast:	Calories	Fat (g)	Sodium (mg)	Exchanges
Low Fat Muffins: Plain	300	3	na	na
Honey Bran	270	3	na	na
Blueberry	270	3	na	na
Banana	330	3	na	na
Low Fat Brownie	280	1	na	na

QUINCYS® FAMILY STEAK HOUSE

Breakfast:	Calories	Fat (g)	Sodium (mg)	Exchanges
Bacon, 1 strip	35	3	100	1FAT
Corned Beef Hash, 4.^{5} oz	210	15	795	1ST+1HFM+1FAT
Scrambled Eggs	95	7	270	1HFM
Country Ham, 1.^{5} oz	90	6	1100	1HFM
Oatmeal, 4 oz	110	2	285	1ST+½FAT
Pancakes, 1.^{5} oz	95	3	250	1ST+½FAT
Syrup, 1 oz	75	0	15	1CHO
Sausage Gravy, 4 oz	70	6	150	1FAT
Sausage Links, 2 oz	225	22	390	1HFM+4½FAT
Sausage Patties, 2 oz	230	23	350	1HFM+4½FAT
Steak Fingers, 3.^{5} oz	360	25	690	2HFM+1ST+2FAT

TACO BELL®

Breakfast:	Calories	Fat (g)	Sodium (mg)	Exchanges
Fiesta Breakfast Burrito	280	16	590	1½ST+1MFM+2FAT
Country Breakfast Burrito	270	14	690	1½ST+1MFM+2FAT
Grande Breakfast Burrito	420	22	1050	3ST+1MFM+2½FAT
Double Bacon & Egg Burrito	480	27	1240	2½ST+1MFM+4½FAT
Breakfast Cheese Quesadilla	390	22	940	2ST+1MFM+3FAT
Breakfast Quesadilla with Bacon	460	28	1130	2ST+2MFM+3FAT
Breakfast Quesadilla with Sausage	440	26	1010	2ST+2MFM+3FAT

WHATABURGER®

Breakfast Items:

	Calories	Fat (g)	Sodium (mg)	Exchanges
Taquito, Potato	446	22	883	2½ST+1HFM+3FAT
Taquito, Sausage	443	26	790	2ST+2HFM+2FAT
Taquito, Bacon	335	16	761	2ST+1½HFM+1FAT
Egg Omlette Sandwich	288	13	602	2ST+1¼HFM+½FAT
Breakfast on a Bun™	455	28	886	2ST+2½HFM+1½FAT
Breakfast on a Bun™ w/Bacon	365	20	815	2ST+2HFM+½FAT
Pancakes, order of 3	259	6	842	3½ST+1FAT
Pancakes, order of 3 w/Sausage	426	21	1127	3½ST+1HFM+2½FAT
Hashbrown	150	9	228	1ST+2FAT
Blueberry Muffin	239	8	538	1ST+1FR+1½FAT
Biscuit, Plain	280	13	509	2½ST+2½FAT
Biscuit w/Bacon	359	20	730	2½ST+4FAT
Biscuit w/Sausage	446	29	794	2½ST+1HFM+4FAT
Biscuit w/Gravy	479	27	1253	2½ST+5½FAT
Biscuit w/Egg and Cheese	434	26	797	2½ST+1HFM+4FAT
Biscuit w/Egg, Cheese & Bacon	511	26	1010	2½ST+1½HFM+3FAT
Biscuit w/Egg, Cheese & Sausage	601	42	1081	2½ST+2HFM+5FAT
Breakfast Platter w/Sausage	785	53	1234	3½ST+2HFM+7FAT
Breakfast Platter w/Bacon	695	44	1162	3½ST+1½HFM+6½FAT
Scrambled Eggs, 2	189	15	211	2MFM+1FAT

Breakfast Accompaniments:

	Calories	Fat (g)	Sodium (mg)	Exchanges
Picante Sauce, 1 pc	5	0	130	FREE
Butter, 1 pc	36	4	42	¾FAT
Margarine, 1 pc	25	3	40	½FAT
Pancake Syrup, 1 pc	180	0	50	3CHO
Honey, 1 pc	25	0	0	½CHO
Strawberry Jam, 1 pc	40	0	15	¾CHO
Grape Jelly, 1 pc	45	0	15	¾CHO

Burgers & Fast Food

Chapter Contents:

- Burgers
- Chicken & Fish
- Roast Beef, Ham, Roast Turkey,& Chicken
- Pitas, Wraps, Potatoes, Chili & Teriyaki Bowls
- French Fries & Onion Rings
- Calculating the Calories and Fat grams in your Fast Food Meal
- Your Favorite Burger & Fast Food Restaurants

Yes, you really can dine lean at a fast food restaurant. The leanest choices include:

- Grilled chicken sandwiches with low fat toppings

- Smaller hamburgers

- Stuffed baked potatoes w/out butter

- Chicken teriyaki bowls

- Chicken fajita pitas

- Smaller "wraps" without dressing

- Salad with fat free dressing

- Low fat soups & chili

- Roast beef, turkey, chicken, or ham sandwiches

- Skinless, roasted chicken with mashed potatoes & gravy

- Barbecue sandwiches made from trimmed lean beef

- Low fat burgers (such as buffalo, turkey and veggie burgers)

Almost anything is acceptable on a lower fat eating program. If you order high fat, high calorie foods, simply balance it by choosing low fat foods throughout the rest of the day so as not to exceed your maximum fat intake as discussed in the *Dining Lean Basics* chapter. Here are some suggestions to follow when you visit a fast food restaurant.

Burgers

Burgers are not the leanest food available at a fast food restaurant, but they are certainly the most popular. While you may be able to select lean ground beef at your local grocery store, this is not typically an option at burger and fast food restaurants. The lowest fat burger meal is a small burger cooked well-done with a minimum of toppings; ask for the buns to be grilled without butter.

✔ **Order the smallest burger available.**

Compare these Burgers:	Calories	Fat (g)
Raw Weight (cooked weight):		
Half Pound (6 oz)	490	35
Third Pound (4 oz)	330	24
Quarter Pound (3 oz)	245	18

Avoid Double Meat Sandwiches:	Calories	Fat (g)
Burger King® Double Whopper® Sandwich	870	56
Burger King® Whopper® Sandwich	640	39
Savings:	**230**	**17**

✔ **Ask for the burger to be cooked well done**. The more you cook the burger, the less fat remains.

Order it Well Done:	Calories	Fat (g)
Third Pound Burger, broiled medium	330	24
Third Pound Burger, broiled well-done	315	22
Savings:	**15**	**2**

✔ **Eliminate the cheese.** Each slice of cheese contains approximately 100 calories. Some burgers have more than one slice. Ask yourself if the taste is worth the calories?

Have it Without Cheese:	Calories	Fat (g)
Jumbo Jack® with Cheese	650	43
Jumbo Jack®	560	36
Savings:	**90**	**7**

✓ **Request the hamburger buns to be grilled without butter or oil**. Many restaurants brush the burger buns with butter or oil before grilling them.

Request the Buns to be Grilled without Butter:		Calories	Fat (g)
Bun with butter		260	12
Bun without butter		160	1
	Savings:	100	11

✓ **Use mustard instead of mayonnaise**. While some restaurants are now offering low fat mayonnaise, few restaurants are offering the fat-free version. Choose mustard instead of mayonnaise for a flavorful, low calorie option. Other low fat dressings include salsa, barbecue sauce, and fat-free salad dressings.

Use Mustard instead of Mayonnaise:		Calories	Fat (g)
1T Mayonnaise		100	11
1T Mustard		15	1
	Savings:	85	10

✓ **Limit the toppings**. Sure they all add flavor, but all these toppings could double the fat grams of your burger. Be selective.

Forget the Extras (or at least some of them):		Calories	Fat (g)
Avocado, ¼		80	8
Bacon, 2 crisp slices		70	6
Cheese, 1 oz slice		90	9
Mushrooms, ¼c sautéed in 1T butter		110	11
	Savings:	350	34

Chicken & Fish

✓ **Skinless, roasted chicken has less than half the fat and calories of fried chicken**. Your fried chicken contains more fat than it appears. Many fats, especially the saturated fats, solidify after cooking and don't look greasy. A wiser choice is to select roasted chicken and remove the skin.

Select Roasted Chicken rather than Fried Chicken:		Calories	Fat (g)
KFC® Original Recipe® Drumstick & Thigh		390	27
KFC® Tender Roast® Drumstick & Thigh,no skin		173	8
	Savings:	217	19

Order Grilled Chicken rather than Fried Chicken:		Calories	Fat (g)
Chick-fil-A Nuggets®, 8 pack		290	14
Chick-fil-A® Chick-n-Strips®, 4		230	8
	Savings:	60	6

✔ **Select a grilled chicken salad with low fat dressing.** Many restaurants offer grilled chicken salad. The salad vegetables and grilled chicken make for a low calorie, low fat meal. If bacon, cheese, avocado, and salad dressing are added they can more than double the calories.

Request Low Fat Dressing for your Salad:

	Calories	Fat (g)
McDonald's® Grilled Chicken Salad Deluxe w/1 pkg Ranch Dressing	350	22.[5]
McDonald's® Grilled Chicken Salad Deluxe w/1 pkg Fat Free Herb Vinaigrette	170	1.[5]
Savings:	180	21

✔ **Request mustard, barbecue sauce, or low fat mayonnaise on your grilled chicken sandwich.**

Get your Grilled Chicken Sandwich plain or with low fat Dressing:

	Calories	Fat (g)
BK Broiler® Chicken Sandwich	530	26
BK Broiler® Chicken Sandwich w/out mayo	390	12
Savings:	140	14

✔ **Avoid the fried chicken or fried fish sandwiches.** Are you choosing chicken or fish because you think they are healthier than beef? Not if they are fried! Unless it says "grilled or broiled" assume they are fried.

Fried Chicken or Fish Sandwiches are not leaner than Hamburgers:

	Calories	Fat (g)
DQ® Homestyle Hamburger	290	12
DQ® Fish Fillet Sandwich (fried)	370	16
DQ® Chicken Breast Fillet Sandwich (fried)	430	20

Order a *Grilled* Fish Sandwich instead of Fried:

	Calories	Fat (g)
Fried Fish Sandwich, average	510	25
Grilled Fish Sandwich w/lettuce, tomato, onion	410	12
Savings:	100	13

✔ **Broiled Fish Lunches are both low fat and filling.** As an alternative to a sandwich, consider a broiled chicken or fish plate which often includes rice, vegetables, bread, and more.

Order a *Broiled* Fish Lunch or Platter such as:

	Calories	Fat (g)
Captain D's® Broiled Fish Lunch	435	7
Captain D's® Broiled Fish Platter	734	7

Roast Beef, Ham, Roast Turkey, & Chicken

The same suggestions apply for select lean roast beef sandwiches, ham, and roast turkey and chicken sandwiches: select a small sandwich and low fat condiments.

✓ **Order a small roast beef sandwich** and keep condiments to mustard or low fat dressing.

Select Small Roast Beef Sandwiches with Low Fat Condiments:		
	Calories	Fat (g)
Arby's® Giant Roast Beef Sandwich	555	28
Arby's® Light Roast Beef Deluxe	296	10
Savings:	259	18

✓ **Ham & Cheese Sandwiches are another remarkably low fat option.** Other submarine sandwiches (such as roast chicken and turkey) offered in fast food restaurants may be low in fat and calories also, check out the nutritional information.

Ham & Cheese has less Calories than a Fried Fish Sandwich:		
	Calories	Fat (g)
Hardee's® Fisherman's Fillet	560	27
Hardee's® Hot Ham'N'Cheese™	310	12
Savings:	250	15

Pitas, Wraps, Potatoes, Chili, & Teriyaki Bowls

Still hungry after your low fat meal? Not surprising. Many people need more than a 300 calorie meal. Here are some higher calorie, but still low fat options.

✓ **Pitas and wraps can be lean option** if lean meats are chosen and a minimal amount of dressing is used.

Order Pitas without Dressing:		
	Calories	Fat (g)
Wendy's® Chicken Caesar Pita	490	18
Wendy's® Chicken Caesar Pita w/out dressing	420	11
Savings:	70	7

✓ **Ask for the stuffed potatoes to be prepared without butter.** Potatoes, by themselves, contain only negligible amounts of fat but are rich in vitamins, minerals, and fiber. Keep the meal healthy by adding only lean meats, vegetables, and low fat toppings to your plain potato. Specialty potato restaurants offer broth as an alternative to butter; they may also offer fat-free sour cream and cheese.

Request the "Lite Potatoes with Broth" instead of Butter:		
	Calories	Fat (g)
1 Potato 2® BBQ Chicken, Cheddar & Bacon	684	43
1 Potato 2® Chicken Fajita Lite (w/broth)	272	2
Savings:	412	41

✔ **Chicken Teriyaki Bowls are low in fat.** They have more calories than a plain grilled chicken sandwich, which makes it an ideal alternative for people who still feel hungry after a lower calorie meal.

Order a Teriyaki Bowl (without the Egg Roll) such as:

	Calories	Fat (g)
Jack in the Box® Chicken Teriyaki Bowl	670	4

✔ **Chili can be a low calorie meal** by itself or an adjunct to a low fat sandwich or potato.

Try these Combinations:

	Calories	Fat (g)
Wendy's Grilled Chicken Sandwich +Small Chili	520	15
Arby's® Plain Baked Potato +Timberline Chili	575	10

French Fries & Onion Rings

French fries and onion rings are the most common accompaniments but are more than 50% fat. If you want something to fill you up, healthier alternatives include: garden salads with low fat dressings, low fat soups, small cup of chili, plain baked potato, low fat ice cream or yogurt cone, steamed vegetables, fresh fruit, and baked chips. While not all restaurants provide each and every one of these options, they are sure to offer at least one.

If you must have the fried vegetables, order the smaller version. Many people, focusing more on their wallet than their waist line, order a combination meal that includes a sandwich, medium or large fries, and a drink. Ways to address this less than ideal combination include:

❶ ask them to substitute a *small* bag of fries instead or

❷ on the way to the table dump half the fries into the trash can. Remember, you can't eat what isn't there to tempt you.

Select Small rather than Large:

		Calories	Fat (g)
Whataburger® *Large* French Fries		442	24
Whataburger® *Junior* French Fries		221	12
	Savings:	**221**	**12**

Have it Without Cheese:

		Calories	Fat (g)
Chili Cheese Krys Kross Fries		625	39
Krystal's Krys Kross Fries		486	29
	Savings:	**139**	**10**

Calculating Calories & Fat grams in your Fast Food Meal

As a group, fast food restaurants are more likely to provide the consumer with nutritional information than any other type of restaurant. The last part of this chapter provides the most current nutritional information from most fast food restaurants. If your favorite burger or fast food restaurant does not provide nutritional information, use the generic information below.

Burgers & Fast Food

	Calories	Fat (g)	Sodium (mg)	Exchanges
Burgers on Buns (w/mustard, ketchup/pickles unless noted):				
Hamburger, 2 oz, small/kid's	286	12	636	1½ST+1½HFM
Cheeseburger, small/kid's	342	16	895	1½ST+2HFM
Quarter Pound Burger	452	22	912	2ST+3HFM
Quarter Pound Burger w/cheese	505	29	1304	2ST+3½HFM
Quarter Pound Burger w/bacon & cheese	540	33	1620	2ST+3½HFM+1FAT
Quarter Pound Burger w/mayo	595	35	967	2ST+3HFM+2FAT
Quarter Pound Burger w/cheese & mayo	660	44	1015	2ST+3½HFM+3FAT
Third Pound Burger, no toppings	640	34	575	3ST+4HFM
Half Pound Burger, no toppings	910	49	845	4ST+6HFM

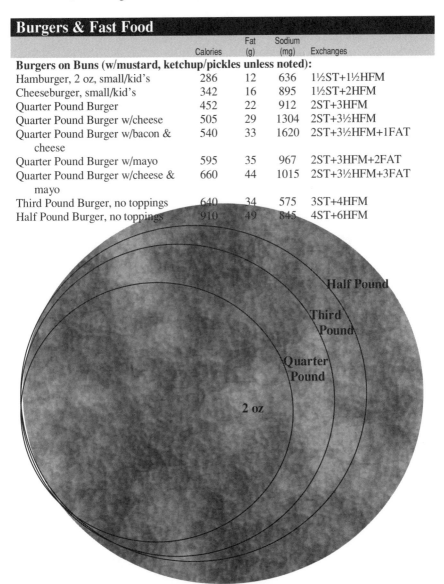

Burgers & Fast Food (continued)

	Calories	Fat (g)	Sodium (mg)	Exchanges
Grilled Chicken & Fish Sandwiches on Buns:				
Grilled Chicken Sandwich, regular	335	9	900	2½ST+3VLM+1FAT
Grilled Chicken, regular, w/out dressing	300	5	850	2½ST+3VLM
Grilled Chicken Sandwich, large	475	21	930	3ST+3½LM+2FAT
Grilled Chicken, large, w/out dressing	385	11	890	3ST+3½LM
BBQ Grilled Chicken Sandwich w/bun	350	9	915	2½ST+3LM
Grilled Fish Fillet w/"no butter on bun"	410	12	na	3ST+3VLM+2FAT
Fried Chicken & Fish Sandwiches on Buns:				
Fried Chicken Sandwich	485	24	1047	2½ST+2HFM+2FAT
Fried Fish Fillet Sandwich	345	15	710	2½ST+1HFM+1½FAT
Fried Fish Fillet SW w/cheese	452	22	967	2½ST+1½HFM+2FAT
Fried Fish Fillet Sandwich w/out cheese, w/out tartar sauce	320	13	800	2½ST+1½HFM
Fried Fish Fillet Sandwich, large	582	31	1091	3ST+2HFM+3FAT
Other Fast Food Sandwiches on Buns:				
Hot Dog, regular	250	14	600	1½ST+1HFM+1FAT
Cheese Dog, regular	290	18	950	1½ST+1HFM+2FAT
Chili Dog, regular	280	16	875	1½ST+1HFM+1½FAT
Chili & Cheese Dog, regular	350	22	1050	1½ST+1½HFM+2FAT
Hot Dog or Sausage, ¼#	460	37	1360	2ST+3HFM
Corn Dog, regular 2½ oz	200	10	620	1¼ST+½HFM+1FAT
Corn Dog, ¼#	330	17	990	1¾ST+1HFM+2FAT
Roast Beef Sandwich, small	325	12	875	2ST+1½MFM+1FAT
Roast Beef Sandwich, regular	375	17	915	2ST+2½MFM+1FAT
Garden Burger on Bun	320	5	610	3ST+1MFM
Other Fast Foods:				
Chicken Pieces, regular order	290	16	697	1ST+2HFM
Chili, Small/regular	214	8	830	1ST+1V+1HFM
Large	318	11	1237	1½ST+2V+1½HFM
Individual Components:				
Half Pound Burger	490	35	350	6MFM+1FAT
Third Pound Burger	330	24	232	4MFM+1FAT
Quarter Pound Burger	245	18	175	3MFM+½FAT
Small Burger, 2 oz	155	11	90	1½HFM
Turkey Burger, 4 oz	210	15	30	3MFM
Grilled Chicken Breast, 4 oz	200	8	70	3LM
Grilled Fish Fillet	220	10	na	3LM
Hot Dog, ¼#	360	36	1170	2HFM+4FAT
Hot Dog, 2 oz	180	16	585	1HFM+1½FAT

Burgers & Fast Food (continued)

	Calories	Fat (g)	Sodium (mg)	Exchanges
Individual Components (continued):				
Sausage, ¼#	360	32	1100	2½HFM+2½FAT
Garden Burger	130	3	340	1ST+½MFM
4 oz Bun (for ½# burger)	320	3	500	4ST+½FAT
3 oz Bun (for 1/3# burger)	240	2.5	375	3ST+½FAT
2¼ oz Bun (for ¼# burger)	190	2	270	2ST+½FAT
1½ oz Bun (for 2 oz burger)	120	1	190	1½ST+¼FAT
Hot Dog Bun, regular	100	1	190	1½ST+¼FAT
Butter/Oil on buns, 1T	100	11	0	2FAT

Hamburger Bun Sizes:

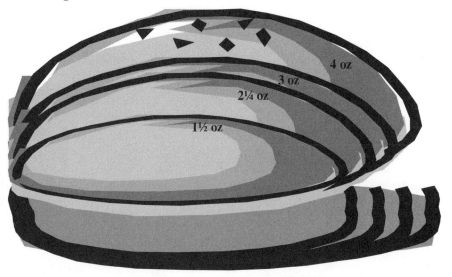

Burgers & Fast Food (continued)

	Calories	Fat (g)	Sodium (mg)	Exchanges
Toppings:				
Avocado, ¼	85	7	5	1½FAT
Bacon, 2 slices crisp	70	6	200	1½FAT
Cheese, American 1 oz	90	9	420	1HFM
Cheddar Cheese, 1 oz	114	9	175	1HFM
Swiss Cheese, 1 oz	107	8	75	1HFM
Lettuce	0	0	0	FREE
Mushrooms, sautéed in 1T butter	110	11	125	2FAT
Onion,	5	0	0	FREE
Pickles, 2 slices	1	0	140	FREE
Tomato, 2 slices	5	0	0	FREE

Burgers & Fast Food (continued)

	Calories	Fat (g)	Sodium (mg)	Exchanges
Condiments (1T) *your sandwich may have more or less*:				
Barbecue Sauce	15	0	250	¼CHO
Chili Hot Dog Sauce	17	1	75	¼CHO
Honey Mustard Sauce	45	$4.^2$	15	1FAT
Ketchup	15	0	180	FREE
Mayonnaise	110	11	80	2FAT
Mustard	15	1	190	FREE
Sweet N'Sour Sauce	30	0	35	¼CHO
Tartar Sauce	70	8	220	1½FAT
Accompaniments:				
Onion Rings, regular	297	16	438	2ST+3FAT
Large	441	27	838	3ST+5½FAT
Onion Rings, each	82	6	150	½ST+1FAT
Potato Puffs, each	14	$0.^7$	30	na
French Fries, small/junior	232	12	204	1½ST+2½FAT
Medium/regular	352	18	254	2½ST+3½FAT
Large	434	21	333	3¼ST+4FAT
Extra Large	540	28	758	4ST+5½FAT
French Fries, 1 c	155	8	170	1ST+1½FAT
Skinny French Fries, 1 @ 2½" long	5	$0.^{25}$	na	na
20 @ 2½" long	100	5	75	¾ST+1FAT

Skinny French Fries

	Calories	Fat (g)	Sodium (mg)	Exchanges
Regular French Fries, 1@ 2½" long	10	$0.^5$	na	na
10 @ 2½" long	100	$4.^1$	na	na
Battered French Fries, 1 @ 2½"	14	$0.^8$	na	na
7 @ 2½" long	100	$5.^3$	na	na

Regular & Battered French Fries

	Calories	Fat (g)	Sodium (mg)	Exchanges
Steak Fries, 1 @ 2½" long	17	$0.^9$	na	na
6 @ 2½" long	100	$5.^2$	na	na

Steak Fries

Your Favorite Burger & Fast Food Restaurants

1 POTATO 2®

	Calories	Fat (g)	Sodium (mg)	Exchanges
Ultra Lites & Lite Potato Entrees (assumes skin not eaten):				
Fresh Mexican Chicken Lite	328	9	833	3ST+1MFM+½FAT
Chicken Caesar and Broccoli Lite	372	12	845	3ST+1LM+1V+1½FAT
Chicken Stir-Fry Lite	330	3	1258	3½ST+1LM+1V
Crab & Broccoli DeLite	335	2	711	3ST+1VLM+1V
Herb Roasted Vegetable Lite	255	6	210	2½ST+1V+1FAT
Spinach Soufflé Lite	315	10	628	2½ST+½HFM+1V+ 1FAT
Chicken Fajita Lite	272	2	na	na
Chicken, Mushroom & Roasted Peppers Lite	242	2	na	na
Gourmet Potato Entrees (assumes skin not eaten):				
Philly Steak & Cheese	676	40	1409	3ST+3HFM+3FAT
Crab, Broccoli, & Cheese	593	35	1299	2½ST+3HFM+1V+ 2FAT
Chicken, Broccoli, & Cheddar	591	37	816	2½ST+3HFM+1V+ 2½FAT
Bacon Double Cheeseburger	766	54	1290	2½ST+3HFM+6FAT
Mexican	669	46	1071	3ST+1HFM+7½FAT
Broccoli & Cheese	545	36	575	2½ST+1½HFM+1V+ 5FAT
Bacon & Cheese	657	47	921	2½ST+2HFM+6FAT
3 Cheese	582	39	753	2½ST+2½HFM+4FAT
BBQ Chicken, Cheddar & Bacon	684	43	1766	2½ST+2½HFM+4½FAT
Chicken Santa Fe	647	41	929	2½ST+2HFM+1V+5FAT
Steak Santa Fe	687	44	965	2½ST+2HFM+1V+ 5½FAT

Tip: If you request broth instead of margarine on Gourmet Potato Entrees, you will reduce calories by 202, fat by 23 g, and sodium by 304 mg. No-Fat Sour Cream is available on all entrees.

	Calories	Fat (g)	Sodium (mg)	Exchanges
Smothered Mashed Potatoes w/chicken tenders, country gravy, roll, & corn	767	39	1220	5ST+2HFM+4½FAT
Potato Skins:				
Bacon n' Cheddar with Sour Cream	1017	57	776	6½ST+1HFM+10FAT
Southwestern with Sour Cream	907	46	1423	6ST+2HFM+6FAT
Fresh Bread Bowl Soups (includes bread bowl):				
Baked Potato Soup	640	26	1630	5ST+1HFM+3½FAT
Broccoli and Cheese Potato Soup	736	35	1549	5ST+2HFM+4FAT

1 POTATO 2® (continued)

	Calories	Fat (g)	Sodium (mg)	Exchanges
Country Skillet Combos:				
Texas BBQ Chicken & Cheddar	890	57	759	5ST+1HFM+10FAT
Bacon, Ranch & Cheddar	1090	74	937	5ST+2HFM+11½FAT
Idaho Nachos	1009	61	838	5ST+2½HFM+8FAT
Fresh Cut Fries:				
Small	612	39	321	4ST+8FAT
Medium	765	49	401	5ST+10FAT
Large	1224	78	642	8ST+15½FAT
Nacho Cheese Fries	838	54	622	5ST+11FAT
Fresh Fries'n Chicken Tenders	917	50	893	5½ST+10FAT

ARBY'S®

	Calories	Fat (g)	Sodium (mg)	Exchanges
Roast Beef Sandwiches:				
Arby's Melt w/Cheddar	368	18	937	2½ST+2HFM
Arby Q	431	18	1321	3ST+2MFM+1½FAT
Bac'n Cheddar Deluxe	539	34	1140	2½ST+2HFM+3½FAT
Beef'n Cheddar	487	28	1216	2½ST+2½MFM+3FAT
Giant Roast Beef	555	28	1561	2½ST+4MFM+1½FAT
Junior Roast Beef	324	14	779	2ST+1½MFM+1½FAT
Regular Roast Beef	388	19	1009	2ST+2½MFM+1½FAT
Super Roast Beef	523	27	1189	3ST+3MFM+2½FAT
Chicken Sandwiches:				
Breaded Chicken Fillet	536	28	1016	2½ST+3MFM+2½FAT
Chicken Cordon Bleu	623	33	1594	2½ST+4MFM+2½FAT
Chicken Fingers, 2 pieces	290	16	677	1½ST+2HFM
Grilled Chicken BBQ	388	13	1002	3ST+2½LM+1FAT
Grilled Chicken Deluxe	430	20	848	2½ST+2½LM+2½FAT
Roast Chicken Club	546	31	1103	2½ST+3½MFM+2½FAT
Roast Chicken Deluxe	433	22	763	2½ST+2½MFM+2FAT
Roast Chicken Santa Fe	436	22	818	2½ST+3MFM+1½FAT
Sub Roll Sandwiches:				
French Dip	475	22	1411	2½ST+3MFM+1½FAT
Hot Ham'n Swiss	500	23	1664	2½ST+3MFM+1½FAT
Italian Sub	675	36	2089	3ST+3HFM+2½FAT
Philly Beef'n Swiss	755	47	2025	3ST+4MFM+5½FAT
Roast Beef Sub	700	42	2034	2½ST+4½MFM+4FAT
Triple Cheese Melt	720	45	1797	2½ST+4MFM+5FAT
Turkey Sub	550	27	2084	3ST+3MFM+2½FAT

ARBY'S® (continued)

	Calories	Fat (g)	Sodium (mg)	Exchanges
Light Menu:				
Roast Beef Deluxe	296	10	826	2ST+2MFM
Roast Chicken Deluxe	276	6	777	2ST+2LM
Roast Turkey Deluxe	260	7	1262	2ST+2LM
Garden Salad	61	0.5	40	2V
Roast Chicken Salad	149	2	418	2V+2½VLM
Side Salad	23	0.3	15	½V
Other Sandwiches:				
Fish Fillet	529	27	864	3ST+2HFM+2FAT
Ham 'n Cheese	359	14	1283	2ST+2½LM+1½FAT
Ham 'n Cheese Melt	329	13	1013	2ST+2½LM+1FAT
Potatoes:				
Cheddar Curly Fries	333	18	1016	2½ST+3½FAT
Curly Fries	300	15	853	2½ST+3FAT
French Fries	246	13	114	2ST+2½FAT
Potato Cakes	204	12	397	1½ST+2½FAT
Baked Potato, plain	355	0.3	26	5ST
Baked Potato w/marg & sour cream	578	24	209	5ST+5FAT
Broccoli'n Cheddar Baked Potato	571	20	565	5ST+1V+4FAT
Deluxe Baked Potato	736	36	499	5ST+1HFM+5½FAT
Soups (8 oz serving):				
Boston Clam Chowder	190	9	965	1ST+1LM+1FAT
Cream of Broccoli	160	8	1005	1V+½WMk+1FAT
Lumberjack Mixed Vegetable	90	4	1150	2V+1FAT
Old Fashioned Chicken Noodle	80	2	850	1ST+½MFM
Potato with Bacon	170	7	905	1ST+½WMk+½FAT
Timberline Chili	220	10	1130	1ST+2MFM
Wisconsin Cheese	280	18	1065	1ST+½WMk+½HFM+2 ½FAT
Desserts:				
Apple Turnover	330	14	180	2CHO+1FR+3FAT
Cherry Turnover	320	13	190	2CHO+1FR+2½FAT
Cheesecake, plain	320	23	240	1½CHO+4½FAT
Chocolate Chip Cookie	125	6	85	1CHO+1FAT
Chocolate Shake, 12 oz	451	12	341	5CHO+2½FAT
Jamocha Shake, 12 oz	384	10	262	4CHO+2FAT
Vanilla Shake, 12 oz	360	12	281	3½CHO+2½FAT
Butterfinger Polar Swirl, 11.6 oz	457	18	318	4CHO+3½FAT
Heath Polar Swirl, 11.6 oz	543	22	346	5CHO+4½FAT
Oreo Polar Swirl, 11.6 oz	482	22	521	4½CHO+4½FAT
Peanut Butter Cup Polar Swirl, 11.6 oz	517	24	385	4CHO+5FAT
Snickers Polar Swirl, 11.6 oz	511	19	351	5CHO+4FAT

ARBY'S® (continued)

	Calories	Fat (g)	Sodium (mg)	Exchanges
Sauces and Dressings:				
Arby's Sauce, ½ oz	15	0.[2]	113	FREE
Barbecue Sauce, ½ oz	30	0	185	½CHO
Beef Stock Au Jus, 2 oz	10	0	440	FREE
Blue Cheese Dressing, 2 oz	290	31	580	6FAT
Cheddar Cheese Sauce, ¾ oz	35	3	139	½FAT
Honey French Dressing, 2 oz	280	23	400	1CHO+4½FAT
Horsey Sauce, ½ oz	60	5	150	1FAT
Ketchup, ½ oz	16	0	143	1=FREE or ¼CHO
Light Chol. Free Mayonnaise, ¼ oz	12	1	64	1=FREE or ¼FAT
Mayonnaise, ½ oz	110	12	80	2½FAT
Mustard, German Style, 0.[16] oz	5	0	70	FREE
Non-Sep. Italian Sub Sauce, ½ oz	70	7	240	1½FAT
Parmesan Cheese Sauce, ½ oz	70	7	130	1½FAT
Red Ranch Dressing, ½ oz	75	6	115	1½FAT
Red. Cal. Honey Mayonnaise, ½ oz	70	7	135	1½FAT
Red. Cal. Italian Dressing, 2 oz	20	1	1000	FREE or ¼FAT
Red. Cal. Buttermilk Ranch Dressing, 2 oz	50	0	710	1CHO
Tartar Sauce, 1 oz	140	15	220	3FAT
Thousand Island Dressing, 2 oz	260	26	420	½CHO+5FAT

BURGER KING®

	Calories	Fat (g)	Sodium (mg)	Exchanges
Burgers:				
Whopper Sandwich®	640	39	870	3ST+2½HFM+4FAT
Mustard Whopper®	490	22	920	3ST+3HFM
Whopper® with Cheese Sandwich	730	46	1350	3ST+3½HFM+3½FAT
Double Whopper® Sandwich	870	56	940	3ST+5HFM+3FAT
Double Whopper® w/Cheese SW	960	63	1420	3ST+6HFM+3FAT
Whopper Jr®	420	24	530	2ST+2HFM+1½FAT
Mustard Whopper Jr®	350	16	640	2ST+2HFM
Whopper Jr® with Cheese	460	28	770	2ST+2½HFM+1½FAT
Big King Sandwich	660	43	920	2ST+5HFM
Hamburger	330	15	530	2ST+2HFM
Cheeseburger	380	19	770	2ST+2½HFM
Double Cheeseburger	600	36	1060	2ST+4½HFM
Double Cheeseburger w/Bacon	640	39	1240	2ST+5HFM

BURGER KING® (continued)

	Calories	Fat (g)	Sodium (mg)	Exchanges
Sandwich/Side Orders:				
BK Big Fish™ Sandwich	720	43	1180	3½ST+2HFM+5½FAT
BK Broiler® Chicken Sandwich	530	26	1060	2½ST+1V+3LM+ 3FAT
BK Broiler® Ch. SW w/out mayo	390	12	360	2½ST+1V+3LM
Chicken Sandwich	710	43	1400	3½ST+2HFM+5½FAT
Chicken Tenders®, 8 pc	350	22	940	1ST+2½MFM+2FAT
Broiled Chicken Salad, no dressing	190	8	500	1V+3LM
Side Salad, without dressing	60	3	55	1V+½FAT
French Fries, medium salted	370	20	240	3ST+4FAT
Garden Salad, without dressing	100	5	110	1V+½HFM
Coated French Fries, med. Salted	400	21	820	3ST+4FAT
Onion Rings	310	14	810	2½ST+3FAT
Dutch Apple Pie	300	15	230	1ST+½CHO+1FR+3FAT
Shakes, medium:				
Vanilla Shake	300	6	230	1LfMk+3CHO+1FAT
Chocolate Shake	320	7	230	1LfMk+3CHO+1FAT
Chocolate Shake, w/syrup added	440	7	430	1LfMk+4CHO+1FAT
Strawberry Shake, w/syrup added	420	6	260	1LfMk+4CHO+1FAT
Sandwich Condiments/Toppings:				
Mayonnaise	210	23	160	4½FAT
Tartar Sauce	180	19	220	4FAT
Land O'Lakes® Wh. Classic Blend	65	7	75	1½FAT
Bull's Eye® Barbecue Sauce	20	0	140	¼CHO
Bacon Bits	15	1	70	FREE or ¼FAT
Croutons	30	1	90	¼ST+¼FAT
Burger King® Salad Dressings:				
Thousand Island Dressing	140	12	190	½CHO+2½FAT
French Dressing	140	10	190	1CHO+2FAT
Ranch Dressing	180	19	170	4FAT
Bleu Cheese Dressing	160	16	260	3FAT
Reduced Calorie Light It. Dressing	15	0.⁵	360	FREE
Dipping Sauces:				
Honey Dipping Sauce	90	0	10	1½CHO
Ranch Dipping Sauce	170	17	200	3½FAT
Barbecue Dipping Sauce	35	0	400	½CHO
Sweet & Sour Dipping Sauce	45	0	50	¾CHO

CAPTAIN D'S® SEAFOOD

	Calories	Fat (g)	Sodium (mg)	Exchanges
Captain's Broilers (Lunch): includes rice w/vegetable medley & breadstick.				
Broiled Chicken Lunch	503	9	na	na
Broiled Fish Lunch	435	7	na	na
Broiled Shrimp Lunch	421	7	na	na
Broiled Fish & Chicken Lunch	478	8	na	na
Captain's Broilers (Platters): includes rice w/veg medley, baked potato, salad, & breadstick.				
(Nutritional info does *not* include condiments for baked potato & salad dressings.)				
Broiled Shrimp Platter	720	8	na	na
Broiled Chicken Platter	802	10	na	na
Broiled Fish Platter	734	7	na	na
Baked Fish & Chicken Platter	777	10	na	na
Sandwiches & Accompaniments:				
Broiled Chicken	451	19	858	2ST+4½LM+1FAT
Baked Potato	278	0	na	3½ST
Salad	20	0	na	1V
French Dressing, 1 oz pkt	111	11	187	2FAT+¼CHO
Blue Cheese Dressing, 1 oz pkt	105	12	101	2½FAT
Ranch Dressing, 1 oz pkt	92	10	230	2FAT
Light Italian Dressing, 1 oz pkt	16	0.^{5}	na	FREE
Rice	184	0	na	2½ST
Vegetable Medley	36	1	na	1V
Breadstick	113	4	na	1ST+1FAT
Cole Slaw	158	12	246	1V+½CHO+2½FAT
Cob Corn	251	2	13	4ST+½FAT
Green Beans, seasoned	46	2	752	1V+½FAT
White Beans	126	0.^{5}	99	1½ST
Fried Okra	300	16	445	2ST+1V+3FAT
French Fried Potatoes	302	10	152	3ST+2FAT
Imitation Sour Cream	29	3	na	½FAT
Margarine	102	12	na	2½FAT
Cracklins, 1 oz (with dinner)	218	17	741	1ST+3½FAT
Hushpuppy, 1	126	4	465	1ST+1FAT
Hushpuppies, 6	756	25	2790	8ST+5FAT
Crackers, 4	50	1	147	½ST+¼FAT
Slice of Cheese	54	5	206	½HFM
Cocktail Sauce, 1 oz side portion	34	0.^{1}	252	½CHO
Tartar Sauce, 1 oz side portion	75	7	158	¼CHO+1½FAT
Sweet & Sour Sauce, side portion	52	0	5	1CHO
Desserts, one piece:				
Pecan Pie	458	20	373	4CHO+4FAT
Chocolate Cake	303	10	259	3CHO+2FAT
Carrot Cake	434	23	414	3CHO+4½FAT
Cheesecake	420	31	480	2CHO+6FAT
Lemon Pie	351	10	135	4CHO+2FAT

CARL'S JR.®

	Calories	Fat (g)	Sodium (mg)	Exchanges
Hamburgers/Sandwiches:				
Famous Big Star™ Hamburger	610	38	890	2½ST+2½HFM+3½FAT
Super Star® Hamburger	820	53	1030	2½ST+5HFM+2FAT
Western Bacon Cheeseburger®	870	35	1490	4ST+3HFM+3FAT
Double Western Bacon ChBurger®	970	57	1810	4ST+6HFM+2FAT
Big Burger	470	20	810	3ST+2½HFM
Hamburger	200	8	500	1½ST+1MFM
BBQ Chicken Sandwich	310	6	830	2½ST+3LM
Chicken Club Sandwich	550	29	1160	2½ST+4LM+3FAT
Santa Fe Chicken Sandwich	530	30	1230	2½ST+3LM+4FAT
Carl's Catch Fish Sandwich™	560	30	1220	3½ST+1HFM+4½FAT
Hot & Crispy Sandwich	400	22	980	2ST+1HFM+3FAT
American Cheese	60	5	270	½HFM
Swiss Cheese	45	4	220	½HFM
Great Stuff™ Potatoes:				
Broccoli & Cheese Potato	530	22	930	4ST+1HFM+3FAT
Bacon & Cheese Potato	630	29	1720	4ST+1HFM+4FAT
Plain Potato	290	0	40	4ST
Sour Cream & Chive Potato	430	14	160	4ST+3FAT
Entrée Salads-To-Go™:				
Char. Chicken Salad-To-Go™	260	9	530	½ST+3LM+1V
Garden Salad-To-Go™	50	3	75	1V+½FAT
Bakery Products:				
Chocolate Chip Cookie	370	19	350	3CHO+4FAT
Chocolate Cake	300	10	260	3CHO+2FAT
Cheese Danish	400	22	390	3CHO+4½FAT
Cheesecake, Strawberry Swirl	300	17	220	2CHO+3½FAT
Sides:				
French Fries, reg.	370	20	240	3ST+4FAT
Onion Rings	520	26	840	4ST+5FAT
Zucchini	380	23	1040	2ST+1V+4½FAT
Hash Brown Nuggets	270	17	410	2ST+3½FAT
CrissCut Fries®, large	550	34	1280	3½ST+7FAT
Salad Dressings (2 oz) portions:				
House Dressing	220	22	440	4½FAT
Blue Cheese Dressing	310	34	360	7FAT
1000 Island Dressing	250	24	540	5FAT
Fat Free Italian Dressing	15	0	800	FREE
Fat Free French Dressing	70	0	760	1FR

CARL'S JR.® (continued)

	Calories	Fat (g)	Sodium (mg)	Exchanges
Breads:				
Croutons	35	1	65	½ST
Breadsticks	35	1	60	½ST
Sauces:				
Salsa	10	0	160	FREE
Mustard Sauce	45	1	150	½CHO
Honey Sauce	90	0	5	1½CHO
BBQ Sauce	50	0	270	1CHO
Sweet N'Sour Sauce	50	0	60	1CHO
Shakes (small):				
Vanilla	330	8	250	1SkM+3CHO+1½FAT
Chocolate	390	7	280	1SkM+4CHO+1½FAT
Strawberry	400	7	240	1SkM+4CHO+1½FAT

Chick-fil-A®

	Calories	Fat (g)	Sodium (mg)	Exchanges
Specialties:				
Chick-fil-A® Chicken Sandwich	290	9	870	2ST+3LM
Chick-fil-A® Chick. Deluxe SW	300	9	870	2ST+3LM
Chick-fil-A® Chargrilled Ch. SW	280	3	640	2ST+3VLM
Chick-fil-A® Chargrilled Chicken Deluxe Sandwich	290	3	640	2ST+3VLM
Chick-fil-A® Chicken Club Sandwich, no dressing	390	12	980	2ST+4LM+1V
Chick-fil-A® Chick-n-Strips®, 4	230	8	380	½ST+4LM
Chick-fil-A Nuggets®, 8 pack	290	14	770	1ST+4LM
Chick-fil-A® Chicken Salad Sandwich, on whole wheat	320	5	810	3ST+2LM
Hearty Breast of Chick. Soup, cup	110	1	760	1V+2VLM
Chick-fil-A® Chargrilled Chicken Garden Salad	170	3	650	2V+2LM
Chick-fil-A® Chick-n-Strips Salad	290	9	430	½ST+4LM+2V
Chick-fil-A ® Chicken Salad Plate	290	5	570	2ST+2LM+2V
Side Orders:				
Tossed Salad	70	0	0	2½V
Cole Slaw, small	130	6	430	2½V+1FAT
Carrot & Raisin Salad, small	150	2	650	2V+1FR+½FAT
Chick-fil-A Waffle Potato Fries®, small, salted	290	10	960	3ST+2FAT
Chick-fil-A Waffle Potato Fries®, small, unsalted by request	290	10	80	3ST+2FAT

Chick-fil-A® continued

	Calories	Fat (g)	Sodium (mg)	Exchanges
Desserts/Beverages:				
Icedream®, small cup	350	10	390	1½CHO+1LfMk+1FAT
Icedream®, small cone	140	4	240	1½CHO+1LfMk
Lemon Pie, slice	280	22	550	½CHO+1FR+4FAT
Fudge Nut Brownie	350	16	650	2CHO+1FR+3FAT
Cheesecake, slice	270	21	510	½CHO+1HFM+3FAT
w/ Strawberry Topping	290	23	580	½CHO+1HFM+3FAT
w/ Blueberry Topping	290	23	550	½CHO+1HFM+3FAT
Chick-fil-A® Lemonade, 9 oz	90	0	4	1½CHO
Chick-fil-A® Diet Lemonade, 9 oz	5	0	4	FREE
Iced Tea, unsweetened, 9 oz	0	0	50	FREE
Iced Tea, sweetened, 9 oz	150	0	50	2½CHO

CHURCH'S FRIED CHICKEN

	Calories	Fat (g)	Sodium (mg)	Exchanges
Fried Chicken:				
Wing, 3.^{1} oz±	250	16	540	½ST+2HFM
Leg, 2 oz±	140	9	160	2MFM
Thigh, 2.^{8} oz±	230	16	520	½ST+2HFM
Breast, 2.^{8} oz±	200	12	510	½ST+2½MFM
Tender Strip™, 1.^{1} oz	80	4	140	1MFM
Side Orders:				
Cajun Rice	130	7	260	1ST+1½FAT
Potatoes & Gravy	90	3	520	1ST+½FAT
Okra	210	16	520	1ST+3FAT
Biscuits	250	16	640	1½ST+3FAT
Corn on the Cob	139	3	15	1½ST+½FAT
Apple Pie	280	12	340	1ST+1½FR+2½FAT
Cole Slaw	92	6	230	1½V+1FAT
French Fries	210	11	60	2ST+2FAT

± Refers to edible portion (without bones, cob, etc.)

DAIRY QUEEN®/BRAZIER®

	Calories	Fat (g)	Sodium (mg)	Exchanges
DQ Homestyle® Hamburger	290	12	630	2ST+2½MFM
DQ Homestyle® Cheeseburger	340	17	850	2ST+3½MFM
DQ Homestyle® Double ChB	540	31	1130	2ST+6MFM
DQ Homestyle® Deluxe Dble HB	440	22	680	2ST+5MFM
DQ Homestyle® Deluxe Dble ChB	540	31	1130	2ST+6MFM
DQ Homestyle® Bacon Dble ChB	610	36	1380	2ST+7MFM
DQ Homestyle® Ultimate Burger	670	43	1210	2ST+6MFM+2½FAT

DAIRY QUEEN®/BRAZIER® continued

	Calories	Fat (g)	Sodium (mg)	Exchanges
Hot Dog	240	14	730	1½ST+1HFM+1FAT
Cheese Dog	290	18	950	1½ST+1HFM+2FAT
Chili Dog	280	16	870	1½ST+1HFM+1½FAT
Chili 'n' Cheese Dog	330	21	1090	1½ST+1½HFM+2FAT
Fish Fillet Sandwich	370	16	630	2½ST+1HFM+1½FAT
Fish Fillet Sandwich w/Cheese	420	21	850	2½ST+1½HFM+2FAT
Chicken Breast Fillet Sandwich	430	20	760	2½ST+2HFM+1FAT
Chicken Breast Fillet SW w/Cheese	480	25	980	2½ST+3HFM
Chicken Strip Basket w/gravy	860	42	1820	5½ST+3HFM+3½FAT
Chicken Strip Basket w/BBQ Sce	810	37	1590	5½ST+3HFM+2½FAT
Grilled Chicken Fillet Sandwich	310	10	1040	2ST+3LM
French Fries, small	210	10	115	2ST+2FAT
French Fries, regular	300	14	160	2½ST+3FAT
French Fries, large	390	18	200	3½ST+3½FAT
Regular Onion Rings	240	12	135	2ST+2½FAT

HARDEE'S®

	Calories	Fat (g)	Sodium (mg)	Exchanges
Sandwiches:				
Hamburger	270	11	670	2ST+2MFM
Cheeseburger	310	14	890	2ST+2MFM+2½FAT
The Boss™	570	33	910	3ST+3MFM+2½FAT
Cravin'Bacon™ Cheeseburger	690	46	1150	2½ST+3½MFM+5FAT
The Works Burger	530	30	1030	2½ST+3MFM+3FAT
Mesquite Bacon Cheeseburger	370	18	970	2ST+2MFM+1½FAT
Quarter-Pound Dble Cheeseburger	470	27	1290	2ST+3MFM+2½FAT
Chicken Fillet Sandwich	480	18	1280	3½ST+3MFM
Regular Roast Beef	320	16	820	2ST+1½MFM+1FAT
Big Roast Beef™ Sandwich	460	24	1230	2½ST+2½MFM+2FAT
Grilled Chicken Sandwich	350	11	950	2½ST+3LM
Mushroom 'N' Swiss™ Burger	490	25	1100	2½ST+3MFM+2FAT
Frisco™ Burger	720	46	1340	3ST+4HFM+3FAT
Hot Ham 'N' Cheese™	310	12	1410	2ST+2MFM
Fisherman's Fillet™	560	27	1330	3½ST+2½MFM+2FAT
Fried Chicken/Sides:				
Breast, 1 piece	370	15	1190	2ST+3MFM
Wing, 1 piece	200	8	740	1½ST+1HFM
Thigh, 1 piece	330	15	1000	2ST+2HFM
Leg, 1 piece	170	7	570	1ST+1½MFM
Cole Slaw, 4 oz	240	20	340	1V+½CHO+4FAT
Mashed Potatoes, 4 oz	70	<1	330	1ST
Gravy, 1.5 oz	20	<1	260	¼ST
Baked Beans, sm, 5 oz	170	1	600	2ST

HARDEE'S® (continued)

	Calories	Fat (g)	Sodium (mg)	Exchanges
Salads & Fries:				
Side Salad	25	<1	45	1V
Garden Salad	220	13	350	2V+1HFM+1FAT
Grilled Chicken Salad	150	3	610	2V+2LM
Fat Free French Dressing	70	0	580	1CHO
Ranch Dressing	290	29	510	1V+6FAT
Thousand Island Dressing	250	23	540	½ST+5FAT
French Fries, small	240	10	100	2ST+2FAT
French Fries, medium	350	15	150	3ST+3FAT
French Fries, large	430	18	190	4ST+3½FAT
Shakes & Desserts:				
Shake, Vanilla	350	5	300	3CHO+1½SkMk+1FAT
Shake, Chocolate	370	5	270	3CHO+1½SkMk+1FAT
Shake, Strawberry	420	4	270	4½CHO+1½SkMk+ 1FAT
Shake, Peach	390	4	290	4CHO+1SkMk+1FAT
Vanilla Cone	170	2	130	2CHO+½SkMk+½FAT
Chocolate Cone	180	2	110	2CHO+½SkMk+½FAT
Cool Twist™ Cone, Vanilla/Choc.	180	2	120	2CHO+½SkMk+½FAT
Hot Fudge Sundae	290	6	310	2½CHO+1SkMk+2FAT
Strawberry Sundae	210	2	140	2½CHO+½SkMk+½FAT
Peach Cobbler, sm 6 oz	310	7	360	4CHO+1FAT
Big Cookie™	280	12	150	3CHO+2½FAT

HARTZ CHICKEN® INC.

	Calories	Fat (g)	Sodium (mg)	Exchanges
Meats & Dinners:				
2 Piece White Dinner	970	47	1440	na
2 Piece Dark Dinner	770	36	1130	na
3 Piece White Dinner	1550	77	2060	na
3 Piece Dark Dinner	1000	54	1440	na
Roasted Chicken Dinner	910	39	460	na
3 Piece Fish Dinner	590	24	450	na
Fish Snack	610	20	550	na
Gizzards, ¾ c	130	4	50	3VLM
Livers, ¾ c	100	3	60	2VLM
Fish Fillet, 1	240	9	280	4LM+½ST
Fried Chicken, 1 average	380	22	120	5MFM
Barbecue Chicken, 5 oz	270	12	880	1CHO+3LM+½FAT
Meatloaf, 3 oz	160	8	420	¼ST+2MFM

HARTZ CHICKEN® INC. (continued)

	Calories	Fat (g)	Sodium (mg)	Exchanges
Vegetables & Starches (½ c):				
Broccoli, average	35	1.^{5}	25	1V+¼FAT
Broccoli & Cauliflower, average	30	1	220	1V+¼FAT
Broc, Caul, & Carrots, average	35	1	430	1V+¼FAT
Cabbage	40	1	200	1V+¼FAT
Candied Carrots, average	70	0.^{5}	155	1V+½CHO
Cauliflower, average	30	1.^{7}	175	1V+½FAT
Corn, average	85	1.^{7}	175	1ST+½FAT
Mexican Corn	100	1.^{5}	180	1ST+¼FAT
Beans	130	2	350	1ST+½FAT
Green Beans, average	40	1.^{3}	455	1V+¼FAT
Corn on Cob, 1	140	1	800	1½ST+¼FAT
Green Beans/Potatoes	60	0	350	¾ST
Green Beans/Onion Casserole	80	5	330	1V+½ST+½FAT
Gr Beans/Mushroom/Cheese Sauce	50	2	440	1V+¼ST+½FAT
Green Bean Supreme	140	11	490	1V+2FAT
Green Peas	50	1.^{5}	180	½ST+¼FAT
Green Peas/Carrots, average	65	1.^{2}	180	½ST+¼FAT
Macaroni & Cheese	270	17	470	1½ST+½HFM+2½FAT
Mustard/Turnip Greens, average	68	4.^{2}	450	1V+1FAT
Okra & Tomatoes	60	2	600	1V+½FAT
Pinto Beans, average	110	1.^{5}	600	1ST+½FAT
Golden Ex Rich Potatoes	160	5	65	1½ST+1FAT
Whipped Potatoes	100	3	300	1St+1FAT
Fry's, 3 oz	190	7	25	1½ST+1½FAT
Rice, average	150	1.^{7}	310	2ST+½FAT
Squash	30	1	28	1V+¼FAT
Squash & Tomato, average	45	1.^{3}	330	1V+¼FAT
Stewed Tomatoes, average	47	1	630	1V+¼FAT
Steamed Red Potatoes	110	7	890	¾ST+1½FAT
Candied Yams	190	2	65	1ST+1½CHO+½FAT
Hot Beets	40	0	320	1V
Baked Beans	170	2	560	1½ST+½FAT
Carrots & Bacon	100	5	380	1V+1FAT
Hominy	80	2	240	1ST+½FAT
Casseroles (½ c):				
Broccoli & Rice Casserole	130	5	400	1V+1ST+1FAT
Broccoli/Rice/Cheese	120	5	470	1ST+1FAT
Cornbread Dressing	270	8	660	3ST+1½FAT
Spanish Rice	150	4	510	1½ST+1FAT
Squash Casserole	300	29	780	1V+6FAT
Derty Rice	150	4	650	1½ST+1FAT

HARTZ CHICKEN® INC. (continued)

	Calories	Fat (g)	Sodium (mg)	Exchanges
Casseroles (1c):				
Chicken & Rice Casserole	300	15	280	2ST+1MFM+2FAT
Chicken & Rice Casserole, steamer	250	4	650	2ST+1MFM
Chicken Spaghetti	370	12	970	3ST+1½MFM+1FAT
Chicken Spaghetti, steamer	210	8	550	1½ST+1MFM+½FAT
Chicken Enchiladas Casserole	400	22	990	2ST+2HFM+1FAT
Chicken Creole	240	13	630	1ST+2½MFM
Chicken Vegetable Stew	230	10	400	1ST+1V+2MFM
Corn & Rice Casserole, average	160	4.^{3}	335	1½ST+1FAT
King Ranch Chicken	350	22	900	1ST+3MFM+1½FAT
Liver & Onions w/Gravy	170	5	740	½ST+2½LM
Macaroni & Tomato Casserole	130	4	460	1ST+1FAT
Green Bean/Onion Casserole	60	2.^{5}	480	1V+½FAT
Chicken & Dumplings	280	13	940	2ST+1MFM+1½FAT
Chicken Cabbage	240	18	430	1V+1½MFM+2FAT
Paella	350	14	900	1ST+1V+3MFM
Spicy Shrimp & Rice	230	2.^{5}	860	2ST+1LM
Breads (1):				
Cornbread Muffins	150	5	240	1½ST+1FAT
Jalapeño Cornbread Muffin	150	5	290	1½ST+1FAT
Yeast Rolls	180	3	260	2ST+½FAT
Dinner Rolls	220	3.^{5}	230	2½ST+½FAT
Soup (1c):				
Cream of Chicken/Rice Soup	210	10	390	1ST+1MFM+1FAT
Cream of Chicken Noodle Soup	210	11	430	1ST+1½MFM+1FAT
Vegetable Soup	80	0	770	1V+½ST
Salad (½ c):				
Beet Salad	60	0	260	1V+½CHO
Broccoli Salad	35	0	115	1V
Carrot/Raisin Salad	380	28	330	1V+1½CHO+5½FAT
Green Pea & Carrot Salad	110	8	210	1½V+1½FAT
Macaroni & Pea Salad	300	23	210	1ST+1HFM+3FAT
Green Bean Salad	160	13	580	1V+2½FAT
Pasta Salad	210	13	210	1½ST+2½FAT
Cole Slaw	220	18	115	1V+3½FAT
Fruit Salad	110	0.^{5}	5	1FR+1CHO
Mexican Salad	90	1	480	1ST+¼FAT
Three Bean Salad	130	3.^{5}	80	1V+1ST+½FAT
Rice & Egg Salad	480	22	330	2ST+2CHO+4½FAT
Garden Salad, 1	130	6	110	1V+1MFM
Croutons, 3T	25	1.^{5}	60	¼ST+¼FAT
Green Pea & Egg Salad	280	23	580	1V+1MFM+3½FAT
Potato Salad	150	3.^{5}	610	1½ST+½FAT

HARTZ CHICKEN® INC. (continued)

	Calories	Fat (g)	Sodium (mg)	Exchanges
Cool Salad	70	0	0	1CHO
Plain Jello	80	0	0	1CHO
Fruit Jello Salad	80	0	0	1CHO
Cold Spicy Pasta Salad	200	7	310	1½ST+1½FAT
Krab Slaw	160	12	380	1V+2½FAT
Sauces & Gravy (2T):				
Cocktail Sauce	30	0	350	½CHO
Hartz Gravy	10	0	135	FREE
Tartar Sauce	220	23	200	4½FAT
White Sauce	40	3	115	½FAT
Cheese Sauce	80	6	260	½HFM+½FAT
White Gravy	0	0	30	FREE
Desserts:				
Apple Cobbler 4 oz	250	2.⁵	280	1FR+2½CHO+½FAT
Pineapple Cobbler, 4 oz	240	2.⁵	280	1FR+2½CHO+½FAT
Bread Pudding, 4 oz	240	8	170	2½CHO+1½FAT
Crunchy Dessert, 4½ oz	330	12	160	3½CHO+2½FAT
Peach Cobbler, 4 oz	250	3	290	1FR+2½CHO+½FAT
Coffee Cake Dessert, 1 pc	240	2.⁵	280	3CHO+½FAT
Cinnamon Rolls, 1	820	8	520	12CHO+1½FAT
Pineapple Dessert, 4 oz	180	2	210	1FR+1½CHO+½FAT
Lemon Apple Cobbler, ½ c	320	7	380	1FR+3CHO+1½FAT
Chocolate Cake, 1 average piece	260	8	245	3CHO+1½FAT
Yellow Cake, 1 average piece	200	7	270	2CHO+1½FAT
Banana Flavored Pudding, ½ c	160	3	340	2CHO+½FAT

JACK IN THE BOX®

	Calories	Fat (g)	Sodium (mg)	Exchanges
Sandwiches:				
Chicken Caesar Sandwich	520	26	1050	2¾ST+2½MFM+2¾FAT
Chicken Fajita Pita	280	9	840	1¾ST+2½LM
Chicken Sandwich	450	26	1030	2ST+2MFM+3FAT
Chicken Supreme	680	45	1500	3ST+2¼MFM+6FAT
Grilled Chicken Fillet	520	26	1240	2¾ST+3½LM+2¼FAT
Spicy Crispy Chicken	560	27	1020	3½ST+2MFM+3FAT
Philly Cheesesteak	520	25	1980	2½ST+3¾LM+2¾FAT
Burgers:				
Hamburger	280	12	560	2ST+1MFM+1FAT
Cheeseburger	330	15	760	2ST+1½MFM+1½FAT
Double Cheeseburger	450	24	970	2ST+2½MFM+2½FAT
Jumbo Jack®	560	36	680	2ST+3¼MFM+3¼FAT

JACK IN THE BOX® (continued)

Burgers continued:	Calories	Fat (g)	Sodium (mg)	Exchanges
Jumbo Jack® with Cheese	650	43	1090	2ST+4MFM+4FAT
Sourdough Jack™	670	43	1180	3ST+4MFM+4FAT
Ultimate Cheeseburger	1030	79	1200	2ST+6MFM+9½FAT
Bacon Ultimate Cheeseburger	1150	89	1770	2¼ST+8MFM+8FAT
¼# Burger	510	27	1080	2½ST+2½MFM+3FAT
Salads:				
Garden Chicken Salad	200	9	420	2MFM+2V+½FAT
Side Salad	50	3	75	¼MFM+½V+½FAT
Bleu Cheese Dressing	210	18	750	4¾FAT
Buttermilk House Dressing	290	30	560	6½FAT
Low Calorie Italian Dressing	25	1.^{5}	670	½FAT
Thousand Island Dressing	250	24	570	5½FAT
Croutons	50	2	105	½ST+¼FAT
Mexican Food:				
Taco	190	11	410	1ST+1MFM+1FAT
Monster Taco	290	18	550	1½ST+1MFM+2FAT
Teriyaki Bowl:				
Chicken	670	4	1620	6ST+3LM+2½V
Soy Sauce	5	0	480	FREE
Finger Foods:				
Egg Rolls, 3 piece	440	24	1020	2¼ST+1MFM+1V+ 3½FAT
Egg Rolls, 5 piece	730	41	1700	3½ST+1¾MFM+1¾V+ 5FAT
Chicken Strips, breaded 5 piece	360	17	970	1ST+3¼MFM+1FAT
Chicken & Fries	730	34	1690	5ST+2½MFM+3¼FAT
Fish & Chips	720	35	1580	5ST+2MFM+4FAT
Stuffed Jalapeños, 7 piece	470	28	1560	2½ST+1HFM+4FAT
Stuffed Jalapeños, 10 piece	680	40	2220	3¼ST+1½MFM+5¾FAT
Bacon & Cheddar Potato Wedges	800	58	1470	3ST+½MFM+10FAT
Barbecue Dipping Sauce	45	0	300	½ST
Buttermilk House Dipping Sauce	130	13	240	2½FAT
Sweet & Sour Dipping Sauce	40	0	160	½ST
Sour Cream	60	6	30	1½FAT
Sides & Desserts:				
Seasoned Curly Fries	420	24	1030	3ST+4FAT
Chili Cheese Curly Fries	650	41	1640	4ST+1HFM+5¾FAT
Regular French Fries	360	17	740	3ST+2½FAT
Jumbo Fries	430	20	890	3¾ST+3FAT
Super Scoop French Fries	610	28	1250	5½ST+4FAT

JACK IN THE BOX® (continued)

Sides & Desserts continued:

	Calories	Fat (g)	Sodium (mg)	Exchanges
Onion Rings	460	25	780	3ST+5FAT
Hot Apple Turnover	340	18	510	2¼ST+3¼FAT
Cheesecake	310	18	210	2ST+3FAT
Double Fudge Cake	300	10	320	3½ST+1FAT
Carrot Cake	370	16	340	3½ST+2FAT

Ice Cream Shakes (reg):

	Calories	Fat (g)	Sodium (mg)	Exchanges
Vanilla Classic	610	31	320	3CHO+1SkMk+6FAT
Chocolate Classic	630	27	330	3½CHO+1LfMk+5FAT
Strawberry Classic	640	28	300	3½CHO+1LfMk+5FAT
Cappuccino Classic	630	29	320	3½CHO+1LfMk+5FAT
Oreo® Cookie Classic	740	36	490	5CHO+1LfMk+6FAT

Condiments:

	Calories	Fat (g)	Sodium (mg)	Exchanges
American Cheese, 1 slice	45	4	200	1FAT
Swiss-style Cheese, 1 slice	40	3	190	1FAT
Ketchup Packet	10	0	100	FREE
Salsa	10	0	200	FREE
Sour Cream	60	6	30	1½FAT
Tartar Dipping Sauce	220	23	240	4½FAT

JACK IN THE BOX, JUMBO JACK, SOURDOUGH JACK and the JACK image are
trademarks of Foodmaker, Inc.

KFC®

Tender Roast® Chicken:

	Calories	Fat (g)	Sodium (mg)	Exchanges
Wing with skin, $1.^8$ oz	121	$7.^7$	331	1½MFM
Breast with skin, $4.^9$ oz	251	$10.^8$	830	5LM
Breast without skin, $4.^2$ oz	169	$4.^3$	797	4½VLM
Thigh with skin, $3.^2$ oz	207	12	504	2½LM
Thigh without skin, $2.^1$ oz	106	$5.^5$	312	2LM
Drumstick with skin, $1.^9$ oz	97	$4.^3$	271	2LM
Drumstick without skin, $1.^2$ oz	67	$2.^4$	259	1½VLM

Original Recipe® Chicken:

	Calories	Fat (g)	Sodium (mg)	Exchanges
Whole Wing, $1.^6$ oz	140	10	414	¼ST+1MFM+1FAT
Breast, $5.^4$ oz	400	24	1116	1ST+4MFM+1FAT
Drumstick, $2.^2$ oz	140	9	422	¼ST+1½MFM
Thigh, $3.^2$ oz	250	18	747	½ST+2MFM+1½FAT

KFC® (continued)

	Calories	Fat (g)	Sodium (mg)	Exchanges
Extra Tasty Crispy™ Chicken				
Whole Wing, 1.^{9} oz	200	13	290	½ST+1MFM+1½FAT
Breast, 5.^{9} oz	470	28	930	1½ST+4MFM+½FAT
Drumstick, 2.^{4} oz	190	11	260	½ST+1½MFM+½FAT
Thigh, 4.^{2} oz	370	25	540	1ST+2½MFM+2½FAT
Hot & Spicy Chicken:				
Whole Wing, 1.^{9} oz	210	15	340	½ST+1MFM+2FAT
Breast, 6.^{5} oz	530	35	1110	1½ST+4MFM+3FAT
Drumstick, 2.^{3} oz	190	11	300	½ST+1½MFM+½FAT
Thigh, 3.^{8} oz	370	27	570	1ST+2MFM+3½FAT
Other KFC Items:				
Colonel's Crispy Strips®, 3 (3¼oz)	261	15.^{8}	658	½ST+2½MFM+½FAT
Chunky Chicken Pot Pie, 13 oz	770	42	2160	4ST+2MFM+6½FAT
Hot Wings™ Pieces, 6 (4.^{8} oz)	471	33	1230	1ST+3½MFM+3FAT
Orig'l Recipe® Chicken SW, 7.^{3} oz	497	22.^{3}	1213	3ST+3MFM+1½FAT
Value BBQ flav. Chick. SW, 5.^{3} oz	256	8	782	1½ST+2LM+½FAT
Side Choices:				
Corn on the Cob, 5.^{7} oz	190	1.^{5}	20	2ST+½FAT
Green Beans, 4.^{7} oz	45	1.^{5}	730	1V+½FAT
BBQ Baked Beans, 5.^{5} oz	190	3	760	2ST+½FAT
Specials:				
Macaroni & Cheese, 5.^{4} oz	180	8	860	1½ST+½MFM+1FAT
Mean Greens®, 5.^{4} oz	70	3	650	1V+½FAT
Red Beans & Rice	130	3	360	1ST+½FAT
Potatoes & Rice:				
Mashed Potatoes with Gravy, 4.^{8} oz	120	6	440	1ST+1FAT
Potato Wedges, 4.^{8} oz	280	13	750	1½ST+2½FAT
Salads:				
Coleslaw, 5 oz	180	9	280	1ST+1V+2FAT
Potato Salad, 5.^{6} oz	230	14	540	1½ST+3FAT
Breads:				
Biscuit, 1 (2 oz)	180	10	560	1½ST+2FAT
Cornbread, 1 (2 oz)	228	13	194	1½ST+2½FAT

KRYSTAL®

	Calories	Fat (g)	Sodium (mg)	Exchanges
Sandwiches:				
Krystal	158	7	324	1ST+1HFM
Double Krystal	277	14	547	1½ST+2HFM
Cheese Krystal	187	10	453	1ST+1HFM+½FAT
Double Cheese Krystal	337	19	815	1½ST+2½HFM
Chili Pup	182	10	597	1ST+½HFM+1½FAT
Chili Cheese Pup	211	13	642	1ST+1HFM+1FAT
Plain Pup	160	9	470	1ST+½HFM+1FAT
Big K	540	35	1283	2ST+3½HFM+1½FAT
Bacon Cheeseburger	521	34	1083	2ST+3HFM+2FAT
Burger Plus	415	26	614	2ST+2HFM+2FAT
Burger Plus w/cheese	473	31	867	2ST+2½HFM+2FAT
Crispy Crunchy Chicken Sandwich	467	24	949	3ST+1HFM+3FAT
Corn Pup	214	14	710	1ST+½HFM+2FAT
Chili and Fries:				
Regular Chili	218	8	855	1ST+1V+1HFM
Large Chili	327	12	1283	1½ST+2V+1½HFM
Small Fries	262	13	115	2ST+2½FAT
Regular Fries	358	18	157	3ST+3½FAT
Large Fries	463	23	203	4ST+4½FAT
Krys Kross Fries	486	29	604	3ST+6FAT
Krys Kross Fries w/cheese	515	31	803	3ST+6FAT
Chili Cheddar Krys Kross Fries	625	39	1111	3ST+1HFM+6FAT
Shakes and Desserts:				
Chocolate Shake	275	10	178	3CHO+2FAT
Apple Pie	300	10	420	2ST+1CHO+2FAT
Lemon Meringue	340	9	190	1ST+3CHO+2FAT
Pecan Pie	450	23	290	1ST+3CHO+4½FAT

LONG JOHN SILVER'S®

	Calories	Fat (g)	Sodium (mg)	Exchanges
Sandwiches:				
Batter-Dipped Fish, w/out sauce	320	13	800	2½ST+2LM+1½FAT
Ultimate Fish™	430	21	1340	3ST+1½HFM+2FAT
Fish, Seafood, Chicken:				
Batter-Dipped Fish, 1 pc	170	11	470	1ST+1½HFM
Batter-Dipped Chicken, 1 pc	120	6	400	1ST+1MFM
Batter-Dipped Shrimp, 1 pc	35	2.5	95	7=1ST+1HFM+2FAT
Clams, 3 oz	300	17	670	2ST+1HFM+2FAT
Popcorn Shrimp, 3.3 oz	280	15	920	2ST+1HFM+1½FAT

LONG JOHN SILVER'S® (continued)

	Calories	Fat (g)	Sodium (mg)	Exchanges
Fish Wraps:				
South of the Border	690	32	1640	5ST+1½HFM+4FAT
Classic	730	36	1730	5ST+1½HFM+5FAT
Caesar	730	37	1810	5ST+1½HFM+5FAT
Ranch	730	36	1780	5ST+1½HFM+5FAT
Cajun	730	35	1820	5ST+1½HFM+4½FAT
Chicken Wraps:				
South of the Border	690	32	1690	5ST+1½HFM+4FAT
Classic	730	36	1780	5ST+1½HFM+5FAT
Caesar	730	37	1880	5ST+1½HFM+5FAT
Ranch	730	36	1810	5ST+1½HFM+5FAT
Cajun	720	35	1860	5ST+1½HFM+4½FAT
Popcorn Shrimp Wraps:				
South of the Border	690	32	1660	5ST+1½HFM+4FAT
Classic	730	36	1750	5ST+1½HFM+5FAT
Caesar	730	37	1820	5ST+1½HFM+5FAT
Ranch	720	35	1830	5ST+1½HFM+4½FAT
Cajun	720	35	1830	5ST+1½HFM+4½FAT
Side Items:				
Fries, 3 oz	250	15	500	1ST+3FAT
Cheese Sticks, 1.^{6} oz	160	9	360	1ST+1HFM
Hushpuppies, 1 pc	60	2.^{5}	25	1=½ST+½FAT`
Corn Cobbette	140	8	0	1ST+1½FAT
Corn Cobbette w/out butter	80	0.^{5}	0	1ST
Rice Pilaf	140	3	210	1½ST+½FAT
Cole Slaw	140	6	260	1V+1CHO+1FAT
Side Salad	25	0	15	1V
Condiments:				
Ketchup, 1	10	0	110	1=FREE
Shrimp Sauce, 1	15	0	180	1=FREE
Tartar Sauce, 1	35	2	35	½FAT
Honey Mustard Sauce, 1	20	0	60	¼CHO
Malt Vinegar, 1	0	0	15	FREE
Sweet'N'Sour Sauce, 1	20	0	45	¼CHO
Margarine	35	4	35	1FAT
Dressings:				
Ranch	170	18	260	3½FAT
Fat-Free Ranch	50	0	380	FREE
Fat-Free French	50	0	360	FREE
Italian	130	14	280	3FAT
Thousand Island	110	10	280	2FAT

McDONALD'S® (Nov 1997)

	Calories	Fat (g)	Sodium (mg)	Exchanges
Sandwiches:				
Hamburger	260	9	580	2ST+1│MFM
Cheeseburger	320	13	820	2ST+1½MFM+1FAT
Quarter Pounder®	420	21	820	2│ST+3MFM+1FAT
Quarter Pounder® w/Cheese	530	30	1290	2│ST+3½MFM+2FAT
Big Mac®	560	31	1070	3ST+3MFM+3FAT
Arch Deluxe™	550	31	1010	2│ST+3MFM+3FAT
Arch Deluxe™ with Bacon	590	34	1150	2│ST+4MFM+3FAT
Crispy Chicken Deluxe™	500	25	1100	3ST+3MFM+2FAT
Filet-O-Fish® Deluxe™	560	28	1060	3½ST+2½MFM+3FAT
Grilled Chicken Deluxe™	440	20	1040	2½ST+3MFM+1FAT
Grilled Chicken Deluxe™, no mayo	300	5	930	2½ST+3LM
French Fries:				
French Fries, Small	210	10	135	1½ST+2FAT
French Fries, Large	450	22	290	3½ST+4FAT
French Fries, Super Size®	540	26	350	4½ST+5FAT
Chicken McNuggets®/Sauces:				
Chicken McNuggets®, 4 piece	190	11	340	1ST+1MFM+1FAT
Chicken McNuggets®, 6 piece	290	17	510	1ST+2MFM+1FAT
Chicken McNuggets®, 9 piece	430	26	770	1½ST+3MFM+2FAT
Hot Mustard Sauce, 1 pkg	60	3.^{5}	240	½CHO+½FAT
Barbecue Sauce, 1 pkg	45	0	250	1CHO
Sweet'N Sour Sauce, 1 pkg	50	0	140	1CHO
Honey, 1 pkg	45	0	0	1CHO
Honey Mustard, 1 pkg	50	4.^{5}	85	1FAT
Light Mayonnaise, 1 pkg	40	4	85	1FAT
Salads:				
Garden Salad	35	0	20	1V
Grilled Chicken Salad Deluxe	120	1.^{5}	240	3LM+1V
Croutons, 1 pkg	50	1.^{5}	80	½ST
Salad Dressings:				
Caesar, 1 pkg	160	14	450	3FAT
Fat Free Herb Vinaigrette, 1 pkg	50	0	330	½CHO
Ranch, 1 pkg	230	21	550	½CHO+4FAT
Red French Reduced Calorie, 1 pkg	160	8	490	1½CHO+1FAT
Desserts/Milk Shakes:				
Vanilla Reduced Fat Ice Cream Cone, 3oz	150	4.^{5}	75	1½CHO+1FAT

McDONALD'S® (Nov 1997) (continued)

Desserts/Milk Shakes continued:	Calories	Fat (g)	Sodium (mg)	Exchanges
Strawberry Sundae, 6 oz	290	7	95	3½CHO+1FAT
Hot Caramel Sundae, 6 oz	360	10	180	4CHO+2FAT
Hot Fudge Sundae, 6 oz	340	12	170	3½CHO+2FAT
Nuts, added to sundaes	40	3.⁵	0	1FAT
Baked Apple Pie	260	13	200	2½CHO+3FAT
Chocolate Chip Cookie	170	10	120	1½CHO+2FAT
McDonaldland® Cookies, 1 pkg	180	5	190	2CHO+1FAT
Vanilla Shake, small	360	9	250	4CHO+2FAT
Chocolate Shake, small	360	9	250	4CHO+2FAT
Strawberry Shake, small	360	9	180	4CHO+2FAT

WENDY'S

Sandwiches:	Calories	Fat (g)	Sodium (mg)	Exchanges
Plain Single	360	16	580	2ST+3MFM
Single with Everything	420	20	920	2ST+3MFM+1FAT
Big Bacon Classic	580	30	1460	3ST+3½MFM+2½FAT
Jr. Hamburger	270	10	610	2ST+1½MFM+½FAT
Jr. Cheeseburger	320	13	830	2ST+1½MFM+1FAT
Jr. Bacon Cheeseburger	380	19	850	2ST+2MFM+2FAT
Jr. Cheeseburger Deluxe	360	17	890	2ST+1½MFM+2FAT
Hamburger, Kid's Meal	270	10	610	2ST+1½MFM+½FAT
Cheeseburger, Kid's Meal	320	13	830	2ST+1½MFM+1FAT
Grilled Chicken Sandwich	310	8	790	2ST+3LM
Breaded Chicken Sandwich	440	18	840	3ST+2½HFM
Chicken Club Sandwich	470	20	970	3ST+3HFM+1FAT
Spicy Chicken Sandwich	410	15	1280	3ST+3MFM
Sandwich Components:				
¼ lb Hamburger Patty	200	14	170	3MFM
2 oz Hamburger Patty	100	7	150	1½MFM
Grilled Chicken Fillet	110	3	450	3VLM
Breaded Chicken Fillet	230	12	490	½ST+3LM+½FAT
Spicy Chicken Fillet	210	9	920	½ST+3LM
Kaiser Bun	190	3	340	2½ST+½FAT
Sandwich Bun	160	2.⁵	280	2ST+½FAT
American Cheese, 1 sl	70	5	320	½HFM
American Cheese, Jr., 1 sl	45	3.⁵	220	½HFM
Bacon, 1 pc	20	1.⁵	65	½FAT
Honey Mustard Red. Cal., 1 t	25	1.⁵	45	½FAT
Mayonnaise, 1½ t	30	3	60	½FAT
Ketchup, 1 t	10	0	75	1t=FREE, 3t=½CHO

WENDY'S (continued)

	Calories	Fat (g)	Sodium (mg)	Exchanges
Fresh Stuffed Pitas™				
Chicken Caesar	490	18	1320	2½ST+4LM+1½FAT
Classic Greek	440	20	1050	2½ST+1V+1HFM+ 2½FAT
Garden Ranch Chicken	480	18	1180	2½ST+1V+3½LM+ 1½FAT
Garden Veggie	400	17	760	2½ST+2V+3½FAT
Pita Dressings (1T):				
Caesar Vinaigrette	70	7	170	1½FAT
Garden Ranch Sauce	50	4.^{5}	125	1FAT
Garden Spot® Salad Bar (for other items, see *Salads* chapter):				
Bananas & Strawberry Glaze, ¼ c	30	0	0	½ FR
Chicken Salad, 2T	70	5	135	½LM+1FAT
Pasta Salad, 2T	35	1.^{5}	180	¼ST+½FAT
Potato Salad, 2T	80	7	180	½ST+1FAT
Fresh Salads to Go (w/out dressing):				
Caesar Side Salad	100	4	820	1MFM+1V
Deluxe Garden Salad	110	6	350	½HFM+1V
Grilled Chicken Salad	200	8	720	3LM+1V
Grilled Chicken Caesar Salad	260	9	1170	1ST+3LM
Side Salad	60	3	180	1V+½FAT
Taco Salad	380	19	1040	2ST+3MFM+1FAT
Taco chips, 15	210	11	180	1½ST+2FAT
Soft Breadstick, 1 ea	130	3	250	1½ST+½FAT
Salad Dressings: 2T (1 oz) =1 ladle, Packets = 2 oz except Italian Caesar=1.^{5} oz				
Blue Cheese, 2T	180	19	190	4FAT
French, 2T	120	10	330	½CHO+2FAT
French Fat Free, 2T	35	0	150	½CHO
Hidden Valley Ranch™, 2T	100	10	220	2FAT
Hidden Valley Ranch™, Red. Fat Red. Cal., 2T	60	5	240	1FAT
Italian Caesar, 2T	150	16	240	3FAT
Italian, Red. Fat, Red. Cal., 2T	40	3	340	½FAT
Thousand Island, 2T	90	8	125	2½FAT
French Fries:				
Small, 3.^{2} oz	270	13	85	2ST+2½FAT
Medium, 4.^{8} oz	390	19	120	3ST+4FAT
Biggie, 6 oz	470	23	150	3½ST+4½FAT

WENDY'S (continued)

	Calories	Fat (g)	Sodium (mg)	Exchanges
Baked Potato:				
Plain	310	0	25	4ST
Bacon & Cheese	530	18	1390	5ST+3½FAT
Broccoli & Cheese	470	14	470	5ST+1V+3FAT
Cheese	570	23	640	4½ST+4½FAT
Chili & Cheese	630	24	770	5ST+½HFM+4FAT
Sour Cream & Chives	380	6	40	4½ST+1FAT
Sour Cream, 1 pkt	60	6	15	1FAT
Whipped Margarine, 1 pkt	60	7	110	1½FAT
Chili:				
Small, 8 oz	210	7	800	1ST+2LM
Large, 12 oz	310	10	1190	1½ST+3LM
Cheddar Cheese, shredded, 2T	70	6	110	½HFM
Saltine Crackers, 2 ea	25	0.^{5}	80	7 crackers=1ST+½FAT
Chicken Nuggets:				
5 pc Nuggets	210	14	480	½ST+1½HFM+1FAT
4 pc Kids	170	11	370	½ST+1HFM+½FAT
Barbecue Sauce, 1 pkt	45	0	160	½CHO
Honey Mustard Sauce, 1 pkt	130	12	220	½CHO+2½FAT
Spicy Buffalo Wing Sauce, 1 pkt	25	1	210	½CHO
Sweet & Sour Sauce, 1 pkt	50	0	120	1CHO
Desserts:				
Chocolate Chip Cookie, 1 ea	270	13	120	2CHO+2½FAT
Frosty Dairy Dessert, sm, 12 oz	330	8	200	3CHO+1WMk
medium, 16 oz	440	11	260	4CHO+1½WMk
large, 20 oz	540	14	320	4½CHO+2WMk

WHATABURGER®

	Calories	Fat (g)	Sodium (mg)	Exchanges
Sandwiches:				
Whataburger®	598	26	1096	4ST+2½HFM+1FAT
on small bun & w/out bun oil	407	19	839	2ST+2½HFM
Whataburger® Double Meat	823	42	1298	4ST+5HFM+1FAT
Whataburger Jr®	300	12	583	2ST+1MFM+1½FAT
Justaburger®	276	11	578	2ST+1MFM+1FAT
Chicken Fajita	272	7	691	2½ST+1½MFM
Beef Fajita	326	12	670	2ST+2½MFM

WHATABURGER® (continued)

	Calories	Fat (g)	Sodium (mg)	Exchanges
Sandwiches continued:				
Grilled Chicken Sandwich	442	14	1103	3ST+3½LM+½FAT
w/out salad dressing	385	9	989	3ST+3½LM
w/out bun oil & w/out dressing	358	6	989	3ST+3½LM
on small bun w/out bun oil & w/mustard instead of dressing	300	3	994	3ST+3½LM
Whatachick'n® Sandwich	501	23	1122	3ST+3MFM+1½FAT
Chicken Strips, 2	120	5	420	½ST+1MFM
Texas Toast, 1 slice	147	5	250	1½ST+1FAT
Chicken Gravy, 3 oz	75	5	375	½ST+1FAT
Whatacatch®	467	25	636	3ST+1HFM+3½FAT
Large Cheese Slice	89	7	338	1HFM
Small Cheese Slice	46	4	176	½HFM
Bacon, 1 slice	38	3	106	½HFM
Baked Potato	310	0	23	4½ST
Baked Potato w/cheese topping	510	16	863	4½ST+1HFM+1½FAT
Baked Potato w/broc. ch. topping	453	10	636	4½ST+1HFM+½FAT
Sour Cream, 2 oz	121	12	30	2½FAT
Salad and Salad Dressings:				
Garden Salad	56	0.[6]	32	½ST+1V
Grilled Chicken Salad	150	1	434	1ST+3VLM
Croutons, 1 pkt	29	1	88	¼ST+¼FAT
Club Crackers, 1 pkt	31	1	72	¼ST+¼FAT
Lite Ranch Dressing, 1 pkt	66	3	607	½CHO+½FAT
Thousand Island Dressing, 1 pkt	160	12	470	1CHO+2½FAT
Ranch Dressing, 1 pkt	320	33	750	6½FAT
Lite Vinegarette Dressing, 1 pkt	37	2	896	¼CHO+½FAT
Fries and Onion Rings:				
French Fries, junior	221	12	139	1½ST+2½FAT
French Fries, regular	332	18	208	2½ST+3½FAT
French Fries, large	442	24	227	3ST+5FAT
Onion Rings, regular	329	19	596	2ST+4FAT
Onion Rings, large	493	29	893	3ST+5½FAT
Accompaniments:				
Ketchup, one pkt	30	0	344	½CHO
Jalapeno Pepper, 1 pc	3	0	190	FREE

WHATABURGER® (continued)

	Calories	Fat (g)	Sodium (mg)	Exchanges
Desserts and Shakes:				
Apple Turnover	215	11	241	1FR+1CHO+2FAT
Vanilla Shake, 12 oz	325	10	172	3½CHO+2FAT
Strawberry Shake, 12 oz	352	9	168	4CHO+2FAT
Chocolate Shake, 12 oz	364	9	172	4CHO+2FAT
Chocolate Chunk Cookie	247	16	75	2CHO+3FAT
Macadamia Nut Cookie	269	16	80	2CHO+3FAT
Oatmeal Raisin Cookie	222	7	70	2CHO+½FR+1½FAT
Peanut Butter Cookie	257	13	36	2CHO+2½FAT

Whataburger's customer service number is **1-800-6 BURGER.**

WHITE CASTLE®

	Calories	Fat (g)	Sodium (mg)	Exchanges
Sandwiches:				
Hamburgers, 2	270	14	270	1½ST+1HFM+1FAT
Cheeseburgers, 2	310	17	480	1½ST+1½HFM+1FAT

Nutritional information for other items vary depending on region of US. For information, call
    1-800-THE-CRAVE.

Delis & Sandwich Shops

Chapter Contents:

■ Bread: bagels, sliced bread, croissant, focaccia, pita bread, rolls
■ Meat, cheese, and other fillings
■ Condiments
■ Accompaniments
■ Your Favorite Deli & Sandwich Shops

Cafes and delicatessens are generally smaller restaurants serving a variety of foods including sandwiches, salads, and soups. Soups and salads are discussed in their own respective chapters in Part 3 of this book. This chapter will focus on the wide variety of sandwiches and typical accompaniments.

Deli sandwiches can be healthy or disastrous depending on how you choose your bread; meat, cheese, or other filling; condiments; and other accompaniments. Take a look at the following example.

A Deli Sandwich Meal Can Be Lean:

		Calories	Fat (g)
3 oz Bagel		240	3
2 oz Turkey		60	1
Mustard, 1T		15	1
Baked Potato Chips, 12		110	1
	TOTAL:	425	6

Or It Can Be a Disaster:

		Calories	Fat (g)
Tuna Salad, ½ c		380	20
Croissant, 3 oz		360	20
Mayonnaise, 1T		100	11
Cheese, 1 oz		100	8
Potato Chips, 1 oz		150	10
	TOTAL:	1090	69

Bread

There are many people that, when *dieting*, skimp on the bread and eat just the meat. If anything, they should be doing the opposite. Breads consist mostly of flour and are very low in fat. Meat and cheese are much higher in both calories and fat.

✓ **Choose a sandwich made with a low fat bread** such as sliced sandwich bread, French or Italian bread, bagels, pita bread, or rolls. Avoid breads made with eggs and additional fat such as croissants.

Bread Calorimeter: Calories & fat per serving

Calories per oz	Bread	Calories & Fat grams (g)				
		1 oz	2 oz	3 oz	4 oz	5 oz
120	Croissants, plain	**120** 7g	**240** 13g	**360** 20g	**480** 26g	**600** 33g
90	Focaccio	**90** 3g	**180** 6g	**270** 9g	**360** 12g	**450** 15g
80	Bagel English Muffin Italian Bread Pita Bread Submarine Roll	**80** 1g	**160** 1g	**240** 2g	**320** 2g	**400** 3g
70	French Roll & Baguette Sandwich Bread Slices	**70** 1g	**140** 2g	**210** 3g	**280** 4g	**350** 5g

How many ounces of bread are you eating? Simply compare the bread in your favorite sandwich with a slice of store-bought sandwich bread which weighs approximately 1 oz. Most deli sandwiches contain at least 2 oz of bread and as much as 5 oz! For ease in calculation, various sizes of bagels, croissants, English muffins, focaccio, French & Italian bread, and French rolls are described and/or illustrated in the *Breads & Spreads* chapter. Pita Bread, Soft Rolls, and Submarine rolls are described below.

Pita Bread

Pita bread is a flat, circular bread that is hollow in the middle. It can be served whole or cut in half. When served whole as a gyro, about 4 oz of high fat meat is wrapped inside the pita bread and served with a high fat cucumber/sour cream sauce. Pita bread can also be cut in half, opened up and stuffed with a variety of meats, cheese, and sauces. One 6½-7" (approximately 1" larger than the width of this page) round pita is about 2½ oz and contains approximately 190 calories.

Soft Bun

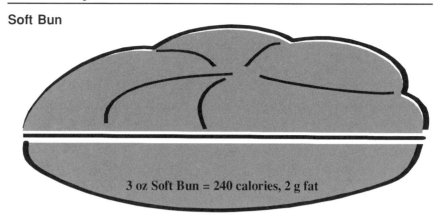

3 oz Soft Bun = 240 calories, 2 g fat

Rolls

A 3¾" crusty French Roll weighs about 3 oz. Submarine rolls are fluffier so the portion size is bigger. A 6" submarine roll (slightly longer than the width of this book) will weigh about 2½ - 3 oz.

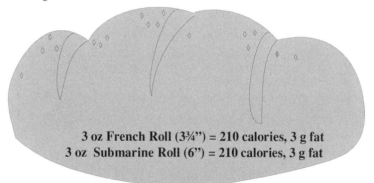

3 oz French Roll (3¾") = 210 calories, 3 g fat
3 oz Submarine Roll (6") = 210 calories, 3 g fat

Sandwich Breads

	Calories	Fat (g)	Sodium (mg)	Exchanges
Bagel, 3 oz, 3½" diameter	240	1	400	3ST
4 oz, 4¼" diameter	320	2	540	4ST+½FAT
5 oz, 5" diameter	400	3	675	5ST+½FAT
Bread, 1 slice ½" thick	70	1	150	1ST
Croissant, 3 oz	360	20	400	2¼ST+4FAT
English Muffin, 3 oz sandwich size	220	2	420	2½ST+½FAT
Focaccio bread, ½ of 9" round loaf	450	10	1000	5ST+2FAT
French Roll, 3 oz	210	3	330	3ST
Italian Bread, 1 oz slice	75	1	150	1ST
Pita Bread, 7" round	190	1.^{5}	410	2½ST
Soft Bun, 3 oz	240	2	450	3ST
Submarine Roll, 3 oz	240	2	450	3ST

Meat, Cheese, & Other Fillings

Deli meat and cheese range from 30-130 calories/ounce with most sandwiches contain anywhere from 2 - 8 ounces.

✓ **Choose sliced turkey, chicken, ham, or roast beef.** Cheeses, specialty deli meats such as salami and pastrami, and prepared tuna or chicken salad are at least twice as high in fat and calories.

✓ **Keep meat portions at 3 oz or less.** Three ounces is the size of a deck of cards. If your sandwich contains more than that, consider splitting a sandwich with a friend and having an extra salad, cup of broth-based soup, or some fruit. In a restaurant that really piles on the meat, ask them to go light on the meat or order just a half of a sandwich along with an extra slice of bread. Split the meat between the two slices of bread to make a whole sandwich.

Deli Meat & Cheese Calorimeter: Calories & fat per serving

Calories per oz	Deli Meat & Cheese	Calories & Fat grams (g)				
		1 oz	2 oz	3 oz	4 oz	5 oz
130	Liver Pate, goose	**130**	**260**	**390**	**520**	**650**
		12g	24g	36g	48g	60g
120	Salami	**120**	**180**	**270**	**360**	**450**
		10g	20g	30g	40g	50g
110	Blood Sausage American, Cheddar, & Swiss Cheese	**110**	**220**	**330**	**440**	**550**
		9g	18g	27g	36g	45g
100	Braunschweiger Meatloaf Provolone Cheese Pastrami	**100**	**200**	**300**	**400**	**500**
		8g	16g	24g	32g	40g
90	Bologna Bratwurst, Brotwurst, Knockwurst, Italian Sausage, Mortadella, Summer Sausage Mozzarella Cheese	**90**	**180**	**270**	**360**	**450**
		8g	15g	23g	30g	38g
60	Headcheese Liver Pate, chicken Corned Beef & Roast Beef, lean	**60**	**120**	**180**	**240**	**300**
		4g	8g	12g	16g	20g
50	Chicken Breast Ham, lean	**50**	**100**	**150**	**200**	**250**
		2g	4g	6g	8g	10g
30	Turkey	**30**	**60**	**90**	**120**	**150**
		$0.^5$g	1g	2g	2g	3g

Sandwich Meats & Cheeses

	Calories	Fat (g)	Sodium (mg)	Exchanges
Per 1 oz unless specified:				
Blood Sausage	108	10	na	1HFM+½FAT
Bologna	89	8	280	1HFM
Bratwurst	85	7	158	1HFM
Braunschweiger	102	9	325	1HFM
Brotwurst	92	8	315	1HFM
Chicken Breast	50	1.^{5}	35	1LM
Chicken Salad, ¼ c	125	9	350	1½LM+1FAT
Corned Beef	72	5.^{4}	325	1MFM
Corned Beef, lean	60	4	270	1MFM
Egg Salad, ¼ c	123	11	170	1MFM+1FAT
Ham	52	3	375	1LM
Headcheese	60	5	355	1MFM
Italian Sausage	92	7	262	1HFM
Knockwurst	87	8	285	1HFM
Liver Pate, chicken	60	4	na	1MFM
Liver Pate, goose	131	12	na	1HFM+1FAT
Meatloaf	100	8	na	1HFM
Mortadella	89	7	355	1HFM
Pastrami	99	8	348	1HFM
Roast Beef, lean	60	3	10	1LM
Salami	116	10	641	1HFM+½FAT
Summer Sausage	94	8	375	1HFM
Tuna Salad, ¼ c	190	10	410	2VLM+½CHO+2FAT
Turkey	31	0.^{5}	407	1VLM
Cheeses (1 oz):				
American	106	9	406	1HFM
Cheddar	114	9	176	1HFM
Mozzarella	90	7	106	1HFM
Provolone	100	8	248	1HFM
Swiss	107	8	74	1HFM

Condiments

✔ **Have the condiments served to you on the side** except for mustard, fat-free mayonnaise, vinegar, and horseradish. The other condiments are high caloric so use them sparingly.

High Fat Condiments can more than Triple the Fat Grams:		
	Calories	Fat (g)
6" Sub with turkey, cheese, mayonnaise, & oil	490	25
6" Sub with turkey, cheese, & mustard	300	7
TOTAL:	**190**	**18**

Condiments

Per 1 Tablespoon:	Calories	Fat (g)	Sodium (mg)	Exchanges
Aioli Sauce, garlic oil	100	10	3	2FAT
Butter	108	12	123	2½FAT
Dijonnaise	15	0	210	FREE
Guacamole	30	3	105	½FAT
Horseradish	6	0	14	FREE
Ketchup	18	0	180	¼CHO
Margarine	100	11	100	2FAT
Mayonnaise	100	11	80	2FAT
Reduced Calorie Mayonnaise	50	5	80	1FAT
Fat Free Mayonnaise	10	0	130	FREE
Mustard	15	1	190	FREE
Oil & Vinegar	70	8	0	1½FAT
Picante Sauce	5	0	110	FREE
Remoulade Sauce	100	11	105	2FAT
Sour cream/cucumber Sauce	45	3.5	na	½FAT
Thousand Island Dressing	60	5	110	1FAT
Vinegar	2	0	0	FREE

Accompaniments

✔ **Request a low calorie accompaniment**. If the meal is typically served with high fat accompaniments ask for a substitute such as a tossed salad with fat-free dressing, sliced tomatoes, pretzels, fresh fruit, or a big pickle. For more details about ordering a salad, see the *Salads* chapter.

Accompaniments

	Calories	Fat (g)	Sodium (mg)	Exchanges
Salads (½ c unless specified):				
Cole Slaw	170	12	200	2V+2½FAT
Fresh Fruit Salad	60	0	2	1FR
Garden Salad	25	1	25	1V
2T Salad Dressing	160	16	300	3FAT
2T Fat-Free Salad Dressing	20	0	270	¼CHO
Macaroni Salad	200	14	360	1ST+3FAT
Potato Salad	200	14	660	1ST+3FAT
Crunchies:				
Baked Potato Chips, 1oz (12 chips)	110	1.5	150	1¼ST+¼FAT
Baked Tortilla Chips, 10	120	1	80	1½ST
Pickles, 3¾" long	7	0	930	FREE
Popcorn, 1 c	55	4	40	¼ST+¾FAT
Potato Chips, 1oz (20 reg/12 ripple)	160	10	180	1ST+2FAT
Pretzels, 1 oz (48 Sticks)	110	0	530	1½ST
Tiny Twists (18) or Regular (8)	100	0	420	1¼ST
Thick Twists (4)	110	1	620	1½ST
Tortilla Chips, 10	180	8	80	1½ST+1½FAT

Your Favorite Deli & Sandwich Shops

AU BON PAIN®

	Calories	Fat (g)	Sodium (mg)	Exchanges
Sourdough Bagels:				
Plain	350	1	540	4½ST
Cinnamon Raisin	390	1	550	5ST
Sesame	380	4	540	4½ST
Honey 9 Grain	360	2	580	4½ST
Everything	360	2.5	710	4½ST
Asiago Cheese	380	6	690	4ST
Spreads:				
Lite Cream Cheese	110	8	240	¾HFM+½FAT
Cream Cheese	170	17	170	½HFM+2½FAT
Sandwich Fillings:				
Country Ham	150	7	1370	3LM
Turkey Breast	120	1	1110	3½VLM
Roast Beef	140	4.5	550	3LM
Tuna Salad	360	29	520	3LM+4FAT
Chicken Tarragon	240	17	170	4VLM+1½FAT
Cracked Pepper Chicken	140	1.6	184	4VLM
Brie Cheese, ½ portion	140	12	270	1HFM+1FAT
Swiss Cheese, ½ portion	160	12	110	1½HFM
Cheddar Cheese, ½ portion	170	14	260	1½HFM+½FAT
Provolone, ½ portion	150	11	355	1½HFM
(½ portion cheese used when adding to meat sandwich)				
Chef's Creation Sandwiches:				
Fresh Mozzarella, Tomato, & Pesto	650	30	1090	4ST+2½HFM+2FAT
Thai Chicken Sandwich	420	6	1320	4ST+2LM
Hot Roast Turkey Club	950	50	2240	5ST+5MFM+5FAT
Arizona Chicken	720	33	1190	4ST+5½MFM+1FAT
Wraps Sandwiches:				
Chicken Caesar	630	31	1140	3ST+4LM+4FAT
w/out dressing	440	12	880	3ST+4LM
Summer Turkey	550	12	1610	4½ST+2½LM+1FAT
w/out dressing	430	4.5	1380	4½ST+2½LM
Fresh Sandwich Breads:				
Hearth Sandwich, 1 roll	140	2	260	1½ST+½FAT
French Sandwich, 1 roll	120	1	320	1½ST
Braided Roll, 1 roll	170	5	320	1½ST+1FAT
Sandwich Croissant, 1 roll	310	16	290	2½ST+3FAT
Multigrain Loaf, 1 slice	130	1	340	1½ST
Rye Loaf, 1 slice	110	2	310	1½ST+½FAT

AU BON PAIN® (continued)

	Calories	Fat (g)	Sodium (mg)	Exchanges
Fresh Loaf Breads:				
Parisienne, 1 slice	120	$0.^5$	300	1½ST
Baguette, 1 slice	140	$0.^5$	350	2ST
Four Grain, 1 slice	130	1	280	1½ST
Fresh Rolls (1 roll):				
Petit Pain	200	1	570	2½ST
Hearth	220	$1.^5$	410	2ST+½FAT
Salad Dressings (3 oz ea):				
Sesame French	370	30	1010	1½CHO+6FAT
Caesar	380	39	410	½HFM+7FAT
Lite Italian	230	20	570	4FAT
Blue Cheese	410	41	910	½ST+8FAT
Fat Free Tomato Basil	70	0	650	1CHO
Lemon Basil Vinaigrette	330	32	460	1CHO+6½FAT
Honey Mustard Lite	280	17	560	1½CHO+3½FAT
Buttermilk Ranch	310	32	270	6½FAT
Fresh Salads:				
Tuna Salad	490	27	750	½FR+1ST+2V+2½LM+ 4FAT
Chicken Tarragon Garden	470	23	500	1ST+2V+3½LM+ 2½FAT
Chicken Caesar Salad	360	11	910	1ST+2V+4LM
Large Garden Salad	160	2	290	3V+1ST+½FAT
Small Garden Salad	100	1	150	2V+½ST
Oriental Chicken Salad	230	5	150	½ST+2V+2½LM
Caesar Salad	270	10	800	1ST+2V+2MFM

Hot Soups per 8 oz (8 oz served w/½ sandwich only, 12 oz served in bread bowl):

	Calories	Fat (g)	Sodium (mg)	Exchanges
Caribbean Black Bean	120	1	770	1½ST+1VLM
NE Potato & Cheese with Ham	150	8	820	1½ST+2½FAT
Corn Chowder	260	16	760	2ST+3FAT
Beef Barley	75	2	660	½ST+½MFM
Vegetarian Chili	139	$2.^5$	1070	1ST+2V+½FAT
Clam Chowder	270	19	730	1ST+1LM+4FAT
Tomato Florentine	61	1	1030	½ST+1V
Garden Vegetable	29	0	820	1V
Chicken Noodle	80	$1.^5$	670	½ST+1LM
Cream of Broccoli	220	18	770	1ST+3½FAT
Bread Bowl alone	640	$3.^5$	1950	8 ST+½FAT
Soup in a Bread Bowl:				
Garden Vegetable	700	$3.^5$	3180	8ST+3V+½FAT
Clam Chowder	1050	32	3040	9½ST+½WhMk+1MFM +4FAT
Tomato Florentine	760	5	3490	8ST+3V+1FAT

AU BON PAIN® (continued)

	Calories	Fat (g)	Sodium (mg)	Exchanges
Soup in a Bread Bowl continued:				
Caribbean Black Bean	830	5	3100	9½ST+1VLM
NE Potato & Cheese with Ham	860	15	3170	9½ST+3FAT
Corn Chowder	1030	28	3090	11ST+5½FAT
Beef Barley	760	7	2940	8½ST+1V+1MFM+ ½FAT
Vegetarian Chili	870	7	3550	10ST+2V+1½FAT
Chicken Noodle	760	6	2950	9½ST+1LM+½FAT
Cream of Broccoli	970	31	3100	8½ST+½WhMk+5½FAT
Hot Croissants:				
Ham & Cheese	380	20	690	2ST+1½LM+3FAT
Spinach & Cheese	270	16	330	1½ST+½MFM+½V+ 2½FAT
Dessert Croissants:				
Plain	270	15	240	2ST+3FAT
Almond	560	37	260	3CHO+7½FAT
Apple	280	10	180	3CHO+2FAT
Chocolate	440	23	230	3CHO+4½FAT
Cinnamon Raisin	380	13	290	1FR+3CHO+2½FAT
Raspberry Cheese	380	19	300	3CHO+4FAT
Sweet Cheese	390	22	330	3ST+4½FAT
Gourmet Cookies:				
Chocolate Chip	280	13	85	2½CHO+2½FAT
Oatmeal Raisin	250	10	240	2CHO+½FR+2FAT
Shortbread	390	25	190	2½CHO+5FAT
Almond Biscotti	200	10	45	1½CHO+2FAT
Chocolate Almond Biscotti	240	13	50	1½CHO+2½FAT

Au Bon Pain's Specialty Drinks can be found in the *Beverage* chapter

BLIMPIE®

	Calories	Fat (g)	Sodium (mg)	Exchanges
6" White Bread Subs (Nutritional info does NOT include toppings and condiments):				
Blimpie® Best	410	13	1480	3ST+2½MFM
Turkey	320	5	890	3ST+2LM
Roast Beef	340	5	870	3ST+2LM
Cheese Trio	510	23	1060	3ST+2½HFM+½FAT
Club	450	13	1350	3ST+2½MFM
Ham & Swiss	400	13	970	3ST+2½MFM
Ham, Salami, Provolone	590	28	1880	3ST+3HFM+1FAT
Tuna	570	32	790	3ST+1½LM+5½FAT
Grilled Chicken Salad	350	12	1190	1ST+5LM
Steak & Cheese	550	26	1080	3ST+2HFM+2FAT
Grilled Chicken	400	9	950	3ST+2LM+½FAT
5 Meatball	500	22	970	3ST+1½HFM+2FAT

BRUEGGER'S BAGEL[SM]

Bagels:	Calories	Fat (g)	Sodium (mg)	Exchanges
Blueberry Bagel, 3.^{6}oz	300	2	480	4ST
Cranberry Orange Bagel, 1.^{7}oz	140	0	220	2ST
Cinnamon Raisin Bagel, 3.^{6}oz	290	2	400	4ST
Egg Bagel, 3.^{6}oz	280	1	510	3½ST
Everything Bagel, 3.^{7}oz	290	2	700	4ST
Garlic Bagel, 3.^{6}oz	280	2	440	3½ST
Honey Grain Bagel, 3.^{6}oz	300	3	390	4ST
Onion Bagel, 3.^{6}oz	280	2	430	3½ST
Pesto Bagel, 3.^{6}oz	280	2	480	3½ST
Plain Bagel, 3.^{6}oz	280	2	430	3½ST
Poppy Seed Bagel, 3.^{6}oz	280	2	440	3½ST
Pumpernickel Bagel, 3.^{6}oz	280	2	390	3½ST
Salt Bagel, 3.^{6}oz	270	2	1670	3½ST
Sesame Bagel, 3.^{6}oz	290	3	440	3½ST
Spinach Bagel, 3.^{6}oz	280	1	490	3½ST
Sun Dried Tomato Bagel, 3.^{6}oz	280	2	490	3½ST
Wheat Bran Bagel, 3.^{6}oz	280	2	410	3½ST
Specialty Sandwiches:				
Chicken Fajita	460	10	830	4ST+2½VLM+1½FAT
Leonardo da Veggie™	420	11	690	4ST+1HFM+½FAT
Herby Turkey™	510	13	1100	4ST+2½VLM+2FAT
Hot Shot Turkey™	450	8	1090	4ST+2VLM+1FAT
Santa Fe Turkey	450	9	1040	4ST+2VLM+1½FAT

D'ANGELO®

D'Angelo D'Lites:	Calories	Fat (g)	Sodium (mg)	Exchanges
Turkey D'Lite Pokket	330	2	490	2ST+3LM+1V
Small Sub	365	4	535	2½ST+3LM+1V
Roast Beef D'Lite Pokket	330	6	710	2ST+3LM+1V
Small Sub	365	7	755	2½ST+3LM+1V
Steak D'Lite Pokket	390	11	735	3ST+2MFM+2V
Spicy Steak D'Lite Pokket	425	11	735	3ST+2MFM+2V
Ginger StirFry Ch. D'Lite Pokket	400	5	1240	2½ST+3LM+1V
Stuffed Turkey D'Lite Pokket	510	8	880	3ST+4LM+1V+1FR
Small Sub	545	9	920	3½ST+4LM+1V+1FR
Classic Vegetable D'Lite Pokket	340	10	960	2ST+1HFM+3V+½FAT
Crunchy Vegetable D'Lite Pokket	350	10	1000	2ST+1HFM+3V+½FAT
Small Sub	385	11	1045	2½ST+1HFM+3V+ ½FAT
Super Salads:				
Turkey D'Lite	355	2	714	2ST+3LM+1V
Roast Beef D'Lite	355	6	935	2ST+3LM+1V
Tuna D'Lite	295	2	853	2ST+2LM+1V
Chicken D'Lite	345	4	980	2ST+2LM+1V

JASON'S DELI®

	Calories	Fat (g)	Sodium (mg)	Exchanges
Healthy Heart Super Combo - Each sandwich is served with your choice of:				
Pretzels	110	1	na	1ST
Baked Lays®	130	2	170	1ST+½FAT
Fruit	50	$0.^3$	na	1FR
German Potato Salad	108	4	na	1ST+1FAT
Steamed Vegetables	7	$0.^2$	na	FREE
Turkey Reuben	335	3	na	2ST+4VLM
"Lite" Tuna Sandwich	324	6	1000	na
"Lite" Chicken Salad Sandwich	324	6	1000	na
Ham It Down™	386	7	na	2ST+6VLM
Garden Sandwich	374	18	500	2ST+3FAT
Heart Healthy Poultry:				
King Ranch Lite	541	5	na	na
Southwestern Pita	266	4	794	2ST+3VLM
Pita Plus	387	13	1000	2ST+3LM+1FAT
Philly Chick™	380	9	852	3ST+4LM (without FF Honey Dijon)
Healthy Heart Super Spuds:				
Pollo Mexicano Lite	650	5	na	na
Spud Lite	499	$1.^3$	na	4ST+3VLM
Slender Jane	375	$2.^5$	621	5ST
Chicken Pepper Sauté "Lite"	529	10	1000	4ST+4LM
Wrap Sandwiches:				
Turkey Wrap	417	15	na	na
Spinach Veggie Wrap	426	17	694	na
Healthy Heart Soups & Salads:				
Gazpacho Soup, cup	53	2	434	1ST
bowl	70	3	579	1ST+1FAT
French Onion Soup, cup	77	5	751	½ST+1VLM+1FAT
bowl	128	9	na	½ST+1VLM+1FAT
Vegetarian Vegetable Soup, cup	75	2	532	1ST
bowl	100	3	710	1ST+1FAT
Salad Bar	na	na	na	Depends on food chosen
Fruit Plate (no dressing), small	100	1	na	3FR
large	200	2	na	4FR
Healthy Heart Desserts:				
Strawberry Shortcake	383	8	341	na
Fat Free Cheesecake	na	na	na	na
Strawb, Rasp, or Choc Brownie	na	na	na	na

SUBWAY®

Nutritional information on regular 6" subs and salads includes the standard vegetables of onions, lettuce, tomatoes, pickles, green peppers, & olives. They do not include cheese (unless noted w/▲) or condiments. These are listed separately below.

	Calories	Fat (g)	Sodium (mg)	Exchanges
6" Cold Subs:				
Veggie Delite™	237	3	593	2½ST+1V
Turkey Breast	289	4	1403	2½ST+1LM+1V
Turkey Breast & Ham	295	5	1361	2½ST+1LM+1V
Ham	302	5	1319	2½ST+1LM+1V
Roast Beef	303	5	939	2½ST+1½LM+1V
Subway Club®	312	5	1352	2½ST+1½LM+1V
Subway Seafood & Crab® a processed seafood & crab blend, made w/light mayo	347	10	884	2½ST+1½LM+1V+1FAT
B.L.T.	327	10	957	2½ST+1HFM+1V
Cold Cut Trio	378	13	1412	2½ST+1½MFM+1V+½FAT
Tuna, made w/light mayo	391	15	940	2½ST+1LM+1V+2FAT
Subway Seafood & Crab® a processed seafood & crab blend	430	19	860	2½ST+1½LM+1V+2½FAT
Classic Italian B.M.T.®	460	22	1664	2½ST+1½HFM+1V+1½FAT
Tuna	542	32	886	2½ST+1LM+1V+5½FAT
6" Hot Subs:				
Roasted Chicken Breast	348	6	978	2½ST+2½VLM+1V
Steak & Cheese▲	398	10	1117	2½ST+2½MFM+1V
Subway Melt™▲	382	12	1746	2½ST+2MFM+1V
Meatball	419	16	1046	3ST+1MFM+1V+1½FAT
Pizza Sub▲	464	22	1621	3ST+1HFM+1V+2FAT
Deli Style Sandwiches:				
Turkey Breast	235	4	944	2ST+1LM+½V
Ham	234	4	773	2ST+½LM+½V
Roast Beef	245	4	638	2ST+1LM+½V
Tuna, made w/light mayo	279	9	583	2ST+½LM+½V+1FAT
Bologna	292	12	744	2ST+½HFM+½V+1FAT
Tuna	354	18	557	2ST+½LM+½V+3FAT
Condiments & Extras:				
Vinegar, 1 tsp	1	0	0	FREE
Mustard, 2 tsp	8	0	0	FREE
Light Mayonnaise, 1 tsp	18	2	33	FREE, 3 tsp=1FAT
Bacon, 2 slices	45	4	182	½HFM *or* 1FAT
Cheese, 2 triangles	41	3	204	½MFM
Mayonnaise, 1 tsp	37	4	27	1FAT
Olive Oil Blend, 1 tsp	45	5	0	1FAT

SUBWAY® (continued)

	Calories	Fat (g)	Sodium (mg)	Exchanges
Salads, without salad dressings:				
Veggie Delite™	51	1	308	2V
Turkey Breast	102	2	1117	1LM+2V
Subway Club®	126	3	1067	1½LM+2V
Roast Beef	117	3	654	1½LM+2V
Ham	116	3	1034	1LM+2V
Turkey Breast & Ham	109	3	1076	1LM+2V
Roasted Chicken Breast	162	4	693	2½VLM+2V
Subway Seafood & Crab® a processed seafood & crab blend, made w/light mayo	161	8	599	1½LM+2V+½FAT
Steak & Cheese▲	212	8	832	2MFM+2V
B.L.T.	140	8	672	½HFM+2V
Subway Melt™▲	195	10	1461	2MFM+2V
Cold Cut Trio	191	11	1127	1½MFM+2V+½FAT
Tuna, made w/light mayo	205	13	654	1LM+2V+2FAT
Meatball	233	14	761	½ST+1MFM+2V+1½FAT
Subway Seafood & Crab® a processed seafood & crab blend	244	17	575	1½LM+2V+2½FAT
Pizza▲	277	20	1336	1HFM+2V+2½FAT
Classic Italian B.M.T.®	274	20	1379	1½HFM+2V+1½FAT
Tuna	356	30	601	1LM+2V+5½FAT
Bread Bowl	330	4	760	4ST
Salad Dressing (per T, each pkt has approx. 4 T):				
Creamy Italian	65	6	132	1FAT
Fat Free Italian	5	0	152	FREE
French	65	5	100	1FAT
Fat Free French	15	0	85	FREE
Thousand Island	65	6	107	1FAT
Ranch	87	9	117	2FAT
Fat Free Ranch	12	0	177	FREE
Cookies (1):				
Oatmeal Raisin	200	8	160	2ST+1FAT
Chocolate Chunk	210	10	140	1½ST+2FAT
Chocolate Chip	210	10	140	1½ST+2FAT
Chocolate Chip M&M®	210	10	140	1½ST+2FAT
Peanut Butter	220	12	180	1½ST+2½FAT
Sugar	230	12	180	1½ST+2½FAT
White Chocolate Macadamia Nut	230	12	140	1½ST+2½FAT
Double Chocolate Brazil Nut	230	12	115	1½ST+2½FAT

Pizza

Chapter Contents

■ Crust
■ Sauce
■ Cheese
■ Toppings
■ Estimating the Calories & Fat in your Pizza
■ Your Favorite Pizza Restaurants

Many people think of pizzas as a high fat dish that one should not eat if they are trying to lose weight or lower their cholesterol. That simply is not true. Pizza can easily fit into a low fat eating program provided you make informed choices.

For the leanest meal, fill yourself up with a green salad and fat-free dressing before eating pizza. Then eat just a few slices of pizza with lower fat toppings such as fresh fruits and vegetables. If you have a hard time stopping at just 2 or 3 slices, buy a small enough pizza so there are no extra slices to tempt you.

Crust

✔ **Pizza crust is generally low in fat and calories.** The pizza crust consists of mostly of flour, yeast, and water so it is very low in fat and has approximately the same amount of calories as bread.

✔ **Choose pizzas cooked in the old fashioned pizza ovens.** When using the old fashioned pizza ovens, the pizza is simply placed on the floor of the oven and baked. The conveyor belt ovens use a higher temperature; therefore, extra fat is required in the dough to allow quick cooking without burning. Thus, pizzas cooked in the conveyor belt ovens are generally higher in calories and fat than those made in the old-fashioned pizza ovens.

✔ **You can have more slices (for the same calories) of the thin crust pizza** than pan pizza or thick crust. The calorie difference is even greater with pizza prepared in a conveyor belt oven. In addition to extra oil added to the crust itself, pan or thick crust pizzas cooked in the conveyor belt ovens usually require well-greased pans to prevent sticking. Generally, the thin crust pizzas are placed on a perforated pizza pan without any additional oil.

If you Want more Slices, Order Thin Crust:	Calories	Fat (g)
Round Table Gourmet Veggie Pan Pizza, 2 sl.	440	15
Round Table Gourmet Veggie Thin Crust, 2 sl.	320	13
Savings:	**120**	**2**

✔ **Avoid Filled or Stuffed Crusts.** The double crusts and the high fat fillings result in a very high fat and calorie content.

Avoid Stuffed Crust:	Calories	Fat (g)
Pizza Hut® Pepperoni Lovers® Stuffed Pizza, 2 slices	960	44
Pizza Hut® Pepperoni Lovers® Thin'n Crispy Pizza, 2 slices	540	24
Savings:	**420**	**20**

Sauce

✔ **Tomato or pizza sauce is low in fat.**

✔ **Ask for "no oil on the crust."** Although not common in pizza parlors, some of the upscale restaurants brush the crust with oil before adding the sauce or *instead of* the tomato sauce. Request that oil not be added.

Cheese

✔ **Cheese is high fat**. Mozzarella cheese is the most frequently used cheese, but Provolone and Feta cheese are also seen. Each of these cheeses contain about 6-8 grams of fat per ounce; each slice has roughly 1 oz of cheese.

✔ **Do not order extra cheese**. Extra cheese increases the fat content of each slice of pizza by another 50%!

Order Regular Cheese rather than "Extra":	Calories	Fat (g)
Pizza w/ Extra Cheese, 2 slices large pizza	370	16
Pizza, 2 slices large pizza	320	11
Savings:	**50**	**5**

✓ **Try pizza with "half the cheese" or even without cheese.** If your favorite part of the pizza is the crust, consider requesting that the pizza parlor add only *half* of the usual amount of cheese on top or request the pizza to be prepared "*light*" on the cheese. Ask the manager of your favorite pizza restaurant which term is more understandable to their cooking staff. Managers say that requesting less cheese has become a frequent request from people watching their weight or cholesterol or those with a lactose-intolerance.

Order Pizza "Light on the Cheese":		
	Calories	Fat (g)
Thin Crust Vegetable Pizza, 2 slices 14" pizza	265	11
Thin Crust Vegetable Pizza, "light on the cheese," 2 slices 14" pizza	215	6
Savings:	**50**	**5**

Toppings

✓ **Choose the leanest toppings of fresh fruits & vegetables:** onions, mushrooms, green and red peppers, broccoli, tomatoes, roasted pepper, spinach, and pineapple.

✓ **Olives are just about pure fat;** a sprinkling of black and green olives will add another 30 calories and 3 grams of fat per 2 slices. If you don't really care much for them, leave them off your Vegetarian Pizza.

✓ **The leanest meats are: grilled chicken, ham, Canadian bacon, tuna, crabmeat, and shrimp.** Each will add only a couple of grams of fat per slice. Hamburger meat will add a bit more. The high fat toppings such as pepperoni, bacon, and sausage can more than double the fat in each slice.

Choose Leaner Toppings:		
(For 2 slices of 12" medium Pizza)	Calories	Fat (g)
Domino's Pizza®, thin crust, 2 slices, sausage & extra cheese	359	19
Domino's Pizza®, thin crust, 2 slices, w/green pepper, onion, mushrooms, banana peppers, pineapple, and ham	295	12
Savings:	**64**	**7**

Estimating the Calories & Fat in Your Pizza Slices

If no nutritional information is available for your favorite pizza restaurant, use these pictures to estimate the calories, fat, and exchanges. On this page is a picture of a slice of large and extra large pizza. The nutritional information for the large pizzas are based on a 7" long slice of pizza with the width shown below (1/6 of a 14" pizza). The extra large size, often sold by-the-slice in malls and airports, is the width of the piece shown below and about 10½ inches long.

Pizza Calorimeter: Large & Extra Large Sliced Pizza			
	Calories	Fat (g)	Exchanges
Large Slice (thin crust):			
Plain, w/low fat Vegetables, or Ham	260	8	2ST+1HFM
Pepperoni, Sausage, Vegetarian, or Lightly Piled Combo	375	15	2ST+2HFM
Extra Cheese & Pepperoni, or Heavily Piled Combo	420	21	2ST+2½HFM
Large Size (thick crust):			
Plain, w/low fat Vegetables, or Ham	375	15	2½ST+2HFM
Pepperoni, Sausage, Vegetarian, or Combo	450	21	2½ST+2½HFM
Extra Large Slice (thin crust):			
Plain, w/low fat Vegetables, or Ham	500	14	3½ST+2HFM
Pepperoni, Sausage, Vegetarian, or Lightly Piled Combo	655	26	3½ST+3½HFM
Extra Cheese & Pepperoni, or Heavily Piled Combo	790	36	3½ST+4½HFM
Extra Large Size (thick crust):			
Plain, w/low fat Vegetables, or Ham	655	25	4½ST+3HFM
Pepperoni, Sausage, Vegetarian, or Deluxe	810	37	4½ST+4½HFM

Large Slice = 7" long

Extra Large Slice = 10½" long

Below are pictures of typical buffet sized and medium sized pizza slices along with average nutritional information.

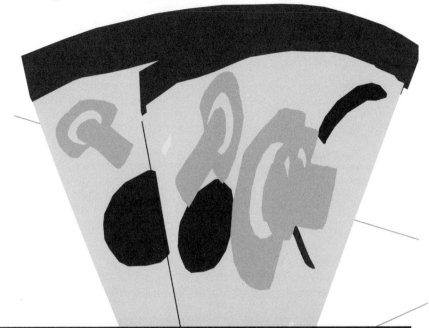

Pizza Calorimeter: Buffet & Medium Sliced Pizza

	Calories	Fat (g)	Exchanges
Buffet Size (thin crust):			
Plain, w/low fat Vegetables, *or* Ham	140	4	1ST+½HFM
Pepperoni, Sausage, Vegetarian, *or* Lightly Piled Combo	190	7	1ST+¾HFM
Extra Cheese & Pepperoni, or Heavily Piled Combo	240	11	1ST+1½HFM
Buffet Size (thick crust):			
Plain, w/low fat Vegetables, *or* Ham	190	6	1½ST+¾HFM
Pepperoni, Sausage, Vegetarian, *or* Combo	240	11	1½ST+1¼HFM
Medium Slice (thin crust):			
Plain, w/low fat Vegetables, *or* Ham	200	6	1½ST+¾HFM
Pepperoni, Sausage, Vegetarian, *or* Lightly Piled Combo	280	11	1½ST+1½HFM
Extra Cheese & Pepperoni, or Heavily Piled Combo	360	18	1½ST+2¼HFM
Medium Size (thick crust):			
Plain, w/low fat Vegetables, *or* Ham	280	10	2ST+1¼HFM
Pepperoni, Sausage, Vegetarian, or Combo	360	18	2ST+2HFM

Your Favorite Pizza Restaurants

BERTUCCI'S

	Calories	Fat (g)	Sodium (mg)	Exchanges
Pizza:				
Plain Cheese Pizza, small	200	7	400	1½ST+1HFM
large	250	9	500	2ST+1HFM
Bertucci Pizza, small	270	12	570	1½ST+1½HFM
large	300	14	650	2ST+1½HFM+½FAT
Romano Pizza, small	160	6	410	1½ST+¾HFM
large	230	8	520	2ST+1HFM
Rigatoni & Ravioli:				
Chicken & Mushroom Ravioli, 1c	320	16	320	1½ST+1½MFM+1½FAT
Rigatoni, Broccoli & Chicken w/wine sauce, 1c	350	17	420	1½ST+1V+1½MFM+ 2FAT
Rigatoni, Broccoli, & Chicken w/cream sauce, 1c	480	35	430	1½ST+1V+1MFM+ 6FAT
Rigatoni Del Rosario	260	13	350	1½ST+1V+2½FAT
Salad Dressings (1 oz or 2 T):				
Bertucci's Low Fat Chianti Italian	40	1.^{5}	470	½CHO+¼FAT
Bertucci's Caesar Dressing	140	15	240	3FAT
Bertucci's Italian Dressing	140	16	380	3FAT

Other tips: All pizzas are prepared with canola/olive oil and romano cheese, but you can request it without. A part-skim mozzarella is used; you can request the pizzas to be prepared with "less cheese." The lowest fat toppings are the fresh vegetable toppings such as peppers, broccoli, plum tomatoes, zucchini, mushrooms, and spinach.

Minestrone Soup is prepared with lots of vegetables. Bertucci's and its suppliers do not use MSG in, or add MSG to, any product. If MSG exists, it is the result of a natural and unintended chemical reaction.

DOMINO'S PIZZA®

	Calories	Fat (g)	Sodium (mg)	Exchanges
2 Slices (¼) of a 12" Medium Pizza:				
Hand Tossed, Cheese only	347	11	723	3ST+1HFM+½FAT
Thin Crust, Cheese only	271	12	808	2ST+1HFM+1FAT
Deep Dish, Cheese only	477	22	1065	3ST+1½HFM+2FAT
"Add A Topping" to 2 Slices Med. Pizza:				
Green Pepper, Onion, Mushrooms, Banana Peppers, or Pineapple	3-10	0	0-92	FREE
Green Olives, Ripe Olives, Ham, or Anchovies	12-23	0.^{8}- 1.^{4}	71- 396	1=FREE, 2=½FAT
Extra Cheese, Beef, Cheddar, Pepperoni, or Italian Sausage	49-62	4-6	88- 199	1=½HFM
Bacon	82	7	226	½HFM+½FAT

DOMINO'S PIZZA® (continued)

	Calories	Fat (g)	Sodium (mg)	Exchanges
2 Slices (1/6) of a 14" Large Pizza:				
Hand Tossed, Cheese only	319	10	660	3ST+1HFM+½FAT
Thin Crust, Cheese only	257	11	757	2ST+1HFM+½FAT
Deep Dish, Cheese only	455	16	1073	3½ST+1HFM+2½FAT
"Add A Topping" to 2 Slices Large Pizza:				
Green Pepper, Onion, Mushrooms, Banana Peppers, *or* Pineapple	2-8	0	0-81	FREE
Green Olives, Ripe Olives, Ham, *or* Anchovies	11-23	0.^{7}-1.^{2}	63-395	1=FREE, 2=½FAT
Extra Cheese, Beef, Cheddar, Pepperoni, *or* Italian Sausage	44-55	3-5	73-177	1=½HFM
Bacon	75	6	207	½HFM+½FAT
6" Deep Dish Pizza:				
Cheese Only	594	27	1208	3ST+1HFM+½FAT
"Add A Topping" to 6" Deep Dish Pizza:				
Green Pepper, Onion, Mushrooms, Banana Peppers, *or* Pineapple	2-5	0	0-73	FREE
Green Olives, Ripe Olives, *or* Ham	10-17	0.^{7}-1.^{1}	57-204	1=FREE, 2=½FAT
Anchovies	45	2	790	1LM
Extra Cheese, Beef, Pepperoni, *or* Italian Sausage	44-59	3-5	123-159	1=½HFM
Bacon	75	6	207	½HFM+½FAT
Cheddar Cheese	86	7	132	1HFM
Domino's Buffalo Wings & Bread:				
Barbecue Wings, 1 wing	50	2.^{5}	175	½MFM
Hot Wings, 1 wing	45	2.^{5}	354	½MFM
Breadsticks, 1 piece	78	3	158	¾ST+½FAT
Cheesy Bread, 1 piece	103	5	182	¾ST+1FAT
Domino's Garden Salads:				
Small Salad, no dressing	22	0.^{3}	14	1V
Large Salad, no dressing	39	0.^{5}	26	1½V
Marzetti Dressings (43 g):				
Thousand Island Dressing	200	20	320	4FAT
Honey French Dressing	210	18	300	1CHO+3½FAT
Light Italian Dressing	20	1	0	FREE
House Italian Dressing	220	24	440	5FAT
Blue Cheese Dressing	220	24	440	5FAT
Ranch Dressing	260	29	380	6FAT
Fat Free Dressing	40	0	560	1FR
Creamy Caesar Dressing	200	22	470	4½FAT

GODFATHERS™ PIZZA

	Calories	Fat (g)	Sodium (mg)	Exchanges
Original Crust, Cheese Pizza, per slice:				
Mini, ¼ of whole pizza	131	3	183	1¼ST+½MFM
Medium, ⅛ of whole pizza	231	5	338	2ST+½MFM+½FAT
Large, ¹⁄₁₀ of whole pizza	258	6	396	2¼ST+1MFM+¼FAT
Jumbo, ¹⁄₁₀ of whole pizza	382	9	580	3¼ST+2MFM
Original Crust, Combo Pizza, per slice:				
Mini, ¼ of whole pizza	176	7	382	1½ST+1HFM
Medium, ⅛ of whole pizza	306	11	660	2¼ST+1½HFM
Large, ¹⁄₁₀ of whole pizza	338	12	740	2½ST+1½HFM
Jumbo, ¹⁄₁₀ of whole pizza	503	18	1096	3½ST+2¼HFM
Golden Crust, Cheese Pizza, per slice:				
Medium, ⅛ of whole pizza	212	8	311	1½ST+1HFM
Large, ¹⁄₁₀ of whole pizza	242	9	363	1¾ST+1¼HFM
Golden Crust, Combo Pizza, per slice:				
Medium, ⅛ of whole pizza	271	12	562	1¾ST+1½HFM
Large, ¹⁄₁₀ of whole pizza	305	14	674	2ST+1¾HFM

LITTLE CAESARS® PIZZA

	Calories	Fat (g)	Sodium (mg)	Exchanges
PIZZA!PIZZA!®, one small slice (14" diameter):				
Cheese only	250	9	359	2ST+1HFM
Pepperoni	280	12	523	2ST+1½HFM
Deep Dish, one large slice:				
Cheese only	210	7	439	1¾ST+1HFM
Pepperoni	280	13	630	1¾ST+1½HFM
Individual Orders:				
Crazy Bread®, 1 piece (1.⁴ oz)	110	3	114	1ST+½FAT
Crazy Sauce®, 3½ oz	40	0.⁵	232	1½V

MAZZIO'S PIZZA®

	Calories	Fat (g)	Sodium (mg)	Exchanges
Appetizers:				
Meat Nachos	500	37	1200	1½ST+2½HFM+3FAT
Garlic Bread w/cheese, approx 2 sl	700	35	1280	5ST+1HFM+5FAT
Sandwiches:				
Ham and Cheese	790	39	1900	4ST+4HFM+1½FAT
Deluxe Submarine	810	43	2240	4ST+4HFM+2FAT

MAZZIO'S PIZZA® continued

	Calories	Fat (g)	Sodium (mg)	Exchanges
Sandwiches continued:				
BBQ Beef & Cheddar	580	24	1260	3ST+4MFM+1FAT
Chicken & Cheddar	570	24	1350	3½ST+3HFM
Pizza (1 slice medium pizza):				
Original Crust Cheese	260	8	450	2ST+1HFM
Thin Crust Cheese	220	9	440	1½ST+1HFM
Deep Pan Cheese	350	13	620	2½ST+1½HFM
Original Crust Pepperoni	280	11	600	2ST+1½HFM
Deep Pan Pepperoni	380	17	740	2½ST+1½HFM+1FAT
Original Crust Sausage	350	16	890	2ST+1½HFM+1FAT
Deep Pan Sausage	430	21	1040	2½ST+2HFM+1FAT
Original Crust Combo	320	13	780	2ST+1½HFM
Deep Pan Combo	410	18	930	2½ST+1½HFM+1FAT
Pasta:				
Chicken Parmesan	590	19	1600	4ST+4MFM
Small Meat Lasagna	460	25	1370	2ST+3HFM
Small Fettuccine Alfredo	440	28	680	2ST+1HFM+4FAT
Small Spaghetti	290	10	800	2ST+2V+2FAT

PAPA JOHN'S

	Calories	Fat (g)	Sodium (mg)	Exchanges
One Slice Original Pizza ($^1/_8$ of a 14" Large Pizza):				
Cheese	286	9	540	2¼ST+1MFM+1FAT
Pepperoni	310	13	760	2¼ST+1MFM+1½FAT
Sausage	340	13	910	2½ST+1MFM+1½FAT
All the Meats™	410	18	1040	2½ST+2MFM+1½FAT
Garden Special™	298	11	570	2¼ST+1MFM+1FAT
The Works™	369	17	840	2¼ST+1½MFM+2FAT
One Slice Thin Pizza ($^1/_8$ of a 14" Large Pizza):				
Cheese	220	11	480	1¼ST+¾MFM+1½FAT
Pepperoni	266	15	580	1¼ST+1MFM+2FAT
Sausage	270	15	730	1¼ST+1¼MFM+1½FAT
All the Meats™	330	20	919	1½ST+1½MFM+2½FAT
Garden Special™	238	12	540	1¼ST+¾MFM+1½FAT
The Works™	319	19	760	1½ST+1½MFM+2½FAT
Sides:				
Cheese Sticks, 2, $^1/_7$ of an order	160	6	290	1½ST+½MFM+1FAT
Bread Sticks, 1, $^1/_8$ of an order	170	3	270	1¾ST+½FAT
Nacho Cheese, 1T	30	2	113	½FAT or ¼HFM
Garlic Sauce, 1 T	75	9	115	2FAT
Pizza Sauce, 1T	10	0.[5]	60	FREE

PETER PIPER™ PIZZA

	Calories	Fat (g)	Sodium (mg)	Exchanges
Based on One Slice (¼ Express Lunch Pizza *or* ELP, $^1/_6$ Sm, $^1/_8$ Med, $^1/_8$ Lg or $^1/_{12}$ XL):				
Cheese, ELP	152	4	152	1½ST+½HFM
small	177	4	179	1½ST+½HFM
medium	203	5	202	2ST+½HFM
large	270	6	271	2½ST+¾HFM
extra large	257	6	260	2½ST+¾HFM
Extra Mozzarella, ELP	174	6	186	1½ST+¾HFM
small	198	6	213	1½ST+¾HFM
medium	236	7	253	2ST+1HFM
large	319	10	349	2½ST+1¼HFM
extra large	300	9	327	2½ST+1¼HFM
Extra Cheddar, ELP	180	6	196	1½ST+¾HFM
small	196	6	208	1½ST+¾HFM
medium	224	6	235	2ST+¾HFM
large	306	9	327	2½ST+1¼HFM
extra large	290	9	311	2½ST+1¼HFM
Salami, ELP	164	5	199	1½ST+½HFM
small	189	5	226	1½ST+¾HFM
medium	216	6	254	2ST+¾HFM
large	288	8	342	2½ST+1HFM
extra large	273	8	322	2½ST+1HFM
Pepperoni, ELP	168	6	293	1½ST+¾HFM
small	198	6	367	1½ST+¾HFM
medium	229	7	431	2ST+1HFM
large	308	9	555	2½ST+1¼HFM
extra large	284	9	507	2½ST+1¼HFM
Beef, ELP	165	5	257	1½ST+½HFM
small	194	5	319	1½ST+¾HFM
medium	222	6	359	2ST+¾HFM
large	296	8	482	2½ST+1HFM
extra large	280	8	446	2½ST+1HFM
Green Pepper, ELP	153	4	152	1½ST+½HFM
small	178	4	179	1½ST+½HFM
medium	204	5	202	2ST+½HFM
large	272	6	272	2½ST+¾HFM
extra large	259	6	260	2½ST+¾HFM
Onion, ELP	153	4	152	1½ST+½HFM
small	177	4	179	1½ST+½HFM
medium	204	5	202	2ST+½HFM
large	271	6	272	2½ST+¾HFM
extra large	258	6	260	2½ST+¾HFM

PETER PIPER™ PIZZA (continued)

Based on One Slice (¼ Express Lunch Pizza or ELP, ¹/₆ Sm, ¹/₈ Med, ¹/₈ Lg or ¹/₁₂ L):

	Calories	Fat (g)	Sodium (mg)	Exchanges
Black Olive, ELP	157	4	198	1½ST+½HFM
small	182	5	230	1½ST+½HFM
medium	209	5	256	2ST+¾HFM
large	279	7	349	2½ST+1HFM
extra large	265	7	331	2½ST+¾HFM
Sausage, ELP	178	6	362	1½ST+¾HFM
small	197	6	342	1½ST+¾HFM
medium	224	6	377	2ST+¾HFM
large	300	8	517	2½ST+1HFM
extra large	284	8	481	2½ST+1HFM
Mushroom, ELP	153	4	152	1½ST+½HFM
small	178	4	179	1½ST+½HFM
medium	204	5	202	2ST+½HFM
large	181	4	182	2½ST+½HFM
extra large	259	6	260	2½ST+¾HFM
Ham, ELP	156	4	191	1½ST+½HFM
small	180	4	218	1½ST+½HFM
medium	207	5	245	2ST+½HFM
large	276	6	330	2½ST+¾HFM
extra large	261	6	311	2½ST+¾HFM
Tomato, ELP	153	4	152	1½ST+½HFM
small	177	4	179	1½ST+½HFM
medium	204	5	202	2ST+½HFM
large	275	6	274	2½ST+¾HFM
extra large	258	6	260	2½ST+¾HFM
Jalapeno, ELP	153	4	198	1½ST+½HFM
small	178	4	219	1½ST+½HFM
medium	205	5	247	2ST+½HFM
large	266	6	336	2½ST+¾HFM
extra large	259	6	314	2½ST+¾HFM
Pineapple, ELP	155	4	152	1½ST+½HFM
small	179	4	179	1½ST+½HFM
medium	206	5	202	2ST+½HFM
large	274	6	273	2½ST+¾HFM
extra large	260	6	260	2½ST+¾HFM
Bacon Pizza, ELP	182	7	237	1½ST+¾HFM
small	217	7	293	1½ST+¾HFM
medium	249	9	330	2ST+1HFM
large	331	11	442	2½ST+1¾HFM
extra large	311	11	411	2½ST+1½HFM

PIZZA HUT®

	Calories	Fat (g)	Sodium (mg)	Exchanges
Personal Pan® Pizza (whole pizza):				
Pepperoni	670	29	1250	4ST+2½HFM+2FAT
Supreme	710	31	1380	4½ST+3HFM+1½FAT
Cheese	630	24	1160	4½ST+2½HFM+1FAT
Thin 'n Crispy® Pizza (1 med slice):				
Cheese	210	9	530	1½ST+1HFM
Beef Topping	240	11	790	1½ST+1¼HFM
Ham	190	6	560	1½ST+1MFM
Pepperoni	220	9	610	1½ST+1HFM
Italian Sausage	300	16	740	1½ST+1½HFM+1FAT
Pork Topping	270	13	780	1½ST+1½HFM
Meat Lovers®	310	16	900	1½ST+1½HFM+1FAT
Veggie Lovers®	170	6	460	1½ST+¾HFM
Pepperoni Lovers®	270	12	780	1½ST+1½HFM
Supreme	250	11	710	1½ST+1¼HFM
Super Supreme	280	13	810	1½ST+1½HFM
Chicken Supreme	220	7	550	1½ST+1½MFM
Hand-Tossed Style (1 med slice):				
Cheese	280	10	770	2ST+1¼HFM
Beef Topping	280	10	860	2ST+1¼HFM
Ham	230	6	710	2ST+¾HFM
Pepperoni	260	9	750	2ST+1HFM
Italian Sausage	300	12	780	2ST+1¼HFM+½FAT
Pork Topping	290	11	850	2ST+1HFM+½FAT
Meat Lovers®	290	11	820	2ST+1¼HFM
Veggie Lovers®	240	7	650	2ST+¾HFM
Pepperoni Lovers®	320	13	910	2ST+1½HFM
Supreme	270	9	760	2ST+1HFM
Super Supreme	290	10	830	2ST+1¼HFM
Chicken Supreme	240	6	660	2ST+1MFM
Pan® Pizza (1 med slice):				
Cheese	300	14	610	2ST+1¼HFM+1FAT
Beef Topping	310	14	720	2ST+1¼HFM+1FAT
Ham	250	9	590	2ST+1HFM
Pepperoni	280	12	640	2ST+1HFM+1FAT
Italian Sausage	350	18	740	2ST+1¼HFM+1½FAT
Pork Topping	300	13	720	2ST+1¼HFM+½FAT
Meat Lovers®	360	19	870	2ST+1½HFM+1½FAT
Veggie Lovers®	240	9	480	2ST+½HFM+1FAT
Pepperoni Lovers®	350	17	800	2ST+1½HFM+1FAT
Supreme	300	13	670	2ST+1HFM+1FAT
Super Supreme	340	16	790	2ST+1¼HFM+1FAT
Chicken Supreme	280	11	570	2ST+1HFM+½FAT

PIZZA HUT® (continued)

	Calories	Fat (g)	Sodium (mg)	Exchanges
Stuffed Crust Pizza (1 med slice):				
Cheese	380	11	1160	3ST+1½HFM
Beef Topping	410	14	1270	3ST+1½HFM+½FAT
Ham	380	14	1250	2½ST+1¾HFM
Pepperoni	410	17	1250	3ST+1½HFM+1FAT
Italian Sausage	430	19	1200	3ST+1½HFM+1½FAT
Pork Topping	420	16	1290	3ST+2HFM
Meat Lovers®	500	23	1510	3ST+2HFM+1½FAT
Veggie Lovers®	390	14	1140	3ST+1¼HFM+1FAT
Pepperoni Lovers®	480	22	1440	3ST+2HFM+1½FAT
Supreme	440	16	1380	3ST+2HFM
Super Supreme	470	20	1440	3ST+2HFM+1FAT
Chicken Supreme	390	13	1130	3ST+1½HFM
Other Menu Items:				
Mild Buffalo Wings, 5 pieces	200	12	510	3MFM
Hot Buffalo Wings, 5 pieces	210	12	900	3MFM
Garlic Bread, 1 piece	150	8	240	1ST+1½FAT
Bread Stick, 1	130	4	170	1¼ST+1FAT
Bread Stick Dipping Sauce, 1 serv	30	0.5	170	1V
Spaghetti w/Marinara	490	6	730	5ST+2V+1FAT
Spaghetti w/Meat Sauce	600	13	910	5ST+2V+1HFM+1FAT
Spaghetti w/Meatballs	850	24	1120	6½ST+2V+2HFM+ 1½FAT
Cavatini® Pasta	480	14	1170	3ST+2V+1½HFM+ ½FAT
Cavatini Supreme® Pasta	560	19	1400	3½ST+2V+2HFM+ ½FAT
Ham & Cheese Sandwich	550	21	2150	3½ST+3MFM+1FAT
Supreme Sandwich	640	28	2150	3¾ST+3HFM+1FAT
Apple Dessert Pizza, 1 sl	250	4.5	230	1ST+2FR+1FAT
Cherry Dessert Pizza, 1 sl	250	4.5	220	1ST+2FR+1FAT

ROUND TABLE® PIZZA

	Calories	Fat (g)	Sodium (mg)	Exchanges
Thin Crust Pizzas ($^1/_{16}$ of large):				
Cheese	160	6.^{2}	240	1ST+½HFM+½FAT
Pepperoni	170	8	240	1ST+1HFM
King Arthur's Supreme	200	10.^{1}	340	1ST+1HFM+½FAT
Guinever's Garden Delight	150	5.^{6}	250	1ST+½HFM+½FAT
Gourmet Veggie	160	6.^{5}	200	1ST+½HFM+½FAT
Chicken & Garlic Gourmet	170	7.^{2}	280	1ST+1HFM
Italian Garlic Supreme	200	10.^{4}	220	1ST+1HFM+½FAT
Garden Pesto	170	7.^{7}	200	1ST+1HFM
Saluté Cashew Chicken	150	4.^{1}	240	1½ST+½HFM
Saluté Chicken & Garlic	150	5.^{4}	250	1ST+1MFM
Saluté Veggie	140	4.^{7}	170	1½ST+1FAT
Alfredo Contempo	170	6.^{5}	210	1ST+1HFM
Classic Pesto	170	7.^{9}	210	1ST+½HFM+1FAT
Zesty Santa Fe Chicken	180	7.^{8}	310	1ST+1HFM
Bacon Super Deli	200	12.^{6}	360	1ST+1HFM+1FAT
Western BBQ Chicken Supreme	170	5.^{6}	330	1ST+½HFM+½FAT
Maui Zaui (Red Pizza Sauce)	170	6.^{5}	350	1ST+1HFM
Maui Zaui (Chili Sauce)	180	6.^{6}	330	1ST+1HFM
Steak Supreme (Red Sauce)	200	9.^{9}	340	1ST+1HFM+½FAT
Steak Supreme (Creamy Garlic Sc)	210	11.^{2}	310	1ST+1HFM+½FAT
Pan Pizza ($^1/_{12}$):				
Cheese	210	7.^{2}	250	1½ST+1HFM+½FAT
Pepperoni	220	8.^{1}	240	1½ST+1HFM+1FAT
King Arthur's Supreme	240	9.^{8}	320	2ST+½HFM+1FAT
Guinever's Garden Delight	200	6.^{2}	250	2ST+½HFM+½FAT
Gourmet Veggie	220	7.^{4}	230	2ST+½HFM+½FAT
Chicken & Garlic Gourmet	230	8.^{1}	310	2ST+1HFM
Italian Garlic Supreme	250	10.^{5}	240	2ST+½HFM+1½FAT
Garden Pesto	230	8.^{6}	230	2ST+½HFM+1FAT
Saluté Cashew Chicken	200	4.^{5}	260	2ST+½HFM
Saluté Chicken & Garlic	200	5.^{8}	270	2ST+½HFM+½FAT
Saluté Veggie	190	5.^{1}	190	2ST+1FAT
Alfredo Contempo	220	7.^{4}	240	2ST+1HFM
Classic Pesto	230	8.^{8}	240	2ST+½HFM+1FAT
Zesty Santa Fe Chicken	240	9.^{2}	360	2ST+1HFM
Bacon Super Deli	260	13.^{5}	380	1½ST+1HFM+1FAT
Western BBQ Chicken Supreme	220	6.^{5}	360	2ST+½HFM+½FAT
Maui Zaui (Red Pizza Sauce)	310	10	490	2½ST+1¼HFM
Maui Zaui (Chili Sauce)	320	10.^{7}	500	2½ST+1½HFM
Steak Supreme (Red Sauce)	350	15	490	2½ST+1½HFM+½FAT
Steak Supreme (Creamy Garlic Sc)	370	16.^{7}	460	2½ST+1½HFM+1FAT

ROUND TABLE® PIZZA (continued)

	Calories	Fat (g)	Sodium (mg)	Exchanges
Personal Size Pizza, thin crust ($^1/_{12}$):				
Cheese	570	24	850	3ST+1V+3HFM
Pepperoni	620	30	830	3ST+1V+3HFM+1FAT
King Arthur's Supreme	710	37	1180	3ST+1V+3½HFM+2FAT
Guinever's Garden Delight	540	20	880	3ST+2V+2HFM+1FAT
Gourmet Veggie	580	23	710	3ST+2V+2½HFM+1FAT
Chicken & Garlic Gourmet	620	26	1030	3ST+1V+3½HFM
Italian Garlic Supreme	730	40	830	3ST+1V+3½HFM+ 2½FAT
Garden Pesto	610	27	710	3ST+2V+2HFM+2FAT
Classic Pesto	610	27	750	3ST+1V+2HFM+2FAT
Bacon Super Deli	690	35	1230	3ST+1V+4HFM+½FAT
Western BBQ Chicken Supreme	590	20	1130	3½ST+1V+3½MFM
Buffalo Chicken	660	31	1410	3ST+1V+3HFM
Personal Size Pizza, pan crust ($^1/_{12}$):				
Cheese	800	26	880	6ST+1V+3HFM+½FAT
Pepperoni	810	29	820	6ST+1V+3HFM+1FAT
King Arthur's Supreme	860	33	1090	6ST+1V+3HFM+2FAT
Guinever's Garden Delight	750	21	840	6ST+2V+2HFM+1FAT
Gourmet Veggie	810	25	780	6ST+2V+2½HFM+1FAT
Chicken & Garlic Gourmet	850	28	1100	6ST+1V+3½HFM
Italian Garlic Supreme	960	42	900	6ST+1V+3½HFM+3FAT
Garden Pesto	830	29	780	6ST+2V+3HFM+1FAT
Classic Pesto	830	29	830	6ST+1V+2HFM+2½FAT
Bacon Super Deli	920	37	1310	6ST+1V+4HFM+1FAT
Western BBQ Chicken Supreme	820	22	1200	6½ST+1V+3½MFM+ 1FAT
Buffalo Chicken	880	33	1480	6ST+1V+4HFM
Sandwiches:				
Garden Vegeable	670	29	990	4ST+2V+2HFM+2½FAT
Turkey Santa Fe	840	44	1360	4ST+1V+4MFM+5FAT
Chicken Club	800	38	1510	4ST+1V+4MFM+ 3½FAT
Ham & Honey Mustard	760	33	1630	4ST+1V+3MFM+ 3½FAT
Turkey Pesto	830	40	1200	4ST+1V+4LM+5½FAT
Other:				
Garlic Parmesan Twists (3)	430	15	690	3½ST+1HFM+1½FAT

For customers with nutritional concerns, please call 1-800-753-2825, extension 1.

Snacks

Chapter Contents:

■ **Candy & Fudge**
■ **Dried Fruits, Nuts, & Seeds**
■ **Pretzels**
■ **Popcorn**

Other popular snacks found elsewhere in this book:

■ **Bagels**, see the *Breads & Spreads* chapter
■ **Cookies**, see the *Desserts* chapter
■ **Doughnuts**, see the *Desserts* chapter
■ **French Fries**, see the *Burgers & Fast Food* chapter
■ **Hot Dogs & Corn Dogs**, see the *Burgers & Fast Food* chapter
■ **Ice Cream/Frozen Yogurt**, see the *Desserts* chapter
■ **Muffins**, see the *Desserts* chapter
■ **Nachos**, see the *Mexican Restaurants* chapter
■ **Pizza**, see the *Pizza* chapter
■ **Potato Chips**, see the *Deli & Sandwich Shops* chapter
■ **Sodas, Milkshakes, and Coffee Drinks**, see the *Beverages* chapter
■ **Tortilla Chips**, see the *Mexican Restaurants* chapter

Candy & Fudge

Stores selling candy in bulk are very popular in shopping malls, amusement parks, theatres, and airports. Since there is no nutritional information on the label, we are likely to consume more calories than we realize. On the next page is a calorimeter for the most popular candies listing the calories and fat grams per 1, 2, and 3 oz portions. Following this chart is more detailed nutritional information per ounce and per individual piece. Since your candy purchase is often shown in pounds rather than ounces, following is a conversion chart.

Conversion Chart:

Ounces	Pounds		Ounces	Pounds		Ounces	Pounds
1	0.06		6	0.38		12	0.75
2	0.13		7	0.44		13	0.81
3	0.19		8	0.5		14	0.88
4	0.25		9	0.56		15	0.94
5	0.31		10	0.63		16	1.0
			11	0.69			

Candy & Fudge Calorimeter: Calories & fat per serving

Calories per oz	Candy & Fudge	1 oz (0.06#)	2 oz (0.13#)	3 oz (0.19#)
160	Chocolate Covered Almonds	**160** 12g	**320** 24g	**480** 36g
160	Hershey® Kisses w/almonds, Semi-Sweet Chocolate, Chocolate w/nuts	**160** 10g	**320** 20g	**480** 30g
150	M&M® Peanut, Nonpareil Chocolate Wafers, Hershey® Kisses, Hershey® Minatures, Reese's Peanut Butter Cups, Milk Chocolate	**150** 9g	**300** 18g	**450** 27g
140	M&M®, Malted Milk Balls, Reese's® Pieces	**140** 6g	**280** 12g	**420** 18g
130	Boston Baked Beans, Chocolate Covered Raisins, Candy Coated Almonds, Fudge w/nuts, Yogurt Cov'd Pretzels	**130** 5g	**260** 10g	**390** 15g
120	Choc Coated Peppermint Patties, Fudge (choc or vanilla), Peanut Brittle	**120** 4g	**240** 8g	**360** 12g
120	Caramels	**120** 2g	**240** 5g	**360** 8g
110	Tootsie Rolls, Caramels w/cream centers	**110** 2g	**220** 4g	**330** 7g
110	Cinnamon Flavored Candies, Drops (lemon & watermelon w/sugar coating), Smarties, Starlight Mints (sugar free & regular), Sweet Tarts	**110** 0g	**220** 0g	**330** 0g
100	Bubble Gum, Candy Corn, Dinner Mints, Gum Drops, Gummy Bears or Worms, Hard Candies, Jaw Breakers, Jelly Beans, Licorice, Orange Slices	**100** 0g	**200** 0g	**300** 0g
70	Gumballs, Sugar Free Gummy Bears & Hard Candies	**70** 0g	**140** 0g	**210** 0g

In the following table, notice that fat, sodium, and exchanges are listed *per ounce*. The calorie column lists the number of calories in each *individual* piece.

Candy Calorimeter: Calories per ounce & per piece

| Candy | PER PIECE | | PER OUNCE | | |
	Calories EACH	Fat (g) EACH	Fat (g) PER OZ	Sodium (mg) PER OZ	Exchanges PER OZ
70 calories/oz:					
Gumballs, regular ½ inch	5	0	0	0	1CHO
Gumballs, larger 1¼ inch	30	0	0	0	1CHO
Gummy bears, sugar-free	6	0	0	0	1CHO
Hard candies, sugar-free	9	0	0	0	1CHO
100 calories/oz:					
Bubble gum	25	0	0	0	1½CHO
Candy corn	6	0	0.^{5}	3	1½CHO
Dinner mints	3	0	0	0	1½CHO
Gum drops, spice drops	11	0	0.^{2}	1	1½CHO
Gummy bears, American or European style	7	0	0	17	1½CHO
Gummy worms	25	0	0	17	1½CHO
Gummy worms, sugar-coated	35	0	0	20	1½CHO
Hard candies	23	0	0	92	1½CHO
Jaw breakers, ½ inch	6	0	0	na	1½CHO
Jaw breakers, 1 inch	40	0	0	na	1½CHO
Jaw breakers, 1¾ inch	200	0	0	na	1½CHO
Jelly beans, regular sized	9	0	0.^{1}	3	1½CHO
Jelly beans, sm gourmet sized	4	0	0.^{1}	3	1½CHO
Licorice sticks, 6"	33	0.^{3}	1	71	1½CHO
Licorice pieces	8	0	1	85	1½CHO
Mints, mini soft non-pareils	2	0	0.^{6}	na	1½CHO
Orange slices	50	0	0	10	1½CHO
110 calories/oz:					
Caramels with cream centers	47	1	2.^{3}	na	1½CHO+½FAT
Cinnamon flav'd candies, sm	2	0	0	0	1½CHO
Drops, lemon or watermelon	15	0	0	3	1½CHO
Smarties	25	0	0	0	1½CHO
Starlight mints	20	0	0	19	1½CHO
Starlight mints, sugar-free	20	0	0	na	1½CHO
Sweet tarts	4	0	0	0	2CHO
Sweet tarts, jumbo	37	0	0	na	2CHO
Tootsie® roll midget	27	0.^{5}	2.^{1}	28	1½CHO+½FAT

Candy Calorimeter: Calories per ounce & per piece (cont.)

Candy	PER PIECE Calories EACH	Fat (g) EACH	PER OUNCE Fat (g) PER OZ	Sodium (mg) PER OZ	Exchanges PER OZ
120 calories/oz:					
Caramels	36	1	2	65	1½CHO+½FAT
Chocolate covered thin mints, small	28	0.[8]	4	na	1¼CHO+1FAT
Fudge, vanilla or chocolate	na	na	4	50	1CHO+1FAT
Peanut Brittle	na	na	3	10	1CHO+½FAT
130 calories/oz:					
Boston baked beans	6	0.[2]	5	0	1½CHO+1FAT
Chocolate covered raisins	6	0.[2]	5	14	1½CHO+1FAT
Candy coated almonds	16	0.[7]	5	na	1½CHO+1FAT
Fudge with nuts	na	na	5	na	1CHO+1FAT
Yogurt-covered pretzels	na	na	5	200	1CHO+1FAT
140 calories/oz:					
M&M®	4	0.[2]	6	17	1¼CHO+1FAT
Malted milk balls, large	40	1.[9]	6	na	1¼CHO+1FAT
Malted milk balls, small	11	0.[4]	5	na	1¼CHO+1FAT
Reese's® pieces	4	0.[2]	6	47	1¼CHO+1FAT
150 calories/oz:					
M&M® peanut	13	0.[7]	9	15	1CHO+1½FAT
Nonpareils, chocolate wafers	21	1	8	na	1CHO+1½FAT
Hershey®'s kisses	26	1.[5]	9	25	1CHO+2FAT
Hershey®'s minatures	46	2.[8]	9	20	1CHO+2FAT
Milk Chocolate	na	na	9	10	1CHO+2FAT
Reese's® peanut butter cups, miniatures	42	2.[4]	9	84	1CHO+2FAT
160 calories/oz:					
Chocolate covered almonds	20	2	12	na	¾CHO+2½FAT
Chocolate w/nuts	na	na	10	20	1CHO+2FAT
Hershey®'s kisses w/almonds	26	1.[6]	10	19	1CHO+2FAT
Semi-sweet Chocolate	na	na	10	5	1CHO+2FAT

Dried Fruit, Nuts & Seeds

Dried fruit, although containing virtually no fat, is high in calories. Fruit, whether dried or fresh, has the same amount of calories. It is easier to eat more calories in the form of dried fruit because the volume is smaller.

Nuts and seeds are also concentrated sources of calories because of their high fat content. If you have purchased the dried fruit, nuts, or seeds from a vendor that weighed your purchase in pounds, refer to the chart in the candy section on how to convert pounds into ounces.

Dried Fruits & Nuts

	Calories	Fat (g)	Sodium (mg)	Exchanges
Dried Fruits (1oz):				
Apple Rings, 4	69	0	25	1FR
Apricots, 8	67	0	2	1FR
Dates, 3½	78	0.[1]	1	1FR
Figs, 1½	72	0.[3]	3	1FR
Mixed Fruit	74	0.[1]	26	1FR
Peaches, 2	68	0.[2]	2	1FR
Pears, 1½	74	0.[2]	2	1FR
Pineapple Ring, 1	30	0	na	½FR
Prunes, 3	67	0.[1]	1	1FR
Raisins, 3T	86	0.[1]	4	1FR
Nuts & Seeds (1 oz):				
Almonds, unsalted, 24	167	15	3	¾VLM+3FAT
Almonds, hickory smoked, 24	166	15	120	¾VLM+3FAT
Almonds, oil roasted, 22	176	16	3	¾VLM+3FAT
Cashews, dry roasted, 18	163	13	4	½VLM+2½FAT
Cashews, oil roasted, 18	163	14	5	½VLM+3FAT
Chestnuts, roasted	70	0.[6]	1	1ST
Coconut, dried sweetened	125	9	6	¾CHO+2FAT
Hazelnuts, dry roasted	188	19	1	4FAT
Hazelnuts, roasted & salted	180	18	40	3½FAT
Macadamia Nuts, dry roasted	193	21	117	4FAT
Macadamia Nuts, oil roasted	204	22	2	4FAT
Mixed Nuts, oil roasted	175	16	3	½ST+3FAT
Peanuts, dry roasted, 3T	164	14	228	1VLM+3FAT
Peanuts, honey roasted	170	13	180	1VLM+2½FAT
Peanuts, Spanish oil roasted	162	14	121	1VLM+3FAT
Pistachio Nuts, dry roasted, 47	172	15	2	½ST+½VLM+3FAT
Pecans, oil roasted, 15 halves	195	20	0	4FAT
Sunflower Seeds, dry roasted	165	14	1	1VLM+3FAT
Sunflower Seeds, ¼ c	180	15	10	1VLM+3FAT
Walnuts	176	17	3	1VLM+3½FAT

Pretzels

A large chewy pretzel (about the width of this book) has been marketed in kiosks at airports, amusement parks, and movie theatres for years. New to the scene is a softer pretzel prepared plain, with butter & salt, and in a variety of other flavors. Freestanding pretzel shops selling the newer varieties are opening all over the country. These latest pretzels are about the same size as the chewy pretzel but weighs less because it is not as dense.

Pretzels	Calories	Fat (g)	Sodium (mg)	Exchanges
Chewy Soft Pretzel, 4 oz	300	1	650	4ST
Tender Soft Pretzel, 3.[1] oz w/out butter *or* salt	270	4	na	3ST+1FAT
w/butter & salt	375	16	na	3ST+3FAT
w/butter, sugar & cinnamon	430	16	na	3ST+1CHO+3FAT
Iced & prepared w/raisins	410	8	na	3ST+1CHO+1½FAT
w/butter & poppyseeds	390	17	na	3ST+3½FAT
w/butter & sesame seeds	400	18	na	3ST+3½FAT

Popcorn

Popcorn is often considered a healthy food due to its high fiber content (about 1 g/cup). When air-popped, popcorn has just 30 calories a cup. Unfortunately, movie theatres, malls, and convenience stores are not using air-popped or "light" popcorn. The end result is a snack that is high in fat and calories (55 calories/cup).

✓ **Select the popcorn prepared with a healthier vegetable oil** (such as cannola or safflower) rather than coconut oil, if you have a choice. Coconut oil is one of the most saturated, "unhealthy" oils available.

✓ **Order it without butter.** The "butter" that is added is usually a butter-flavored oil and contains 125 calories per tablespoon. A medium popcorn may contain more than four tablespoons!

Ask for Popcorn without Butter:	Calories	Fat (g)
10 cups Popcorn w/3T butter	925	80
10 cups Popcorn Plain	550	38
Total:	**375**	**42**

Popcorn

	Calories	Fat (g)	Sodium (mg)	Exchanges
Popcorn (without butter):				
1 cup	55	4	40	¼ST+¾FAT
3 cups	154	11	120	¾ST+2FAT
8 cups	440	30	320	2ST+6FAT
12 cups	660	46	480	3ST+9FAT
20 cups	1100	76	800	5ST+15FAT
24 cups	1320	91	960	6ST+18FAT
Butter-Flavored Oil:				
1 Tablespoon (approx. 1 squirt)	125	14	0	3FAT
4 Tablespoon	600	56	0	11FAT

Popcorn is sold in cups, bags, and boxes. Here are some tips to determine how many cups of popcorn is in your serving.

CUPS:

If your popcorn was served in a cup, estimate how many fluid ounces it holds. Compare it to the cup sizes shown under the *Beverages* chapter or look for a size printed on the cup. The ounces may be labeled on the outside of the cup or on the bottom band (a code of "NO. 22P" is 22 oz). Then divide the number of ounces by 8 to see how many cups it will hold. For example, a 22 oz cup holds nearly three cups (22/8=2.75 cups).

Ounces	Cups		Ounces	Cups
8	1		22	2¾
12	1½		44	5½
16	2		64	8

BOXES:

The small, standard size found in many stores and in most airports measures 5½" wide X 8½"high X 2" deep (the size of the front cover of this book and two inches deep). This contains approximately 8 cups of popcorn when the cover is closed. If it is open and overflowing, count on at least 9 cups.

BAGS:

Watch out, it's easy to overstuff bags. The measurements below are when the bag is filled, not overfilled.

Cups	Height		Width		Depth
12	9"	X	5"	X	3½"
20	9¾"	X	7½"	X	3½"
24	12"	X	7¼"	X	3½"

For visual assistance, the 12 cups bag is about the size of the front cover of this book, but three and a half inches thick.

PART

3

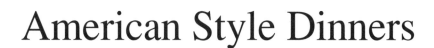

American Style Dinners

Appetizers

Appetizers are small samples of foods designed to pacify your appetite until your meal arrives. But, how many of us can afford the calories of both an appetizer *and* an entrée? If the appetizers appear enticing, consider having an appetizer instead of the entrée.

✓ **Avoid fried appetizers or make the fried appetizer your entrée.** If you enjoy fried foods, ask if there is an appetizer portion (or half portion) available. Appetizers are smaller than the entrée portion and, therefore, have fewer calories.

✓ **Have the leaner appetizers as your entrée**. Think about ordering a lean appetizer such as shrimp cocktail, crabmeat cocktail, or oysters on the half shell with a salad instead of an entrée. Cocktail sauce is also low in fat.

Making Appetizers into Lower Calorie Meals:	Calories	Fat (g)
6 Shrimp Cocktail w/2T Cocktail Sauce	220	3
Garden Salad w/fat-free dressing	80	1
2 oz Italian Bread w/2t Whipped Margarine	210	8
Total:	**510**	**12**
Marguerita Pizza, ½ of 12" ("no oil & light on the cheese")	450	9
Minestrone Soup, 8 oz	95	3
Total:	**545**	**12**

✓ **Limit the sauces** that come with appetizers. Most sauces are high in fat and calories. Order them on the side; dip your fork into the sauce and then into the food for a taste with every bite. For nutritional information on sauces not found in this chapter, refer to the *Entrees and Sauces* chapter.

Appetizers

	Calories	Fat (g)	Sodium (mg)	Exchanges
Artichoke, 1 med cooked	55	0	80	1½V
Bruschetta (1 oz bread grilled w/ olive oil)	198	15	154	1ST+3FAT
Buffalo Wings, 6	420	30	180	2HFM+3FAT
Blue cheese dressing, 2T	160	16	310	3FAT
Calamari, fried, 3 oz	200	8	250	3LM
Caviar, 2T	80	4	480	1MFM
Melba toast, 4	40	0	90	½ST
Ceviche, 4 oz	150	5	na	4VLM
Chicken Quesadillas, 6½"	465	26	1010	2ST+2HFM+1LM+ 1FAT
Clams, raw, 3	50	1	110	2VLM
Crostini (thin French bread toast rounds with pate), 2	170	10	190	½ST+1LM+1½FAT
Egg Rolls, 1 med	240	17	490	1ST+1V+3½FAT
Sweet and Sour Sauce, 2T	55	0	70	1CHO
Fried Mozzarella Sticks, 4 (3 oz)	300	21	950	3HFM
Marinara sauce, ¼ c	50	1	300	1V
Fried Whole Onion	895	68	900	1V+3ST+13½FAT
Fried Zucchini, Mushrooms, ½ c	190	10	200	1V+1ST+2FAT
Herbed Pork Pâté, 2T	70	3	110	1MFM
Butter Crackers, 3	80	4	110	¾ST+½FAT
Liver Pate, 2T	80	7	190	½HFM+½FAT
Nachos w/ beans & cheese, 6 lg	480	30	630	1ST+2HFM+3FAT
Nachos w/ beans, cheese, & meat, 6 lg	690	48	1200	1ST+3HFM+5FAT
Nuts, 1 oz (about ¼ c)	180	14	180	1VLM+3FAT
Olives, 10 lg pickled green	45	5	926	1FAT
10 med pickled, ripe, greek style	65	7	na	1½FAT
1 super colossal ripe	13	1.[1]	145	¼FAT
Oysters Rockefeller, 3	85	6	150	1V+1FAT
Oysters, raw, 6	120	2	150	4VLM
Marguerita Pizza, 12" (thin crust w/vegetables, sauce & cheese)	1100	46	3000	7ST+1V+4HFM+3FAT
Popcorn, 1c	55	4	40	¼ST+¾FAT
Quesadillas, 6½" diameter	430	24	760	2ST+2HFM+1FAT
Roasted Peppers marinated in olive oil	45	3	na	½V+½FAT
Shrimp Cocktail, 4 large	120	2	172	3VLM
Cocktail sauce, 2T	40	0	320	½CHO
Stuffed Jalapenos	70	4	200	½ST+1FAT
Stuffed Mushrooms, 1 regular	40	3	175	¼ST+½FAT
Porcini, 1 lg	150	15	200	½HFM+2FAT
Stuffed Potato Skins, 4 skins (6 oz)	560	40	600	2ST+1HFM+6½FAT
Sour cream, ¼ c	104	10	24	2FAT

Appetizers (continued)

	Calories	Fat (g)	Sodium (mg)	Exchanges
Tortilla Chip, 1 regular-sized	18	1	8	na
Tortilla Chip, 7 regular	126	7	56	1ST+1FAT
Nacho Cheese Sauce, 2T	100	8	580	½HFM+1FAT
Guacamole, ¼ c	110	10	420	2FAT
Salsa, ¼ c	20	0	440	1V

Beverages

Chapter Content:
■ Cold Beverages: Sodas, Juices, Milk, Iced Tea, Lemonade, Eggnog, & Shakes
■ Coffee, Coffee Beverages, & other Hot Beverages
■ Your Favorite Coffee Shops
■ Alcoholic Beverages

Beverages vary greatly in calorie content anywhere from 0 - 125 calories per ounce. The total caloric difference is very significant as a result of the quantity consumed. Notice that alcoholic beverages top the list. That's because alcohol has 7 calories per gram, rather than the 4 calories per gram for all other carbohydrates.

Beverage Calorimeter: Calories per fluid ounce

125	Creme de Menthe
100	Coffee Liqueurs
85	100 Proof Liqueurs
60	Manhattan, Martini
40	Nonalcoholic Eggnog, Table Wines
30	Ice Cream Shake, Sherry
25	Champagne, Dry White Wine, Frozen Yogurt Shakes
20	Whole Milk, Fruit Juices (Cranberry, Grape, Prune)
17	Fruit Punches
15	2% Low Fat Milk, Fruit Juices (Apple, Grapefruit, Orange), Orange Sodas, Lemonade, Orange Breakfast Drinks
12	Regular Colas, 1% Low Fat Milk, Beer
10	Skim Milk & Buttermilk (made with skim milk) Flavored Coffees, Sweetened Tea, Coffee with cream & sugar
0	Water, Sparkling Waters without added sugar, Club Soda, Perrier, Diet Sodas, Unsweetened Tea & Coffee

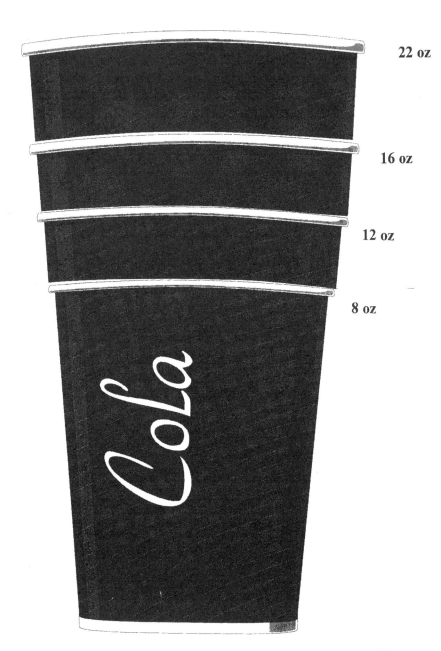

22 oz

16 oz

12 oz

8 oz

Don't know the serving size of your favorite beverage? Use these actual beverages cup sizes for comparison.

Cold Beverages

Fountain Beverages

✓**All sodas are fat-free but only the diet sodas are calorie-free.** A can of soda has about 150 calories - all derived from sugar! While 150 calories may not sound like much, the calories can have a cumulative effect. All other things being equal, if you are currently drinking six cans of regular soda a day and switch to diet soda, you will be consuming 900 calories a day less. That amounts to a weight loss of almost two pounds each week!

If you drink 6 cans of soda/day & switch to diet:	Calories	Fat (g)
12 oz Soda X 6	900	0
12 oz Diet Soda X 6	0	0
Savings:	900	0

900 calories X 365 days in a year = 328,500 calories
328,500/3500 = weight loss of 94 pounds of fat in a year

How many calories do you consume from soda? The exact calories consumed by *you* are determined by the beverage chosen, size of cup, and the amount of ice put into the glass. To quickly assess the calories in your favorite fountain beverage, refer to the following calorimeter.

Fountain Beverage Calorimeter: Calories per serving

Calories/ 12 oz Can	Fountain Beverages	Calories Per Cup with 20% Ice				
		8 oz	12 oz	16 oz	22 oz	32 oz
210	Orange Sunkist® Soda	110	170	225	310	450
195	Mandarin Orange Slice®	105	155	210	285	415
180	Hawaiian Punch®	95	145	190	265	385
170	A&W® Root Beer, Mountain Dew®, Surge®	90	135	180	250	365
160	Barq's® Root Beer, RC® Cola	85	130	170	235	340
150	Big Red®, Dr. Pepper®, Pepsi®, Lemon Lime Slice®	80	120	160	220	320
140	Coca Cola®, Mr. Pibb®, 7Up®, Sprite®	75	110	150	205	300
0	Diet Sodas	0	0	0	0	0

* For fat, sodium, and exchanges per 12 oz can, refer to the nutritional information on the next page.

Milk

✓ **Many restaurants provide skim or low fat milk**, even if it is not listed on the menu. Making this healthy change is recommended for everyone over the age of two.

Request Skim Milk instead of Whole Milk:	Calories	Fat (g)
8 oz Whole Milk	150	8
8 oz Skim Milk	90	0
Savings:	60	8

Fruit Juice

✓ **Fruit juice contains just as many calories as soda.** It may be healthier to switch from drinking soda to fruit juice because, unlike soda, fruit juices contain vitamins and minerals. But fruit juice doesn't contain fewer calories than non-diet soda. So don't expect the change to cause a weight loss. If you want to lose weight, eat *fresh* fruit for vitamins, minerals, and fiber. Then drink a non-caloric beverage such as water or a diet beverage.

Compare these Two Beverages:	Calories	Fat (g)
12 oz Cola Beverage	140	0
12 oz Orange Juice	170	0

Shakes

✓ **Shake made with skim milk are still high in calories**. Even the fat-free shakes are high in calories because of their high sugar content! A 12 oz shake contains almost 10 teaspoons worth! Can you afford the extra calories?

Order a Fat Free Shake:	Calories	Fat (g)
12 oz Ice Cream Shake	385	8
12 oz Fat-Free Shake	275	0
Savings:	110	8

COLD BEVERAGES

	Calories	Fat	Sodium	Exchanges
12 oz can (w/out ice):				
A&W Root Beer	170	0	45	2¾CHO
Barq's® Root Beer	160	0	70	2½CHO
Big Red®	150	0	30	2½CHO
Coca Cola®	140	0	50	2½CHO
Diet Coke®	0	0	40	FREE
Diet Dr. Pepper®	0	0	55	FREE
Diet Pepsi®	0	0	35	FREE
Diet Rite Cola	0	0	0	FREE
Diet 7Up®	0	0	35	FREE
Diet Sprite®	0	0	40	FREE
Dr. Pepper®	150	0	55	2½CHO
Hawaiian Punch®	180	0	170	3CHO
Mr. Pibb®	140	0	45	2¼CHO
Mountain Dew®	170	0	70	2¾CHO
Pepsi®	150	0	35	2½CHO
RC Cola	160	0	50	2½CHO
7Up®	140	0	75	2¼CHO
Slice®, Mandarin Orange	195	0	55	3¼CHO
Slice ®, Lemon Lime	150	0	55	2½CHO
Sprite®	140	0	70	2¼CHO
Sunkist Orange Soda	210	0	60	3½CHO
Surge	170	0	40	2¾CHO
Fruit/Vegetable Juices (6 oz):				
Tomato Juice	40	0	0	1FR
Apple Juice	85	0	13	1½FR
Cranberry Juice	110	0	8	2FR
Grape Juice	120	0	5	2FR
Grapefruit Juice	70	0	2	1FR
Orange Juice	85	0	1	1½FR
Prune Juice	130	0	8	2FR
Milk (8 oz):				
Skim Milk	90	0	120	1SkMk
2% Low Fat Milk	120	5	120	1LfMk
Whole Milk	150	8	120	1WhMk
Other Cold Beverages (12 oz):				
Iced Tea, sweetened	120	0	80	2CHO
Lemonade	130	0	130	2CHO
Shakes & Egg Nog:				
Ice Cream Shakes, 22 oz	625	29	320	4CHO+1WhMk+4FAT
12 oz	385	8	270	3CHO+½WhMk+1FAT
Fat-Free Yogurt Shakes, 12 oz	275	0	160	3CHO+½SkMk
Egg Nog, non-alcoholic, 4 oz	190	13	75	½CHO+½MFM+¼WhMk+2FAT

Coffee and other Hot Beverages

✓ **Coffee, espresso, and tea have negligible calories**. It is what you add to these drinks, however, that will impact your weight and waist!

✓ **Know what's in your beverage** so you'll know what substitutions to ask for.

- ■ Espresso - Strong coffee brewed under pressure
- ■ Cappuccino - Espresso and steamed milk
- ■ Latte - Espresso and steamed milk (but more milk than w/cappuccino)
- ■ Mocha - Espresso, steamed milk, and chocolate syrup

✓ **Ask for your beverage to be prepared with skim or low fat milk.** Nearly every restaurant and coffee shop offers these lower fat alternatives for your coffee and espresso drinks.

Whiten your Coffee with Milk:	Calories	Fat (g)
1 oz Coffee Cream	60	6
1 oz Non-Dairy Creamer	45	3
1 oz Whole Milk	20	1
1 oz Skim Milk	10	0
Savings:	15-50	1-6

Have your Latte Prepared with Skim Milk:	Calories	Fat (g)
12 oz Latte made with whole milk	195	10
12 oz Latte made with skim milk	115	0.5
Savings:	80	9.5

✓ **Enjoy your beverage without whipping cream**. Depending on whether skim, 2% or whole milk is used in the preparation of the drink, the addition of whipping cream can double the calories!

Skip the Whipped Cream:	Calories	Fat (g)
12 oz Mocha (2% milk) w/ ¼ c whipping cream	280	18
12 oz Mocha (2% milk) w/out whipping cream	180	6
Savings:	100	12

✓ **There are sixteen calories in a teaspoon of sugar**. That may not sound like a whole lot of calories, but consider this. If you add just a teaspoon of sugar in every cup you drink, and you drink 3 cups a day, that adds up to an extra 48 calories each day. Multiply that by 365 days in the year and you end up with 17,520 calories (365 X 48) coming from sugar or an extra five pounds of fat (17,520/3500) each year. Can you afford the extra calories?

Get used to the Taste of Sweetners:	Calories	Fat (g)
3 t of sugar a day	48	0
3 t sugar/day X 365 days in a year	17,520	0

17,520 calories / 3500 calories in a pound = 5 pounds of fat!

✔ **For those of you concerned about the dangers of non-caloric sweetners, consider this.** There *may* be risks associated with the excess consumption of non-caloric sweetners - we just don't know enough yet. But researchers do know of *definite risks* associated with carrying around too much weight such as increased risk of heart disease, high blood pressure, diabetes, and certain types of cancer. If you are still concerned about the safety of non-caloric sweeteners, cut out the sugar and sweeteners completely. The coffee or tea may taste different initially, but by the end of two weeks your taste buds will have adjusted to the difference.

Hot Beverages Calorimeter: Calories per ounce & serving size

Calories per oz	Hot Beverages	Calories & Fat grams (g)			
		8 oz	12 oz	16 oz	20 oz
18	Latte (whole)	**145** 6g	**215** 10g	**290** 12g	**360** 16g
17	Mocha (whole)	**135** 5g	**205** 8g	**270** 10g	**340** 14g
15	2% Latte, 2% Mocha, Hot Chocolate	**120** 4g	**180** 6g	**240** 7g	**300** 9g
12	Mocha (skim)	**100** 1g	**145** 2g	**190** 3g	**240** 4g
10	Flavored Coffees (sugar sweetened)	**80** 1g	**120** $1.^5$g	**160** 2g	**200** $2.^5$g
9	Latte (skim)	**72** 0g	**110** $0.^5$g	**145** $0.^6$g	**180** $0.^8$g
7	Cappuccino (whole)	**55** 3g	**85** 5g	**110** 6g	**140** 8g
6	Cappuccino (2%)	**50** 2g	**70** 3g	**100** 4g	**120** 5g
5	Cappuccino (skim)	**40** 0g	**60** 0g	**80** 0g	**100** 0g
0	Coffee, Espresso, Tea (plain)	**0** 0g	**0** 0g	**0** 0g	**0** 0g

Hot Beverages

	Calories	Fat (g)	Sodium (mg)	Exchanges
Coffee & Espresso:				
Coffee, black, 8 oz	5	0	0	FREE
Coffee, decaf, black, 8 oz	5	0	0	FREE
Coffee, flavored w/ sugar, 8 oz	72	1	4	1CHO
Espresso, 1 shot	5	0	0	FREE
Latte:				
Latte w/skim milk, 8 oz	65	0	95	¾SkMk
12 oz	115	$0.^5$	160	1¼SkMk
16 oz	140	$0.^6$	190	1½SkMk
20 oz	190	$0.^8$	250	2SkMk
Latte w/2% milk, 8 oz	95	4	90	¾LfMk
12 oz	155	6	155	1¼LfMk
16 oz	190	7	185	1½LfMk
20 oz	250	9	245	2LfMk
Latte, w/whole milk, 8 oz	120	6	90	¾WhMk
12 oz	195	10	155	1¼WhMk
16 oz	235	12	185	1½WhMk
20 oz	310	16	245	2WhMk
Cappuccino:				
Cappuccino w/skim milk, 8 oz	40	0	50	½SkMk
12 oz	60	0	80	½SkMk
16 oz	80	0	95	¾SkMk
20 oz	100	0	125	1LfMk
Cappuccino w/2% milk, 8 oz	50	2	50	½LfMk
12 oz	75	3	80	½LfMk
16 oz	100	4	95	¾LfMk
20 oz	125	5	125	1LfMk
Cappuccino, w/whole milk, 8 oz	55	3	50	½WhMk
12 oz	85	5	80	½WhMk
16 oz	110	6	95	¾WhMk
20 oz	140	8	125	1WhMk
Mocha (w/out whipping cream):				
Mocha, w/skim milk, 8 oz	100	1	75	½SkMk+¾CHO
12 oz	150	2	125	¾SkMk+1CHO+½FAT
16 oz	200	3	175	1SkMk+1½CHO+½FAT
20 oz	230	4	200	1SkMk+2CHO+ 1FAT
Mocha, w/2% milk, 8 oz	120	4	75	½LfMk+¾CHO
12 oz	180	6	125	¾LfMk+1CHO+½FAT
16 oz	240	7	175	1LfMk+1½CHO+½FAT
20 oz	280	10	200	1LfMk+2CHO+ 1FAT
Mocha, w/whole milk, 8 oz	130	5	75	½WhMk+¾CHO
12 oz	210	8	125	¾WhMk+1CHO+½FAT
16 oz	280	10	175	1WhMk+1½CHO+½FAT
20 oz	320	14	200	1WhMk+2CHO+ 1FAT

Hot Beverages (continued)

	Calories	Fat (g)	Sodium (mg)	Exchanges
Other Hot Beverages:				
Tea, 1 bag	2	0	5	FREE
Hot Chocolate, 8 oz	110	2	130	½LfMk+1CHO
Hot Chocolate, made w/2% milk	120	4	120	½LfMk+1CHO+¼FAT
Condiments:				
Half & half, 1T	20	1.^{7}	6	1/3 FAT
Honey, 1 tsp	21	0	0	1/3 CHO
Honey, 1T	64	0	0	1CHO
18% Butterfat Cream, 1 T	30	2.^{5}	5	½FAT
Light Table Cream, 1T	30	3	6	½FAT
Milk, skim, 1T	5	0	8	FREE
Milk, 2%, 1T	7.^{5}	0.^{3}	8	FREE
Milk, whole, 1T	10	0.^{5}	8	FREE
Nondairy lightener, liquid, 1T	22	1.^{5}	7	1/3 FAT
Nondairy lightener, powdered, 1tsp	10	1	3	FREE
Sugar, 1t	16	0	0	¼CHO
Heavy Cream, 1T	50	6	6	1FAT
Whipping Cream, whipped, 2T	50	6	6	1FAT
Whipped Topping, pressurized, 2T	23	1.^{8}	4	½FAT
Whipped Topping, pressurized, ¼ c	46	3.^{6}	8	1FAT
Accompaniments:				
Biscotti, 7" long, $^7/_8$" wide, 1.^{3} oz	112	5	41	1ST+1FAT

How Much Caffeine am I Consuming?

Coffee provides 75% of all the caffeine consumed in America. Caffeine is also found in tea, caffeinated fountain beverages, chocolate, and some drugs. Although there is no hard evidence to support these concerns, some people are concerned about its possible connections to cancer, high blood pressure, and coronary heart disease. Caffeine is a stimulant; if you are sensitive to its effects you may want to limit your intake.

	Caffeine (mg)		Caffeine (mg)
Coffee Beverages:		**Other Beverages:**	
Espresso, 1 oz	35	Chocolate milk, 1 oz	5
Double	70	Cocoa or hot chocolate, 8 oz	5
Espresso, decaf, 1 oz	5	Cola, 12 oz	50
Double	10	Tea, decaf, 8 oz	5
Coffee, 8 oz	100	Tea, 8 oz	50
Coffee, Gourmet, 8 oz	150	Tea, green or instant, 8 oz	30
Caffè Latte, Cappuccino, *or* Mocha, 8 oz	35	Tea, bottled, 12 oz or from instant mix, 8 oz	15
Caffè Latte, Cappuccino, *or* Mocha, 16 or 20 oz	70	Chocolate, dark, bittersweet, or semi-sweet, 1 oz	20

Your Favorite Coffee Shops

AU BON PAIN®

	Calories	Fat	Sodium	Exchanges
Specialty Drinks:				
Hot Mocha Blast, small	160	4	120	½LfMk+1CHO+½FAT
medium	260	6	180	¾LfMk+2CHO+½FAT
large	310	8	230	1LfMk+2¼CHO+½FAT
Hot Raspberry Mocha Blast, small	180	4	115	½LfMk+1½CHO+½FAT
medium	300	6	170	¾LfMk+3CHO+½FAT
large	350	8	220	1LfMk+3CHO+½FAT
Iced Raspberry Mocha Blast, small	160	3.⁵	100	½LfMk+1¼CHO+½FAT
medium	210	5	140	¾LfMk+1½CHO+½FAT
large	330	7	200	1LfMk+2½CHO+½FAT
Peach Iced Tea, small	90	0	na	1½CHO
medium	130	0	na	2CHO
large	170	0	na	3CHO
Iced Specialty Drinks:				
Iced Cocoa, small	200	6	160	½LfMk+1½CHO+½FAT
medium	280	6	190	¾LfMk+2CHO+½FAT
large	440	11	320	1LfMk+3½CHO+½FAT
Iced Mocha Blast, small	180	4.⁵	135	½LfMk+1¼CHO+½FAT
medium	260	6	180	¾LfMk+2CHO+½FAT
large	360	10	280	1LfMk+2½CHO+1FAT
Iced Caffe Latte, small	130	5	130	½LfMk+½CHO+½FAT
medium	150	6	150	¾LfMk+½CHO+½FAT
large	270	10	270	1LfMk+1½CHO+1FAT
Iced Cappuccino, small	110	4	110	½LfMk+¼CHO+¼FAT
medium	150	6	150	¾LfMk+½CHO+½FAT
large	270	10	270	1LfMk+1CHO+1FAT
Raspberry Breeze, small	130	0	0	2CHO
medium	190	0	0	3CHO
large	260	0	0	4CHO

DENNY'S®

	Calories	Fat (g)	Sodium (mg)	Exchanges
Flavored Beverages:				
Hazelnut Coffee	66	1	4	1CHO
French Vanilla Coffee	76	1	4	1CHO
Irish Cream	73	1	4	1CHO
Raspberry Iced Tea w/ice	78	0	0	1½CHO

STARBUCKS COFFEE

	Calories	Fat (g)	Sodium (mg)	Exchanges
Drip Coffee:				
Tall, 12 oz	10	0	10	FREE
Grande, 16 oz	10	0	15	FREE
Frappuccino® Blended Beverages (coffee, ice, & milk):				
Tall	200	3	170	½LfMk+2½CHO
Grande	270	4	230	½LfMk+3CHO+½FAT
add Venti™, 20 oz	340	4.^{5}	280	½LfMk+4CHO+½FAT
Mocha Frappuccino® blended beverage (coffee, ice, milk, chocolate syrup & flavoring):				
Tall	230	3	180	½LfMk+2½CHO
Grande	310	4.^{5}	240	½LfMk+3½CHO+½FAT
add Venti™, 20 oz	390	5	300	½LfMk+4½CHO+½FAT
Espresso:				
Solo	5	0	0	FREE
Doppio	10	0	0	FREE
Espresso Con Panna (espresso w/whipped cream on top):				
Solo	30	3	0	1FAT
Dopio	35	3	0	1FAT
Espresso Macchiato (espresso dotted w/foamed milk):				
Solo, nonfat milk	10	0	10	FREE
Solo, lowfat milk*	10	0	10	FREE
Solo, whole milk	15	0.^{5}	5	FREE
Doppio, nonfat milk	15	0	10	FREE
Doppio, lowfat milk*	15	0	10	FREE
Doppio, whole milk	20	0.^{5}	5	¼CHO
Caffè Americano (espresso & water):				
Tall	10	0	10	FREE
Grande	15	0	10	FREE
Cappuccino:				
Tall, nonfat milk	80	0	110	¾SkMk+¼CHO
Tall, lowfat milk*	110	4	110	¾LfMk+¼CHO
Tall, whole milk	140	7	105	¾WhMk+¼CHO
Grande, nonfat milk	110	0.^{5}	140	¾SkMk+½CHO
Grande, lowfat milk*	140	5	140	¾LfMk+½CHO
Grande, whole milk	180	9	135	¾WhMk+½CHO

STARBUCKS COFFEE (continued)

	Calories	Fat (g)	Sodium (mg)	Exchanges
Caffè Latte:				
Tall, nonfat milk	120	0.5	170	1¼SkMk+¼CHO
Tall, lowfat milk*	170	6	170	1¼LfMk+¼CHO
Tall, whole milk	210	11	160	1¼WhMk+¼CHO
Grande, nonfat milk	160	1	220	1½SkMk+¼CHO
Grande, lowfat milk*	220	8	220	1½LfMk+¼CHO
Grande, whole milk	270	14	210	1½WhMk+¼CHO
Caffè Mocha (w/whipping cream):**				
Tall, nonfat milk	260	12	170	¾SkMk+1CHO+2½FAT
Tall, lowfat milk*	300	16	160	¾LfMk+1CHO+2½FAT
Tall, whole milk	340	21	160	¾WhMk+1CHO+3FAT
Grande, nonfat milk	320	13	210	1SkMk+1½CHO+ 2½FAT
Grande, lowfat milk*	370	18	200	1LfMk+1½CHO+ 2½FAT
Grande, whole milk	410	24	200	1WhMk+1½CHO+3FAT

 * **Lowfat milk is 1 part whole milk to 1 part nonfat milk.**
** **All Caffé Mocha beverages are available without whipping cream upon request.**

Alcoholic Beverages

In the second chapter we mentioned that carbohydrates and proteins have 4 calories per gram, while fats have 9. Where does alcohol fit it? Alcohol, a fermented carbohydrate, is a concentrated source of calories at 7 calories per gram. Although most alcoholic beverages are fat-free, the calories from alcohol can still be damaging to your weight! Here are some general guidelines for Dining Lean with alcoholic beverages.

✔ **Save the alcoholic drinks for special occasions** if you can't afford the extra calories.

Drink Calorie-free Beverages instead of Mixed Drinks:			
		Calories	Fat (g)
8 oz Screwdriver, Gin & Tonic, Bloody Mary, *or* Bourbon & Soda		200	0
8 oz Diet Soda, Coffee, Tea, Water, Club Soda, *or* Mineral Water		0	0
	Savings:	**200**	**0**

Skip the Liqueurs in Coffee:			
		Calories	Fat (g)
Coffee + 1½ oz Creme de Menthe		180	0
Black Coffee		0	0
	Savings:	**180**	**0**

✔ **Choose the lighter versions of your favorite beverages.**

Order Light Beer:			
		Calories	Fat (g)
12 oz Beer		150	0
12 oz Light Beer		100	0
	Savings:	**50**	**0**

Instead of a Wine Cooler, Order Club Soda/Wine:			
		Calories	Fat (g)
8 oz Wine Cooler		160	0
4 oz Wine + 4 oz Club Soda		80	0
	Savings:	**80**	**0**

✔ **Find another favorite beverage – one with fewer calories.**

Order Simple rather than Fancy:			
		Calories	Fat (g)
8 oz Margarita *or* Piña Colada		320-480	0 - 6
1 oz Rum + 7 oz Cola		190	0
	Savings:	**130-290**	**0 - 6**

Use the Calorimeter below to learn more about the calories in your favorite alcoholic beverages. There is no fat in most alcoholic beverages. If there is fat, it is noted on the Calorimeter and in the nutritional information that follows.

Alcoholic Beverage Calorimeter: Calories & fat per serving

Calories per oz	Alcoholic Beverages	Calories & fat (g)			
		1½ oz	4 oz	8 oz	12 oz
125	Creme de Menthe	188	500	1000	1500
120	Southern Comfort	180	480	960	1440
110	Drambuie	165	440	880	1320
105	Coffee w/Cream*	155	420	840	1260
		7g	19g	38g	57g
100	Liqueurs: Anisette Liqueurs, Crème d'Amande, Crème de Banana, Crème de Cacao	150	400	800	1200
95	Liqueurs: Benedictine, B&B, Rock & Rye, Tía Maria	145	380	760	1140
85	100 Proof Liquor Liqueurs: Kirsch, Sloe Gin, Peppermint Snapps	125	340	680	1020
80	Tequila Liqueurs: Amaretto, Pernod, Triple Sec, Apricot Brandy, Cherry Heering, Creme de Cassis, Grand Marnier	120	320	640	960
75	90 Proof Liquor Liqueurs: Curaçao	115	300	600	900
70	Brandy	105	280	560	840
65	80 Proof Liquor	100	260	520	780
60	Manhattan, Martini	90	240	480	720
58	Piña Coladas*, Grasshopper*, Golden Cadillac*, Velvet Hammer*, Brandy Alexandra*	85	230	465	700
		3g	7g	14g	21g
55	SloeGin Fizz, Old Fashioned	85	220	440	660
50	Glögg*	75	200	400	600
		1g	2g	4g	6g
45	Hot Buttered Rum*, Irish Coffee*	70	180	360	540
		3g	7g	14g	21g
45	Wines: Muscatel, Port, Vermouth (sweet), Dessert Wines (sweet)	70	180	360	540

* These alcoholic beverages contain fat. The others do not.

Alcoholic Beverage Calorimeter (continued)

Calories per oz	Alcoholic Beverages	Calories & fat (g)			
		1½ oz	4 oz	8 oz	12 oz
40	Margarita, Whiskey Sour, Mexican Sunset Wines: Dessert Wines (dry), Madeira Tokay, Dubonnet, Sweet Wines	**60**	**160**	**320**	**480**
38	Brandy Cream*	**60** 3g	**150** 7g	**300** 14g	**450** 21g
35	Tequila Sunrise, Daquiri, Dry Vermouth	55	140	280	420
30	Sherry Wines: Cold Duck, Sparkling Burgundy, Sauterne	45	120	240	360
25	Bourbon/Soda, Bloody Mary, Campari/Soda, Gin/Tonic, Screwdriver Wines: Beaujolais, Champagne, Chablis, Chianti, Rhine, Rhone, Bordeaux, Burgundy, Rosé, White Burgundy, Cabernet Sauvignon, Chardonnay, French Colombard, Riesling, Sylvaner, Red Zinfandel	40	100	200	300
20	Tom Collins, Highball, Mint Julep, Sparkling Wine Coolers Wines: Sauvignon Blanc, White Zinfandel, Chablis, Chenin Blanc, Table Wines, Liebfraumilch	30	80	160	240
15	Wine Spritzer	25	60	120	180
13	Dark Beer & Ale, Malt Liquors	20	50	104	156
12	Beer	20	50	96	144
9	Light Beer	15	35	72	108

* These alcoholic beverages contain fat. The others do not.

Alcoholic Beverages containing fat

	Calories	Fat (g)	Sodium (mg)	Exchanges
Brandy Alexander, 5 fl oz	275	10	15	na
Brandy Cream, 4 fl oz	150	7	na	na
Coffee w/cream, 1½ fl oz	155	7	na	na
Glögg, 4 fl oz	190	2	na	na
Golden Cadillac, 4 fl oz	230	7	na	na
Grasshopper, 4 fl oz	230	7	na	na
Hot Buttered Rum, 6 fl oz	255	9	na	na
Irish Coffee, 6 fl oz	280	11	na	na
Piña Colada, 4½ fl oz	260	3	na	na
Velvet Hammer, 4 fl oz	230	7	9	na

Soups

You've just arrived at the restaurant and you're feeling famished. What can you order that will be served fast? Soups, if chosen wisely, can stave off your appetite until your main course arrives. The following guidelines are for your consideration when ordering soups.

✓ **Choose broth-based soups.** Broth-based soups have fewer calories than cream-based soups and can help satiate you so that you don't overeat during the rest of the meal. Unfortunately, all restaurant soups are high in sodium.

✓ **Milk-based soups are significantly lower in calories than cream-based soups.** Be sure to ask the composition of the soup. You are more likely to find the higher fat cream based soups at the more upscale restaurants than at a salad bar. Some restaurants are serving healthy "cream" soups made with skim milk and pureed vegetables. These would be acceptable low fat options.

✓ **Thicker soups (such as gumbo) may have be prepared with roux** (a thickener made from fat and flour). The fat increases the caloric content more than it would appear by sight.

✓ **Don't garnish the soup.** Some soups, in upscale restaurants, are "garnished" with a dollop of sour cream (50 calories and 5 grams fat) or a swirl of light cream (30 calories and 3 grams of fat per tablespoon). Your Tortilla soup may have fried tortilla strips and avocado cubes added prior to being served. Baked potato soup might be topped with crumbled bacon. You may want to consider asking for your soup to be served plain!

✓ **Do not eat the bread bowl.** In some restaurants, soup is served in a bread bowl, a round loaf of bread with the top removed and the inside partially scooped out. This bowl, though low in fat, contains over 600 calories!

✓ **Select a cup, not a bowl.** Save the calories for other courses you want to enjoy.

✓ **Select a larger bowl of one of the lower calorie soups and make it a meal!**

Make Soup into a Meal:

	Calories	Fat (g)
12 oz Vegetable Soup	120	5
2 oz Focaccio bread w/1t olive oil	220	11
TOTAL:	**340**	**16**

Soup Calorimeter: Calories & fat per serving

Calories per oz	Soup	Calories & Fat (g)		
		8 oz	12 oz	16 oz
45	French Onion Soup (topped with melted cheese), Cheese Soup (thick), Baked Potato Soup	360 22g	540 33g	720 44g
39	Chile con Carne (w/beans & meat)	310 13g	465 20g	620 26g
33	French Onion Soup (simple), New England Clam Chowder, Fish Chowder, Seafood Gumbo, Vichyssoise	260 15g	390 23g	520 30g
29	Cheese Soup (w/milk), Oyster Stew, Cream of Chicken, Lobster Bisque, Tomato Bisque, Tortilla Soup	225 14g	340 21g	450 28g
25	Manhattan Clam Chowder, Split Pea w/ham, Cream of Potato	200 8g	300 12g	400 16g
23	Black Bean, Chili w/beans (no meat), Bouillabaisse, Lentil Cream of: Asparagus, Broccoli, Celery, *or* Mushroom	180 7g	270 11g	360 15g
15	Chicken Noodle, Chicken Rice, Tomato	120 3g	180 5g	240 6g
13	Minestrone	100 3g	150 5g	200 6g
10	Vegetable, Gazpacho	80 3g	120 5g	160 6g

Soups* (1 c)

	Calories	Fat (g)	Sodium (mg)	Exchanges
Baked Potato Soup	350	22	na	½WhMk+1ST+1HFM+ 2FAT
Bean Soup or Black Bean Soup	180	6	na	1½ST+1VLM+1FAT
Bouillabaisse, w/out rice	155	5	na	2VLM+1V+1FAT
Cheese Soup, made w/milk	230	15	na	½ST+½WhMk+½HFM+ 1FAT
Cheese Soup (thick)	360	27	na	½WhMk+1V+1½HFM+ 2FAT
Chicken Noodle or Chicken Rice	120	3	na	1ST+½LM
Chili Con Carne w/Beans	310	13	na	2ST+2MFM+½FAT
Chile w/Beans, no meat	180	6	na	1½ST+1MFM
Clam Chowder, Manhattan	210	9	na	2V+½ST+1LM+1FAT
Clam Chowder, New England or Fish Chowder	260	13	na	½WhMk+½ST+1LM+ 2FAT
Cream of Asparagus, Broccoli, Celery, or Mushroom	180	9	na	¾ST+½WhMk+1FAT
Cream of Chicken	185	12	na	¼ST+½WhMk+½LM+ 1½FAT
Cream of Potato Soup	190	10	na	1ST+2FAT
French Onion Soup	260	15	na	1ST+1V+1HFM+1½FAT
French Onion Soup w/melted cheese	380	22	na	2ST+1HFM+3FAT
Gazpacho	90	2	na	2V+½FAT
Gumbo, Seafood	250	16	na	½WhMk+1VLM+3FAT
Lentil	190	5	na	1½ST+1VLM+1FAT
Lobster Bisque	220	15	na	1V+1LM+3FAT
Minestrone	95	3	na	3V+½FAT
Oyster Stew	220	15	na	½WhMk+1VLM+2FAT
Pasta e Fagioli	280	8	na	2ST+1V+1MFM+½FAT
Split Pea w/Ham	190	6	na	2ST+1FAT
Tomato	135	3	na	1ST+1V+½FAT
Tomato Bisque	225	12	na	½ST+1V+½WhMk+ 1½ FAT
Tortilla Soup	240	14	na	1V+¾ST+½HFM+2FAT
Vegetable Soup	70	2	na	2V+½FAT
Vichyssoise (chilled potato soup)	270	18	na	1ST+½WhMk+2½FAT
Bread Bowl (size to fit 12 oz of soup)	625	3	na	8ST+½FAT

* Sodium content varies greatly depending on the recipe. Most average 1000 mg/8 oz.

Salads

People watching their weight often have the misconception that all salads are low calorie, low fat meals. Salad *can* be low fat, but often the dieter chooses the wrong items and ends up with far more calories than a hamburger and fries. Let's examine how a plate of salad increases in calories and grams of fat as items are selected.

A Healthy Meal:

	Calories	Fat (g)
Raw Vegetables, 2 c	100	0
Cottage Cheese, ¼ c	60	5
Chickpeas, 2T	20	0
Shredded Cheese, 2T	60	5
Fat Free Salad Dressing, 2T	40	0
Croutons, 1 Spoon	45	3
Fresh Fruit, ½ c	50	0
TOTAL:	**375**	**13**

Can Double in Calories *Fast*:

	Calories	Fat (g)
All of the above, without the fat-free dressing	335	13
plus Regular Salad Dressing (2 ladles or 4T)	320	32
TOTAL:	**655**	**45**

And Get Even Higher in Calories:

	Calories	Fat (g)
All of the above, plus…	655	45
Potato Salad, ¼ c	100	7
Broccoli/Cauliflower in Ranch dressing, ¼ c	80	8
Blueberry Muffin, 2 oz	200	8
Margarine, 1½ t	53	6
TOTAL:	**1088**	**74**

The final result is a meal with nearly as much fat as you would find in a stick of butter. Keep reading to find out the calories and fat grams in all your favorite salad components.

Salad Bars

✓ **At the salad bar, pile on the raw vegetables, beans (non-marinated), and fresh fruit**. These are all low in fat and calories. These selections lead people to mistakenly believe that all salads are low calorie. It's the mayonnaise and oil that converts a healthy meal into a harmful meal.

✓ **Keep the prepared salads to a minimum.** While plain pasta, cabbage, potatoes, chicken, and tuna fish are low in calories, the addition of mayonnaise (at 100 calories a tablespoon) will more than double the calories. This also applies for oil-prepared salads.

Look at how the Mayonnaise affects the Total Calories:	Calories	Fat (g)
Cole Slaw prepared w/mayonnaise, ½ c	85	6
Cabbage, ½ c	8	0
Savings:	**77**	**6**

✓ **Select unadulerated lean protein.** There are many high-fat protein selections on the salad bar: cheese, eggs, and tuna fish salad. If you want to add healthy protein to your meal, think about adding cottage cheese or non-marinated beans. You may also want to order grilled chicken to top your salad.

Eat Your Protein Plain:	Calories	Fat (g)
Chicken Salad, ¼ c	125	9
Grilled Chicken Breast, ¼ c	50	1
Savings:	**75**	**8**

✓ **Select only small amounts of nuts and seeds.** Did you know that just a small handful of nuts or seeds (¼ c) contains 200 calories? As a healthy alternative, add water chestnuts or raw jicama for crunch. Jicama is a low calorie white vegetable that looks much like raw potato.

Choose Jicama instead of Nuts:	Calories	Fat (g)
Nuts, ¼ c	200	18
Jicama, ¼ c	12	0
Savings:	**188**	**18**

✓ **Request fat-free salad dressings**. Salad bars and restaurants typically stock them. Other low calorie, no-fat options for a salad include picante sauce, salsa, lemon, and flavored vinegars (such as red wine, balsalmic, or tarragon vinegar).

✓ **How big is that ladle?** Most salad dressing ladles contain two tablespoons of dressing. Some hold four! And how many ladles of salad dressing are you using?

✓ **Keep in mind that all portions listed are for level measures** – not heaping! Generally, a heaping tablespoon contains two level tablespoons.

Salads

	Calories	Fat (g)	Sodium (mg)	Exchanges
Vegetables:				
Raw Vegetables & Sprouts, 1c	25	0	5	1V
Avocado, ¼	85	7	5	1½FAT
Green Peas, 2T	15	0	50	¼ST
Jicama, ¼ c	12	0	1	½V
Olives, Black, 2	10	1	80	FREE, 10=1FAT
Green, 2	9	1	180	FREE, 10=1FAT
Pickles, 2 slices	1	0	60	FREE
Pickle, 1 medium	7	0	928	FREE
Pimento Stuffed Green Olives, 5	25	3	470	½FAT
Meats & Protein (2T unless noted):				
Chopped Egg	30	2	30	½MFM
Whole Boiled Egg, 1	80	6	70	1MFM
Cottage Cheese	25	1	100	½LM
Ham	25	1	250	½LM
Parmesan Cheese	50	3	290	½HFM
Pepperoni, sliced, 6 pc	30	3	70	½FAT, 9 pc=1FAT
Shredded Cheese	50	4	250	½HFM
Garnishes (2T):				
Bacon Bits	45	3	570	¼ST+½FAT
Chickpeas (Garbanzo beans)	20	0	75	¼ST
Chow Mein Fried Noodles	20	1	15	¼ST
Croutons	30	1	75	½ST
Granola	65	2	35	½ST+½FAT
Kidney Beans	27	1	73	½ST
Nuts, unsalted	200	18	0	3½FAT
Raisins	56	0	2	1FR
Sunflower Seeds	80	7	1	1½FAT
Salad Dressings (1T):				
Blue Cheese	80	8	155	1½FAT
French	80	9	200	2FAT
Honey Mustard	85	9	150	2FAT
Italian	80	9	145	2FAT
Oil and Vinegar	70	8	0	1½FAT

Salads (continued)

	Calories	Fat (g)	Sodium (mg)	Exchanges
Salad Dressings (1T) continued:				
Olive Oil	120	14	0	3FAT
Ranch	60	5	130	1FAT
Thousand Island	60	5	110	1FAT
Vinaigrette	90	9	8	2FAT
Low Calorie Dressings	30-50	3-5	120	½-1FAT
Fat-Free Salad Dressing	6-30	0	135	FREE
Picante Sauce or Salsa	5	0	110	FREE
Vinegar	2	0	0	FREE
Lemon, ¼	4	0	0	FREE

Prepared Salads

✔ **Ask about the salad's components.** You may want to request that some of the higher calorie ingredients such as avocado, anchovies, bacon, croutons, boiled egg, or cheese not be added.

Be Picky about What is in your Salad:	Calories	Fat (g)
Cobb Salad w/dressing	465	31
Cobb Salad w/dressing, No Bacon	330	27
Savings:	**35**	**4**

✔ **Ask for your salad to be served in a plate or bowl rather than in a taco shell.** Taco salads are frequently served in a fried tortilla shell. The regular sized fried tortilla, without the filling, can contain about 400 calories. A lower calorie/fat alternative is to have the salad served on a plate.

Ask for a Plate Instead of the Taco Shell:	Calories	Fat (g)
Taco Salad in Taco Shell	930	69
Taco Salad served on a Plate	510	39
Savings:	**420**	**30**

✔ **Request salad dressings** *on the side* so that you can control the amount of dressing that is added. Restaurants add anywhere from an average of three tablespoons (240 calories) of dressing on a small salad to as much as a half cup (640 calories) on a large salad meal.

✔ **Request low calorie dressing** rather than the dressing the salad is typically prepared with. Salad dressings, to prevent wilting, are not added until just prior to serving. Consider ordering the Spinach salad with a lowfat Honey Mustard dressing instead of the usual hot bacon dressing.

Prepared Salads

	Calories	Fat (g)	Sodium (mg)	Exchanges
Prepared Salads (¼ c):				
Ambrosia Salad	75	3	170	¾FR+½FAT
Broccoli/Cauliflower/Ranch	80	8	175	1V+1½FAT
Carrot Raisin Salad	80	5	95	1FR+1FAT
Chicken Salad	125	9	350	1½LM+1FAT
Cole Slaw w/mayonnaise	85	6	100	1V+1FAT
Cole Slaw w/vinaigrette	55	4	5	1V+1FAT
Egg Salad	123	11	170	1MFM+1FAT
Fruit Delight	55	2	2	½FR+½FAT
Kidney Bean Salad	55	2	155	½ST+½FAT
Macaroni Salad	100	7	180	½ST+1½FAT
Marinated Mixed Vegetable Salad	60	4	150	1V+1FAT
Oriental Fruit Salad	80	3	30	1FR+½FAT
Pea Salad	70	6	90	1V+1FAT
Potato Salad w/ mayo	100	7	330	½ST+1½FAT
Potato Salad w/vinaigrette	75	4	130	½ST+1FAT
Rotelli Pasta Salad	120	6	150	1ST+1FAT
Snow Salad	70	4	20	½FR+1FAT
Spaghetti Salad	125	7	2	¾ST+1½FAT
Three Bean Salad	90	4	180	½ST+1FAT
Tuna Salad	190	10	410	2VLM+½CHO+2FAT
Waldorf Salad	70	5	70	½FR+1FAT
Fresh Tossed Salads (per 1 c):				
Caesar Salad w/ dressing	170	13	550	¼ST+1V+½MFM+2FAT
Caesar Salad w/out dressing	90	4	475	¼ST+1V+½MFM
Chicken Caesar w/ dressing	260	20	750	¼ST+1V+2MFM+2FAT
Chicken Caesar w/out dressing	140	7	450	¼ST+1V+1MFM+½FAT
Cobb Salad w/ dressing	365	31	675	1V+1½HFM+4FAT
Crab Louis w/ dressing	290	21	410	1V+2LM+3FAT
Crab Louis w/out dressing	150	5	455	1V+2LM
Garden Salad w/out dressing	50	2	45	1V+½FAT
Green Side Salad w/out dressing	50	3	75	1V+½FAT
Greek Salad w/ dressing	120	9	320	1V+2FAT
Oriental Chicken w/out dressing	160	5	150	½ST+1V+2LM
Oriental Chicken w/ dressing	275	17	725	½ST+1V+2LM+2FAT
Roma Tomato, Mozzarella, & Basil	120	9	180	1V+½HFM+1FAT
Spinach Salad w/dressing	120	10	210	1V+2FAT

Breads & Spreads

Chapter Contents:

■ Estimating the Calories & Fat Grams in Bread
■ Bread Portion Sizes: Bagels, Biscuits, Bread, Breadsticks, Cornbread, Ginger-bread, Croissants, English Muffins, Foccacio, French & Italian Bread, French Roll, and Rolls
■ Nutritional Information: Breads & Spreads

Breads and muffins contain anywhere from 70-125 calories per ounce. That doesn't sound like much until you realize how fast an ounce goes down! Most of us eat far more than a single ounce serving. Here are some suggestions to help you keep your weight down.

✓ **Unbuttered breads such as sliced bread or toast, English muffins, bagels, and French bread have 70-80 calories per ounce and little or no fat.** Biscuits and croissants are higher in fat and calories.

Order the English Muffin rather than a Biscuit:

		Calories	Fat (g)
Biscuit, 1½ oz		190	11
English Muffin, 1½ oz		130	1
	Savings:	**60**	**10**

Have a Bagel instead of a Croissant:

		Calories	Fat (g)
Croissant, 3 oz		360	20
Bagel, 3 oz		240	2
	Savings:	**120**	**18**

✔ **Limit the amount of bread you eat**. A 1 oz unbuttered breadstick has just 80 calories and 1 gram of fat. However, most restaurants are serving larger breadsticks in the range of 1½ to 2 oz each. And do you stop at just one breadstick? Can your body afford all those calories?

✔ **Just take the portion you can healthily afford to eat and then ask that the rest of the bread be taken away** or simply move it from your end of the table. Don't torture yourself by staring at the bread basket all evening!

✔ **Always order your bread** *dry* so you can decide how much of the toppings to add. Ask for that roll or breadstick *plain* (without the butter glaze on the top). In time, your taste buds will adjust to the unbuttered taste.

✔ **Add only small amounts of fat to your bread.** Use thin slivers of fat rather than hunks. A thin layer of jelly or jam has less calories and fat than a comparable portion of butter or margarine.

Put Jelly on your Toast instead of Margarine:		Calories	Fat (g)
2 Pieces Toast with 1 T margarine		240	12
2 Pieces Toast with 1 T jelly		195	1
	Savings:	45	11

✔ **Vegetable margarine or oil has as many calories as butter, but is a healthier fat** because it is mostly unsaturated. This means that it is lower in saturated fats. Like all other non-animal foods, vegetable margarine and oil contains no cholesterol.

✔ **Watch the cream cheese**. Are you spreading your bagel with cream cheese because of the promotion that "cream cheese has half the calories of butter or margarine"? While it is true that cream cheese has half the calories of butter or margarine, we tend to use more than twice as much!

Caution on the Cream Cheese:		Calories	Fat (g)
Bagel with 2T cream cheese		340	13
Bagel with 1T margarine		340	13
	Savings:	0	0

Estimating the Calories & Fat grams in Bread

How many calories are in the breads that you enjoy? To find out you'll need two nuggets of information found in this chapter:

❶ Calories per ounce found on the Bread Calorimeter below and

❷ Portion size of the bread you ate. The most accurate way to find this out is to take the food back to the home or the office and weigh your portion on a postage scale. Since that is not always practical, many portion sizes of your favorite breads are described or depicted on the next few pages.

Bread Calorimeter: Calories & fat per serving

Calories per oz	Breads	Calories & Fat (g)				
		1 oz	2 oz	3 oz	4 oz	5 oz
125	Biscuits	125	250	375	500	625
		8g	15g	23g	30g	38g
120	Croissants, plain	120	240	360	480	600
		7g	13g	20g	26g	33g
110	Gingerbread Muffins (lemon poppy seed, chocolate chip)	110	220	330	440	550
		6g	11g	17g	22g	28g
100	Muffins (fruit or grain)	100	200	300	400	500
		4g	8g	13g	17g	21g
90	Buttered Breadsticks Cornbread Focaccio Yeast Rolls, glazed w/butter	90	180	270	360	450
		3g	6g	9g	12g	15g
90	Bagel (chocolate chip)	90	180	270	360	450
		2g	4g	7g	9g	11g
80	Bagel (except chocolate chip) Breadstick English Muffin Hamburger & Hot Dog Bun Italian Bread Low Fat Muffins Pita Bread Submarine Roll Yeast Rolls, unbuttered	80	160	240	320	400
		1g	1g	2g	2g	3g
70	French Roll & Baguette Sandwich Bread Slices	70	140	210	280	350
		1g	2g	3g	4g	5g

Bread Portion Sizes

How many ounces are you eating? The descriptions and depictions below should help you to determine your portion size:

Bagels

While bagels in your grocery store usually weigh 2 - 3 ounces, gourmet bagels are 4 - 5 ounces! Mini bagels are 1 ounce in size. The outline of the 5 ounce bagel, at almost five inches in diameter, wouldn't even fit in the borders of this printed page. Compare your bagel to the diameter of the bagels shown here.

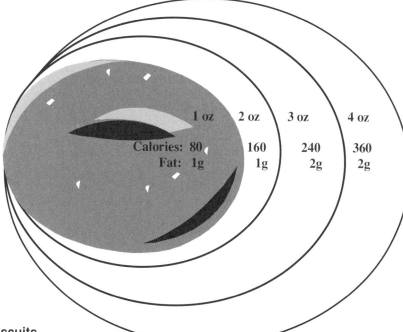

	1 oz	2 oz	3 oz	4 oz
Calories:	80	160	240	360
Fat:	1g	1g	2g	2g

Biscuits

Biscuits are very heavy; therefore, portion sizes are deceptively smaller than you may think. A 1 oz biscuit is about the size of a small biscuit packed in the smallest tubes in the refrigerated section in the grocery store. Most restaurant biscuits weigh at least 2 oz.

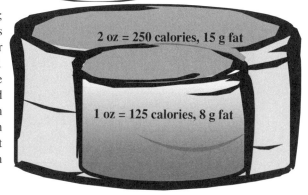

2 oz = 250 calories, 15 g fat

1 oz = 125 calories, 8 g fat

Bread

Most of us are familiar with the standard 1 oz slice of bread (½" thick) at the grocery store. Compare the bread slices at the restaurant to this size. Restaurants also serve a thicker, 1½ oz slice of bread (¾" thick) that is often referred to as "Texas Toast." Figure on the mini loaf of bread to contain 3 - 4 ounces.

Breadsticks

Depicted here are the two most common sizes of breadsticks served in restaurants. The 1 oz breadstick is about 5½" long while the 1½ oz breadstick is 7½" long and thicker.

1 oz	1½ oz
Buttered: 90 calories **3 g fat**	**135 calories** **5 g fat**
Plain: 80 calories **1 g fat**	**120 calories** **1 g fat**

Cornbread

1 oz = 90 calories
3 g fat

Gingerbread

1 oz = 110 calories
6 g fat

Cornbread & Gingerbread

Portion sizes for both cornbread and gingerbread are about the same:
    1 oz = 2" X 1¾" (1" high)
    2 oz = 2" X 3½" (1" high)

1" thick

Croissants

The 1 oz dinner croissant is very small – just 3½" long. The 3 oz croissant is more sandwich sized at 5½" long. This is how they may look from a side view.

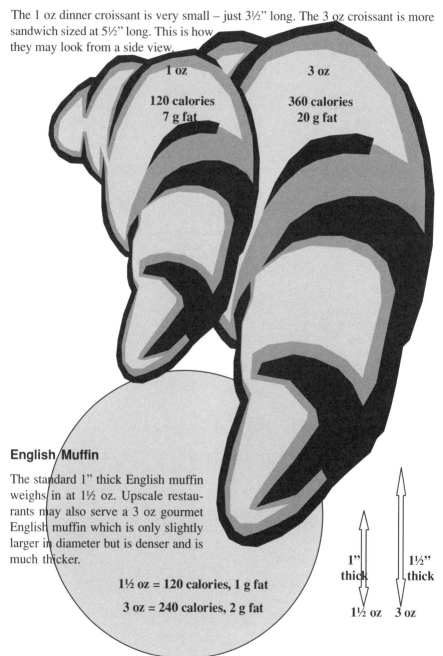

1 oz

**120 calories
7 g fat**

3 oz

**360 calories
20 g fat**

English Muffin

The standard 1" thick English muffin weighs in at 1½ oz. Upscale restaurants may also serve a 3 oz gourmet English muffin which is only slightly larger in diameter but is denser and is much thicker.

1½ oz = 120 calories, 1 g fat

3 oz = 240 calories, 2 g fat

**1"
thick**

**1½"
thick**

1½ oz   3 oz

A new 3 oz English muffin (4¼" diameter & 1" thick) is sized for sandwiches.

Focaccio

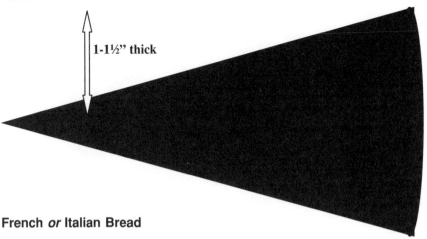

1-1½" thick

French *or* Italian Bread

A baguette is a long and thin French bread. A 1½" slice of this bread will weigh about 1 oz . A ¾" slice of the regular French or Italian bread would also be 1 oz.

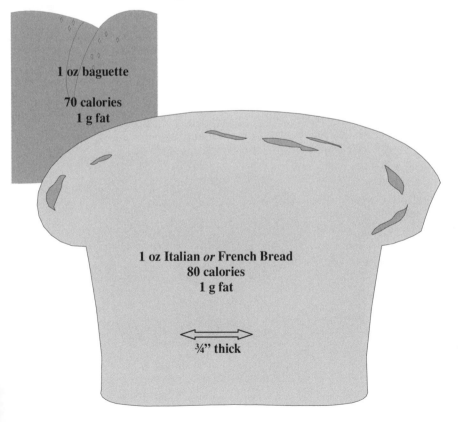

1 oz baguette

**70 calories
1 g fat**

**1 oz Italian *or* French Bread
80 calories
1 g fat**

¾" thick

French Roll

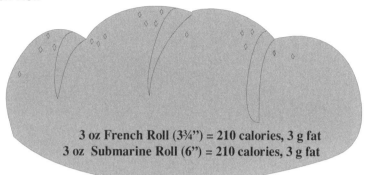

3 oz French Roll (3¾") = 210 calories, 3 g fat
3 oz Submarine Roll (6") = 210 calories, 3 g fat

Pita Bread & Submarine Rolls – see the *Delis & Sandwich Shops* chapter.

Hamburger Bun – see the *Burgers & Fast Foods* chapter.

Muffins – see the *Desserts* chapter.

Rolls

Yeast rolls are light and fluffy dinner rolls. A 1 oz roll is quite small – about the size of the "brown and serve" rolls found in the bread section of your local grocery store. Most restaurants serve rolls about 1½ to 2 oz in size. Compare your favorite yeast rolls to the ones pictured here.

2 oz Glazed: 180 calories, 6 g fat
Plain: 160 calories, 1 g fat

1 oz Glazed: 90 calories, 3 g fat
Plain: 80 calories, 1 g fat

Your Favorite Breads & Spreads

Breads & Spreads

	Calories	Fat (g)	Sodium (mg)	Exchanges
Breakfast Breads:				
Bagel, 1 oz, 2½" diameter	80	0	135	1ST
2 oz, 3" diameter	160	0.⁵	270	2ST
3 oz, 3½" diameter	240	1	400	3ST
4 oz, 4¼" diameter	320	2	540	4ST+½FAT
5 oz, 5" diameter	400	3	675	5ST+½FAT
Chocolate chip, 5 oz	450	11	675	5ST+2FAT
Poppy seed, 5 oz	415	4	675	5ST+1FAT
Sesame seed, 5 oz	427	5	675	5ST+1FAT
Biscuits, 1 oz, 2" around	125	8	275	¾ST+1½FAT
1½ oz, 2" X 2¾" square	190	11	400	1¼ST+2FAT
2 oz, 3" around	250	17	533	1½ST+3½FAT
3 oz	375	22	750	2ST+4½FAT
Bread, regular slice ½" thick, 1 oz	70	1	150	1ST
Thicker slice ¾" thick	110	1	225	1½ST
Small loaf, 4 oz	280	5	640	3½ST+1FAT
Breadstick, 1 oz plain	80	1	120	1ST
1 oz buttered	116	5	160	1ST+1FAT
1½ oz plain	120	2	180	1½ST
1½ oz buttered	175	8	240	1½ST+2FAT
Cornbread, 1¾" X 2"X 1", 1 oz	90	3	480	1ST+½FAT
1½ oz piece, 2½" X 2"X1"	135	5	720	1¼ST+1FAT
2 oz piece, 3½" X 2"X1"	180	6	960	1¾ST+1FAT
Cracker, Butter Crackers, 3	80	4	110	¾ST+½FAT
Melba Toast, 2	20	0	45	¼ST
Saltine Cracker, 2	24	1	70	¼ST
Sesame Breadstick, 1	15	0	20	¼ST
Croissant, 1 oz dinner	120	7	130	¾ST+1½FAT
2 oz	240	13	260	1½ST+2½FAT
3 oz sandwich-sized	360	20	400	2¼ST+4FAT
English Muffin, regular, 1½ oz	130	1	140	1½ST
Gourmet *or* Sandwich size, 3 oz	220	2	420	2½ST+½FAT
Focaccio Bread, 1 oz	90	2	200	1ST+½FAT
French Baguette, 1 oz	70	1	110	1ST
French Roll, 2 oz, 4" long	140	2	220	2ST
3 oz, 6" long	210	3	470	2½ST+½FAT
Gingerbread, 1¾" X 2"X 1", 1 oz	90	3	480	1ST+½FAT
1½ oz piece, 2½" X 2"X1"	135	5	720	1¼ST+1FAT
2 oz piece, 3½" X 2"X1"	180	6	960	1¾ST+1FAT
Italian Bread, 1 oz	75	1	150	1ST
Spoon Bread, ½ c	150	6	260	1ST+½WhMk+½FAT
Yeast Roll, small, 1oz	80	2	140	1ST+½FAT
Yeast Roll, large, 2 oz	160	4	280	2ST+1FAT

Breads & Spreads (continued)

	Calories	Fat (g)	Sodium (mg)	Exchanges
Spreads:				
Apple Butter, 1T	20	0	0	¼FR
Butter, 1t	36	4	41	1FAT
Butter, 1T	108	12	123	2½FAT
Country Gravy, ¼ c	85	7	250	¼ST+1½FAT
Cream Cheese, 2T	100	10	85	2FAT
Cream Cheese, 2T low fat	70	5	150	½MFM+½FAT
Honey Butter, 1t	28	2	20	½FAT
Honey Butter, 1T	84	6	60	½CHO+1FAT
Honey, 1t	21	0	0	¼CHO
Honey, 1T	64	0	1	1CHO
Jelly, Jams, *or* Preserves, 1t	18	0	1	¼CHO
Jelly, Jams, *or* Preserves, 1T	54	0	2	1CHO
Margarine, 1t	35	3	45	¾FAT
Margarine, 1T	100	11	100	2½FAT
Oil, 1t	40	5	1	1FAT
Oil, 1T	120	14	6	3FAT
Whipped Butter, 1T	81	9	93	2FAT
Whipped Margarine, 1T	70	7	70	1½FAT

Entrees & Sauces

Chapter Contents:

■ Estimating the Calories & Fat Grams in Your Entree
■ Beef, Pork, & Lamb
■ Chicken & Other Poultry
■ Seafood
■ Other Meats
■ Fats, Gravies, and Sauces

Most of the calories and fat grams in a single meal are found in the entree. Here are some general guidelines for dining lean during this course.

✓ **Select fish, chicken, and turkey** that have been grilled, baked, or roasted.

Order Fish, Poultry (remove skin) or Lean, Trimmed Beef:		
	Calories	Fat (g)
Per 6 oz portion:		
Sausage	600	48
Fried Catfish, Red Snapper, *or* Shrimp	540	30
Fried Chicken Thigh	480	30
Sirloin Steak, untrimmed	480	28
Fried Chicken Breast	420	20
Roasted Dark Chicken *or* Turkey, w/skin	420	20
Roasted White Chicken *or* Turkey, w/skin	360	16
Roasted Dark Chicken, w/out skin	360	16
Sirloin Steak, trimmed	360	16
Grilled Orange Roughy	300	13
Roasted White Chicken, w/out skin	300	8
Roasted White Turkey, w/out skin	270	6
Grilled Pollock	180	2

✓ **Remove the skin off poultry.**

✓ **Trim all visible fat off meats and poultry.** Leaner cuts of beef that have been trimmed of all visible fat can be as low in fat and calories as chicken.

Trim all Visible Fat:	Calories	Fat (g)
8 oz Brisket, lean & fat	800	72
8 oz Brisket, lean only	550	30
Savings:	250	42

✓ **Request little or no oil when preparing the meat.** Steaks, fajitas, chicken, and fish are often brushed with oil during cooking (some *may* be necessary to prevent sticking on the grill) and before serving (for appearances only). Ask them to use as little as necessary.

Have your Meat, Poultry, & Seafood prepared without Added Oils:	Calories	Fat (g)
Grilled Chicken Breast, 6 oz brushed with 2t oil	360	20
Grilled Chicken Breast, 6 oz with "no oil"	300	8
Savings:	60	12

✓ **Ask for sauces on the side**, including barbecue sauce. Most sauces are either very high in fat or high in sugar. Leaner sauces include salsas, black bean sauce, and those made from chicken stock and pureed vegetables.

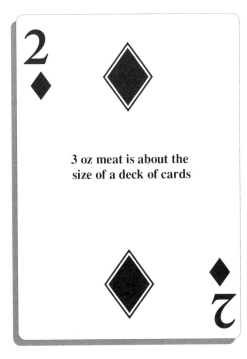

3 oz meat is about the size of a deck of cards

✓ **Eat half the meat.** Health authorities recommend we eat no more than 6 oz of meat, poultry, and seafood a day. That's two portions of 3 oz (the size of a deck of cards) each. This recommendation is based upon the need to replace our daily protein losses as well as our need to cut back on our fat and cholesterol intake. Restaurants often serve protein portions much larger than 6 oz so be prepared to split the entree with another person or request a "doggie bag" to take half of the meat home.

Estimating the Calories & Fat Grams in your Entrée

To calculate the calories and fat grams of your meat entrée, follow these 3 steps:

❶ **Find your entrée in the next four calorimeters.** Note that menu items may be detailed as fried, untrimmed, trimmed, with skin, and w/out skin. *Italicized print* denotes fried items. The calories and fat of the all other entrees are considered to be baked, roasted, or grilled without any additional fat. Unless you requested otherwise, the restaurant probably added some fat as described in step 3. The four calorimeters include:

■ Beef, Pork, & Lamb

■ Poultry – Chicken, Turkey, Duck, Goose, Pheasant, & Quail

■ Seafood – Shellfish & Fish

■ Other Meats – Organ meats, Variety cuts, Wild game, & Exotic meats

❷ **Read across the calorimeter to find the number of calories and fat gram for *your* cooked portion size.** The *cooked* portion size will be significantly smaller than the uncooked portions quoted on the menu or by the server. The following are some expected weights for the most commonly served portions after cooking losses. Trimming the fat and bone as well as removing the skin will reduce the portion size further.

Boneless Meats			
Raw Wt (oz)	Cooked Wt (oz)	Raw Wt (oz)	Cooked Wt (oz)
4	3	12	9
6	4½	14	10½
8	6	16	12
10	7½	20	15

Meat with Bones		Ribs, Chops	
Raw Wt (oz)	Cooked Wt (oz)	Raw Wt (oz)	Cooked Wt (oz)
8	4	8	2
12	6	16	4
16	8	20	5
20	10	24	6

❸ **Account for the fat or sauces that were added to your entrée.** Unless you have requested otherwise, most restaurants are adding butter, margarine, or oil to your entrée. Expect a teaspoon of these fats to be added for every 3 oz cooked portion. See the Gravies, Sauces, & Spread Calorimeter, that follows the four entrée calorimeters, for more details on these and other sauces.

Beef, Pork, & Lamb

Did you know that lean, trimmed beef and pork are in the same caloric range as skinless dark poultry? Beef and pork also have the same amount of cholesterol as poultry. The nutritional difference is that beef and pork are higher in saturated fat, the unhealthy kind of fat. However, lean beef and pork can still be part of a healthy diet, if they are consumed just a few times a week and in moderate portions.

✓ **Order a lean cut.** At the grocery store you can recognize the leanest cuts of beef and pork by the use of "round" or "loin" in the name. In restaurants different names are used:

Club	Kabob	Medallions	Sirloin Steak
Delmonico	Kansas City	New York	Strip Steak
Filet Steak	London Broil	Roast Beef	Tenderloin, pork
Filet Mignon (without the bacon)			

✓ **Order a boneless cut of beef, pork, or lamb.** Typically, bone-in cuts are higher in fat than boneless cuts.

✓ **Order a smaller cut.** A smaller beef cut of 3-4 oz may be available as an appetizer or on a sandwich plate. A petite steak of 4 oz would fit nutritional guidelines better than a typical 8-10 oz entrée portion. Since many upscale restaurants cut their own beef they may be able to cut a steak any size that you request.

✓ **Avoid *Prime* cuts of beef.** There are three grades of beef based on the fat content of the meat. Select is the leanest, choice is in the middle, and prime is the fattiest cut. If you are buying lean meat in the grocery store, you are probably getting the select grade. You'll be hard pressed to find the select grade in many restaurants; choice is far more common. Upscale steakhouses often buy prime cuts of beef because they feel that the extra marbling of fat adds more flavor. The extra fat contributes an additional 5-10 % more calories and 10-25% more fat than the choice grade.

✓ **Request your steak or fajitas grilled without butter or oil**. The fats make the meat look shiny but can you afford the extra 100 calories or more?

✓ **Trim off all the visible fat** before you bite into your steak. Yes, much of the fat is marbled into the meat, but look at what a difference you can make in total calories and fat grams when you trim your steak.

Trim your Meat:		
12 oz Prime Rib, lean & fat	810	56
12 oz Prime Rib, lean only	560	35
Savings:	**250**	**21**

Beef, Pork, & Lamb Calorimeter: Calories & fat per cooked portion

Calories per oz	Beef, Pork, & Lamb	Calories & Fat (g)			
		3 oz	4½ oz	6 oz	7½ oz
130	**Beef,** untrimmed: Short Ribs	**390** 36g	**585** 54g	**780** 72g	**975** 90g
110	**Beef,** untrimmed: Brisket	**330** 28g	**495** 42g	**660** 56g	**825** 70g
100	**Beef & Pork**: Sausage **Beef,** untrimmed: Beef Ribs, Meatloaf **Lamb,** untrimmed: Lamb Chops **Pork**, untrimmed: Pork Chops, Pork Ribs, Spareribs	**300** 24g	**450** 36g	**600** 48g	**750** 60g
90	**Beef:** *Chicken Fried Steak* **Beef,** untrimmed: Porterhouse Steak, T-bone, Prime Rib, Filet Mignon **Pork**, untrimmed: Pork Loin, Tenderloin	**270** 19g	**405** 28g	**540** 37g	**675** 47g
80	**Beef,** untrimmed: Sirloin Steak **Beef,** trimmed: Beef Short Ribs **Pork,** trimmed: Ribs	**240** 14g	**360** 21g	**480** 28g	**600** 34g
70	**Lamb,** untrimmed: Leg of Lamb **Veal,** untrimmed: Roast **Beef,** untrimmed: London Broil, Roast Beef, Kabobs **Beef,** trimmed: Prime Rib, Rib Steak, Rib Eye Steak, Brisket, Corned Beef, Fajitas, Ribs, Porterhouse, T-bone **Pork**, trimmed: Pork Loin, Pork Chop	**210** 13g	**315** 20g	**420** 26g	**525** 33g
60	**Beef,** trimmed: Sirloin Steak, New York, Club, Demonico, Strip Steak, Kansas City, Filet Mignon, Filet Steak, Medallions, London Broil, Kabob, Roast Beef, Pot Roast, Stew & Soup Meat, Stir Fry Meat **Pork**, trimmed: Ham, Pork Tenderloin	**180** 8g	**270** 12g	**360** 16g	**450** 20g
50	**Lamb,** trimmed: Chops, Leg of Lamb	**150** 6g	**225** 10g	**300** 13g	**375** 16g

* Add 10% to calories and fat grams if meat is labeled as a *prime* cut.

Entrees

	Calories	Fat (g)	Sodium (mg)	Exchanges
Beef, trimmed (3 oz):				
Corned Beef, trimmed	210	13	945	3MFM
Fajitas	210	13	750	3MFM
London Broil, Kabob, Roast Beef, Pot Roast, Stew, Soup, & Stir Fry Meat	180	8	20	3LM
Short Ribs	240	14	15	3MFM
Prime Rib, Rib & Rib Eye Steak, Brisket, Ribs, Porterhouse, T-bone	210	13	20	3MFM
Steaks: Sirloin, New York, Club, Delmonico, Strip, Kansas City, Filet Mignon, Filet	180	8	20	3LM
Beef & Veal, untrimmed (3 oz):				
Beef Stroganoff, 3 oz beef	410	27	620	3MFM+1V+ 2½FAT
Brisket	330	27	20	3HFM
Chicken Fried Steak	270	19	500	1ST+2½HFM
London Broil, Roast Beef, Kabobs	210	13	20	3MFM
Meatballs, 6 - 1½" balls	400	25	632	1ST+3MFM+2FAT
Pepper Steak, 3 oz steak + veggies	275	13	485	3LM+2V+1FAT
Porterhouse, T-bone, Prime Rib, Filet Mignon	270	19	20	3HFM
Ribs	300	24	15	3HFM
Sauerbraten	240	14	160	3MFM
Sausage	300	24	960	3HFM
Short Ribs	390	36	15	3HFM+2½FAT
Sirloin Steak	240	14	20	3MFM
Steak au Poivre, 3 oz	220	12	120	3MFM
Swiss Steak, 3 oz steak w/veggies	240	10	400	3LM+1½ST+1V+½FAT
Veal, untrimmed: Roast	210	13	20	3MFM
Weiner Schnitzel, 3 oz breaded veal w/sauce	335	17	550	1ST+3LM+2FAT
Pork (3 oz):				
Pork, untrimmed: Chops, Spareribs	300	24	25	3HFM
Pork, untrimmed: Loin, Tenderloin	270	19	20	3HFM
Pork, trimmed: Ribs	240	14	20	3MFM
Loin Chop	210	13	20	3MFM
Pork Ham, trimmed	180	8	1190	3LM
Pork Tenderloin, trimmed	180	8	20	3LM
Lamb (3 oz):				
Lamb Chops, untrimmed	300	24	15	3HFM
Lamb, untrimmed: Leg of Lamb	210	13	20	3MFM
Lamb, trimmed: Chops, Leg of Lamb	150	6	20	3LM

Chicken & Other Poultry

Chicken is one of the leaner meats, but the calories increase substantially when eaten with the skin on, fried, or mixed with high fat foods such as mayonnaise. In this next calorimeter, you will notice three commonalties with all poultry.

✔ **White meat is lower in fat than dark meat.**

✔ **Removing the skin off poultry will save you calories** – about 60 calories of almost pure fat for each portion.

✔ **Roasted poultry is leaner than fried.**

Chicken & Poultry Calorimeter: Calories & fat per cooked portion

Calories per oz	Chicken & Poultry	Calories & Fat (g)			
		3 oz	4½ oz	6 oz	7½ oz
100	**Chicken**: *Fried Chicken Wing*	**300**	**450**	**600**	**750**
	Duck w/skin	24g	36g	48g	60g
90	**Goose** w/skin	**270**	**405**	**540**	**675**
		19g	28g	37g	47g
80	**Chicken**: *Fried Dark Chicken*	**240**	**360**	**480**	**600**
		15g	23g	30g	38g
70	**Chicken**: Dark Chicken w/skin, *Fried Chicken Fingers, Fried White Chicken* **Goose** w/out skin **Turkey**: Dark Turkey w/skin	**210** 10g	**315** 15g	**420** 20g	**525** 35g
60	**Pheasant**: w/skin **Turkey**: White Turkey w/skin **Chicken**: White Chicken w/skin, Dark Chicken w/out skin **Duck**: w/out skin **Squab** (pigeon) w/out skin	**180** 8g	**270** 12g	**360** 16g	**450** 20g
55	**Turkey**: Dark Turkey w/out skin **Quail** w/out skin	**165** 6g	**250** 9g	**330** 11g	**415** 15g
50	**Chicken**: Breast w/out skin **Pheasant** w/out skin	**150** 4g	**225** 6g	**300** 8g	**375** 10g
45	**Turkey**: White Turkey w/out skin	**135** 3g	**205** 5g	**270** 6g	**340** 8g
40	**Guinea Hen** w/out skin	**120** 3g	**180** 5g	**240** 6g	**300** 8g

Chicken & Other Poultry

	Calories	Fat (g)	Sodium (mg)	Exchanges
Fried Chicken (per average piece):				
Wing	190	12	385	¼ST+1½HFM
Thigh	310	21	575	½ST+4MFM
Breast	360	18	760	1ST+3½MFM
Drumstick	150	10	265	¼ST+1¾MFM
Chicken Fingers, 5 (9oz)	620	34	1450	1½ST+6MFM+1FAT
Buffalo Wings, 1	70	5	300	½MFM+½FAT
Ranch Dressing, 1T	75	8	80	1½FAT
Fried Chicken (3 oz):				
Dark w/skin	244	15	440	¼ST+3MFM
Dark w/out skin	205	10	160	2½MFM
White w/skin	211	10	440	2¾MFM
White w/out skin	165	5	140	3LM
Roasted Chicken (per average piece):				
Dark w/skin	330	22	765	4½MFM
Dark w/out skin	210	10	725	4LM
Breast and wing w/skin	370	19	1160	6½LM
Breast w/out skin	160	4	800	5VLM
Roasted Chicken (3 oz):				
Dark w/skin	217	14	75	3MFM
Dark w/out skin	174	8	81	3LM
White w/skin	190	9	64	3LM
White w/out skin	148	4	66	3VLM
Other Poultry (3 oz cooked, without added salt):				
Duck, w/skin	288	24	60	3HFM
Duck, w/out skin	171	10	56	3LM
Dark Turkey w/skin	189	10	65	3LM
Dark Turkey w/out skin	160	6	66	3LM
White Turkey w/skin	169	7	54	3LM
White Turkey w/out skin	135	3	55	3VLM
Goose w/skin	270	19	23	3HFM
Goose w/out skin	204	11	65	3MFM
Guinea Hen w/out skin	126	3	na	3VLM
Pheasant w/out skin	152	4	42	3LM
Quail w/out skin	153	5	58	3LM
Squab (pigeon) w/out skin	162	9	na	3LM
Other Chicken Dishes:				
Chicken and Dumplings, 2 c	410	20	470	1½ST+1V+3LM+2FAT
Chicken Divan, 1¼ c	350	22	390	½ST+1V+3LM+2½FAT
Chicken Tetrazzini, ½ c spaghetti + ½ c chicken with sauce	490	23	505	1½ST+1V+3LM+3FAT

Seafood

Fish and shellfish, as a group, comprise the leanest "meat" category, however, the calories and fat grams ranges widely within this group. Specific fish and shellfish are often referred to as either lean fish or fatty fish. Even the fattiest fish are fairly low in calories and are considered healthy. They simply have *more* fat than the white fishes like cod, flounder, and snapper. The fat found in raw fish (fish oil) is very unsaturated and is one of the "healthy" fats. One class of fats present in fish, omega-3 fatty acids, appears to be able to lower serum cholesterol and triglycerides.

What about cholesterol? Isn't shellfish high in cholesterol? The recent refinement of measuring procedures has demonstrated that shellfish does not have as much cholesterol as was once thought. The cholesterol content of clams, mussels, oysters, scallops, Alaska King crab, and lobster are in the same range as chicken and beef. Shrimp and squid *are* higher in cholesterol (see the cholesterol chart in the next section), but they are so low in fat that they can still be included in a low fat/low cholesterol diet once or twice a week.

✔ **Order broiled or grilled seafood instead of fried.** Some fat is usually added when seafood is broiled or grilled, but not as much as when the seafood is fried.

Fried Seafood is Often Twice as High in Calories:		
	Calories	Fat (g)
6 oz Fried Scallops	510	26
6 oz Broiled Scallops w/2t butter	252	10
Savings:	**258**	**16**

✔ **Request your fish to be prepared with little or no butter or oil.** It's not uncommon for restaurants to use a tablespoon or two of butter or oil to grill, blacken, or pan-fry fish. Consider asking for your fish to be seasoned with lemon, wine, and spices.

Fats can Double the Calories:		
	Calories	Fat (g)
6 oz Cod, Pollock, or Scrod	180	2
Plus 1T butter	108	12
Total:	**288**	**14**

✔ **Send the melted butter back.** Enjoy the sweet taste of lobster – without the butter dip. Clarified butter contains 120 calories per tablespoon!

✔ **Ask for sauces on the side or substitute a lower calorie sauce.**

Ask for Lower Calorie Sauces:		
	Calories	Fat (g)
Po Boy: Roll, *Fried* Shrimp+¼c ***Tartar Sauce***	890	54
Po Boy: Roll, *Grilled* Shrimp+¼c ***Cocktail Sauce***	535	11
Savings:	**355**	**43**

Seafood Calorimeter: Calories & fat per cooked portion

Calories per oz	Seafood	Calories & Fat (g)			
		3 oz	4½ oz	6 oz	7½ oz
100	Bass (stuffed & baked)	**300**	**450**	**600**	**750**
	Fried Eel, Fried Mackerel, Fried Smelt	16g	24g	32g	40g
90	*Fried: Catfish, Ocean Perch, Red Snapper, Shrimp*	**270**	**405**	**540**	**675**
		15g	23g	30g	38g
85	*Fried: Croaker, Pomfret, Scallops*	**255**	**385**	**510**	**640**
		13g	20g	26g	33g
75	Greenland Halibut, Shad, Pacific Herring, Atlantic Mackerel, Sablefish	**225**	**340**	**450**	**565**
		16g	23g	31g	39g
75	*Fried: Clams, Oysters*	**225**	**340**	**450**	**565**
		13g	20g	26g	33g
75	*Fried: Bass*	**225**	**340**	**450**	**565**
		10	15g	20g	25g
70	*Fried Abalone*	**210**	**315**	**420**	**525**
		8g	12g	16g	20g
65	Pompano, Chinook & Sockeye Salmon	**195**	**295**	**390**	**490**
	Fried: Fish Cakes, Squid	10g	15g	20g	25g
60	Atlantic Herring, Other Mackerel, Whale	**180**	**270**	**360**	**450**
	Fried: Haddock, White Perch	8g	12g	16g	20g
55	Milkfish, Coho & Atlantic Salmon, Trout (other varieties), Bluefish Tuna, Yellowtail	**165**	**250**	**330**	**415**
		7g	11g	14g	18g
	Fried: Cuddlefish				
50	Halibut, Carp, Orange Roughy, Spot, Whitefish, Shark	**150**	**225**	**300**	**375**
		6g	10g	13g	16g
45	Freshwater Bass, Bluefish, Catfish, Mullet, Chum & Pink Salmon, Sturgeon, Swordfish, Rainbow Trout	**135**	**205**	**270**	**340**
		4g	6g	8g	10g
40	Abalone, Cisco, Halibut, Spiny Lobster, King Mackerel, Sea Trout, Sheepshead, Shrimp, Smelt, Yellowfin & Skipjack Tuna	**120**	**180**	**240**	**300**
		2g	3g	4g	6g
35	Striped Bass, Mussels, Northern Lobster, Oysters, Pacific Rockfish, Perch, Red Snapper, Sea Bass, Squid, Tilefish, Turbot, White Sucker, Whiting, Wolfish	**105**	**160**	**210**	**265**
		2g	3g	4g	5g
30	Clams, Cod, Crab, Crayfish, Cuttlefish, Ling, Lingcod, Monkfish, Ocean Pout, Octopus, Pike, Pollock, Scallops, Scrod, Skate, Sunfish	**90**	**135**	**180**	**225**
		1g	2g	2g	3g

Fish & Shellfish

	Calories	Fat (g)	Sodium (mg)	Exchanges
4 oz Raw Fish/3 oz cooked (no fat added):				
Abalone	120	0.[8]	340	3VLM
Bass, Freshwater	128	4	80	3VLM
Bass, Striped	108	3	80	3VLM
Bluefish	140	5	68	3LM
Carp	144	6	56	3LM
Catfish, Channel	132	5	72	3VLM
Clams	84	1	64	3VLM
Cisco	112	2	64	3VLM
Cod	92	0.[8]	68	3VLM
Crab, Alaska King	96	0.[8]	948	3VLM
Crab, Blue & Dungeness	96	1	336	3VLM
Crab, Queeen	100	1	612	3VLM
Crayfish	100	1	60	3VLM
Cuttlefish	88	0.[8]	420	3VLM
Halibut	124	3	60	3VLM
Halibut, Greenland	212	16	92	3MFM
Herring, Atlantic	180	10	100	3LM
Herring, Pacific	220	16	84	3MFM
Ling	100	0.[8]	152	3VLM
Lingcod	96	1	68	3VLM
Lobster, Northern	104	1	336	3VLM
Lobster, Spiny	128	2	200	3VLM
Mackerel, Atlantic	232	16	104	3MFM
Mackerel, King	120	2	180	3VLM
Mackerel, other varieties	176	9	100	3LM
Milkfish	168	8	92	3LM
Monkfish	84	2	20	3VLM
Mullet, Striped	132	4	72	3VLM
Mussels, Blue	96	2	324	3VLM
Ocean Pout	88	1	68	3VLM
Octopus	92	1	260	3VLM
Orange Roughy	144	8	72	3LM
Oysters	88	3	124	3VLM
Perch	104	2	72	3VLM
Pike	100	0.[8]	48	3VLM
Pollock	92	1	80	3VLM
Pompano	188	11	72	3LM
Red Snapper	112	2	72	3VLM
Rockfish, Pacific	108	2	68	3VLM
Salmon, Atlantic & Coho	164	7	48	3LM
Salmon, Chinook & Sockeye	196	11	52	3LM
Salmon, Chum & Pink	136	4	60	3LM
Sablefish	220	16	64	3MFM
Scallops	100	0.[8]	184	3VLM
Scrod, Atlantic	92	0.[8]	60	3VLM
Sea Bass	108	2	76	3VLM

Fish & Shellfish (continued)

	Calories	Fat (g)	Sodium (mg)	Exchanges
SeaTrout	116	4	64	3VLM
Shad	220	16	60	3MFM
Shark	148	5	88	3LM
Sheepshead	124	3	80	3VLM
Shrimp (½ c cooked)	120	2	172	3VLM
Smelt, Rainbow	112	3	68	3VLM
Spot	140	6	32	3LM
Squid	104	2	52	3VLM
Sturgeon	120	4	92	3VLM
Sucker, White	104	3	44	3VLM
Sunfish	100	0.8	92	3VLM
Swordfish	136	4	100	3LM
Tilefish	108	3	60	3VLM
Trout, Rainbow	132	4	32	3VLM
Trout, other varieties	168	8	60	3LM
Tuna, Bluefish	164	6	44	3LM
Tuna, Yellowfin & Skipjack	120	1	40	3VLM
Turbot, European	108	3	168	3VLM
Whitefish	152	7	56	3LM
Whiting	104	2	80	3VLM
Wolfish	108	3	96	3VLM
Yellowtail	164	6	44	3LM
Fried Fish, 3 oz:				
Abalone, Fried	216	8	668	3LM
Bass, Striped, Fried	224	10	280	3LM
Bass, Stuffed & Baked	296	18	na	3MFM
Catfish, Breaded & Fried	260	15	316	3MFM
Clams, Breaded & Fried	228	12	412	3MFM
Croaker, Breaded & Fried	252	14	396	3MFM
Cuddlefish, Fried	168	9	180	3LM
Eel, Fried	288	16	104	3MFM
Fish Cakes, Fried	196	9	200	3LM
Haddock, Breaded & Fried	188	7	200	3LM
Mackerel, Fried	312	16	192	3MFM
Ocean Perch, Breaded & Fried	260	15	172	3MFM
Oysters, Breaded & Fried	224	14	472	3MFM
Pomfret, Fried	256	12	160	3MFM
Red Snapper, Fried	260	14	104	3MFM
Scallops, Breaded & Fried	244	12	528	3MFM
Shrimp, Fried	276	14	388	3MFM
Smelt, Breaded & Fried	284	14	608	3MFM
Squid, Fried	200	8	248	3LM
White Perch, Fried	188	9	200	3LM
Other Fish Dishes:				
Shrimp Paella, 2 c	430	10	685	3ST+4LM

Other Meats

Variety cuts of beef, pork, and lamb are considered delicacies. Many are comparable in calories and fat grams to other meat cuts, but some organ meats have very high amounts of cholesterol. For that reason, it is suggested that these organ meats be consumed only once a month. The American Heart Association recommends no more than 300 mg of cholesterol each day.

Cholesterol/3 oz	Animal Protein (3 oz)	Cholesterol (mg)
<100	Fish, Clams, Crab, Mussels, Sardines, Salmon, Scallops	20-70
	Lobster	60-90
	Chicken	70
	Beef: steak, roast, ear, feet, jowl, tail, tongue, tripe	80
100-199	Caviar, 1T or Roe, 1 oz	100
	Crayfish	120
	Pork Chitterlings, Pork Tongue	125
	Shrimp	130
	Beef & Pork Hearts, Pork Stomach	170
200-299	Squid	200
	Beef Lungs, Beef Thymus	240
	Pork Pancreas	270
300-399	Pork Liver, Beef Spleen	300
	Beef Kidney & Liver, Pork Lungs	330
400-499	Pork Kidney	410
	Pork Spleen	430
>500	Beef Brains	1700
	Pork Brains	2200

Other Meats Calorimeter: Calories & fat per cooked portion

Calories per oz	Other Meats	Calories & Fat (g)			
		3 oz	4½ oz	6 oz	7½ oz
110	**Pork:** Tail	**330**	**495**	**660**	**825**
		31g	46g	61g	77g
90	**Beef:** Sweetbreads, Thymus **Pork:** Chitterlings **Sheep:** Tongue	**270**	**405**	**540**	**675**
		22g	33g	44g	55g
80	**Beef:** Pancreas, Tongue **Pork:** Tongue	**240**	**360**	**480**	**600**
		16g	24g	32g	40g
80	**Chicken:** *Fried Giblets*	**240**	**360**	**480**	**600**
		12g	18g	23g	30g
70	**Lamb:** Liver, Tongue	**210**	**315**	**420**	**525**
		14g	21g	28g	35g

Other Meats Calorimeter (continued)

Calories per oz	Other Meats	Calories & Fat (g)			
		3 oz	4½ oz	6 oz	7½ oz
70	**Lamb:** Heart	**210**	**315**	**420**	**525**
	Other Meats: Beaver, Eel, Raccoon	12g	54g	72g	90g
60	**Beef:** Brains	**180**	**270**	**360**	**450**
	Pork: Pickled Pig's Feet	13g	20g	26g	33g
60	**Beef:** *Panfried Liver* **Pork:** Pancreas **Squab (pigeon):** Giblets **Other Meats:** Opossum, Rabbit	**180** 8g	**270** 12g	**360** 16g	**450** 20g
55	**Pork:** Pig's Feet	**165**	**250**	**330**	**415**
		11g	17g	22g	28g
55	**Chicken:** Heart **Duck:** Liver **Goose:** Gizzard **Turkey:** Heart **Pheasant:** Giblets	**165** 6g	**250** 9g	**330** 12g	**415** 15g
50	**Beef:** Brains **Pork:** Stomach, Ears	**150** 10g	**225** 15g	**300** 20g	**375** 25g
50	**Beef:** Heart, Liver **Calf:** Sweetbreads, Tongue **Goose:** Liver **Lamb:** Sweetbreads **Pork:** Liver **Turkey:** Giblets, Gizzard, Liver	**150** 4g	**225** 6g	**300** 9g	**375** 11g
45	**Chicken:** Giblets, Gizzard, Liver **Other Meats**: Muskrat, Reindeer, Turtle, Venison	**135** 4g	**205** 6g	**270** 8g	**340** 10g
40	**Pork:** Brains	**120** 8g	**180** 12g	**240** 16g	**300** 20g
40	**Beef:** Kidneys, Spleen, Tripe **Lamb** Spleen **Pork:** Heart, Kidneys, Spleen	**120** 4g	**180** 5g	**240** 7g	**300** 9g
35	**Beef:** Lungs	**105** 3g	**160** 5g	**210** 6g	**265** 8g
30	**Pork:** Lungs **Lamb:** Lungs **Other Meats**: Frog Legs, Snail	**90** 2g	**135** 3g	**180** 5g	**225** 6g

Variety Cuts & Other Meats

	Calories	Fat (g)	Sodium (mg)	Exchanges
Poultry Variety Cuts (3 oz cooked):				
Giblets: Chicken, fried	237	12	97	4LM
Chicken, simmered	135	4	50	3LM
Pheasant	159	6	na	3LM
Squab (pigeon)	176	8	na	3LM
Turkey, simmered	143	4	51	3LM
Gizzard: Chicken, simmered	131	3	57	3VLM
Goose	159	6	na	3LM
Turkey, simmered	140	3	46	3VLM
Heart: Chicken, simmered	159	7	41	3LM
Turkey, simmered	152	5	47	3LM
Liver: Chicken, simmered	135	5	44	3LM
Duck	155	5	na	3LM
Goose	143	5	151	3LM
Turkey, simmered	145	5	55	3LM
Beef Variety Cuts (3 oz cooked):				
Brains, simmered	138	11	103	2MFM
Brains, pan fried	168	14	135	2MFM+½FAT
Heart	150	5	54	3VLM
Kidney, simmered	123	3	41	3VLM
Liver, braised	132	4	60	3VLM
Liver, pan fried	186	7	100	½ST+3LM
Lungs, braised	103	3	87	3VLM
Pancreas, braised	231	15	51	3MFM
Spleen, braised	123	4	49	3VLM
Sweetbreads, cooked	272	20	99	3HFM
Calf Sweetbreads, cooked	143	3	na	3VLM
Thymus, braised	273	21	99	3HFM
Tongue, simmered	243	18	51	3MFM+½FAT
Calf Tongue, braised	135	5	na	3LM
Tripe	112	5	53	2LM
Pork Variety Cuts (3 oz cooked):				
Chitterlings, simmered	261	25	33	3HFM
Ears, simmered	141	9	141	3LM
Feet, cured, pickled	174	14	na	2HFM
Feet, simmered	165	11	na	2MFM
Brains, braised	117	8	78	1HFM
Heart, braised	126	4	31	3½VLM
Jowl	748	80	30	1HFM+14FAT
Kidney, braised	129	4	69	3VLM
Liver, braised	141	4	42	3VLM
Lungs, braised	84	3	69	2VLM
Pancreas, braised	189	9	36	3LM
Spleen, braised	129	3	na	3VLM
Stomach	135	11	59	3MFM

Other Meats (continued)

	Calories	Fat (g)	Sodium (mg)	Exchanges
Pork Variety Cuts (3 oz cooked):				
Tail, simmered	339	31	na	2HFM+3FAT
Tongue, braised	231	16	93	3MFM
Sheep & Lamb Variety Cuts (3 oz cooked):				
Lamb Heart, braised	222	12	na	3LM
Lamb Liver, broiled	222	11	71	3LM
Lamb Lungs	87	2	na	2VLM
Lamb Spleen	132	5	na	3LM
Lamb Sweetbreads, cooked	149	5	na	3LM
Lamb Tongue, braised	216	15	na	3MFM
Sheep Tongue, braised	276	22	na	3HFM
Other Meats (3 oz cooked):				
Beaver	211	12	na	3MFM
Eel	200	13	55	3MFM
Frog Legs	83	0.3	na	3VLM
Muskrat	131	4	na	3LM
Opossum	189	9	na	3LM
Rabbit	185	9	35	3LM
Raccoon	219	12	na	3MFM
Reindeer	145	4	na	3LM
Snail	75	1	na	3VLM
Turtle	120	4	na	3LM
Venison	143	5	na	3LM

Fats, Gravies, & Sauces

✔ **Always ask for your entrée to be prepared with as little fat as necessary.** Most of the cooked meats, poultry, and seafood listed in the previous calorimeters were calculated without the typical addition of fats. Unless you requested otherwise, estimate that an additional teaspoon (t) of butter, margarine, or oil has been used for the preparation of each cooked 3 oz portion of non-fried entrée. For reference there are three teaspoons in a tablespoon.

If you found your entrée on the calorimeter preceded by the italicized word "*fried*," there is no need to any fats and calories. However, if you consumed a meat fried and the calorimeter did not list it as fried, assume that each 3 oz portion has an added one tablespoon (T) of fat.

✓ **Request the use of a non-stick spray whenever possible.** Ounce for ounce, non-stick sprays have just as many calories as the oil it is derived from. But is sprayed in such a thin layer that the non-stick spray adds on fewer calories. Each typical five-second spray contains about 12 calories.

✓ **Ask for the sauces to be served on the side** where you can control the amounts used.

✓ **Request low fat sauces.** Plain butter, margarine, and oil are commonly used in cooking and glazing meats, poultry, and fish. In addition, sauces, spreads, or gravies may be added. There are six types of sauces from highest fat and calorie to the lowest:

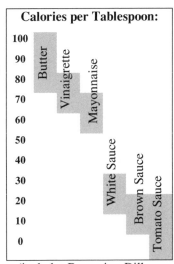

Calories per Tablespoon:

■ Butter – melted butter or margarine to which seasonings are added (includes herb butter, lemon butter, pesto sauces).

■ Vinaigrette – blend of oil, vinegar, and seasonings (includes Beurre Blanc, Beurre Noir, Vinaigrettes, and Italian dressing).

■ Mayonnaise-Type – created from an emulsion of margarine, butter, or oil and eggs (includes Bearnaise, Dill sauce, Hollandaise, Lemon Caper sauce, Roumoulade, Tarragon sauce, and Tartar sauce).

■ White Sauce – roux-based sauce made from margarine or butter, flour, and milk, cream, or light stock (includes Bechamel sauce, Cheese sauce, Mornay sauce, and Veloute).

■ Brown Sauce – roux-based sauce made with margarine or butter, flour, and brown stock (includes Bordelaise, Brown gravy, and Mushroom sauce).

■ Tomato – tomato sauce seasoned with spices and herbs (includes Cocktail Sauce, Barbecue sauce, Marinara, Salsas, and Veracruz sauce).

Sauces, Spreads, & Gravies Calorimeter

Calories per t	Fats, Gravies, Sauces & Spreads	Calories & Fat (g)			
		1T	2T	3T	4T
40	Oil (all types), Clarified Butter	**120** 14g	**240** 28g	**360** 42g	**480** 56g
37	Butter	**110** 12g	**220** 24g	**330** 37g	**440** 48g
33	Aioli, Herb Butter sauce, Mayonnaise, Margarine, Rémoulade sauce	**100** 11g	**200** 22g	**300** 33g	**400** 44g
27	Lemon Butter sauce, Whipped Butter, Salad Dressings	**80** 9g	**160** 18g	**240** 28g	**320** 37g
25	Beurre Blanc, Buerre Noir, Butter Wine sauce, Hollandaise, Meuniere, Pesto, Tartar sauce, Whipped Margarine	**75** 8g	**150** 15g	**225** 23g	**300** 30g
20	Béarnaise, Creamy Dill sauce, Creamy Horseradish sauce	**60** 6g	**120** 12g	**180** 18g	**240** 24g
15	Creamy Dijon sauce, Tarragon sauce, Honey Mustard Cream sauce	**45** 4g	**90** 8g	**130** 12g	**185** 16g
12	Alfredo sauce, Lemony Dill sauce, Chili Cream sauce	**35** 4g	**70** 7g	**110** 11g	**145** 14g
10	Au Jus (drippings), Béchamel, Caper sauce, Cheese sauce, Cream sauce, Guacamole, Mornay sauce, Newburg sauce, Oyster sauce, Sour Cream	**30** 3g	**60** 5g	**90** 8g	**120** 10g
8	Chutneys, Cranberry sauce, Orange sauce, Sweet & Sour sauce	**25** 0g	**50** 0g	**75** 0g	**100** 0g
7	Bolognese (cream based), Mustard sauce, Gravy, Mushroom sauce, Veracruz	**20** 2g	**42** 3g	**65** 5g	**85** 6g
6	Chili sauce, Cocktail sauce, Ketchup, Sweet Pickle Relish, White Sauce-thin	**20** 0g	**40** 0g	**60** 0g	**75** 0g
5	Bolognese (tomato based), Mustard, Veloute, Tomato Coulis	**15** 1g	**30** 2g	**45** 3g	**60** 4g
5	Barbecue, Steak sauce, Teriyaki sauce	**15** 0g	**30** 0g	**45** 0g	**60** 0g
4	Bordelaise, Marinara	**12** 0.^{7}g	**24** 1g	**36** 2g	**48** 3g
3½	Soy sauce, Worcestershire	**10** 0g	**20** 0g	**30** 0g	**40** 0g
2½	Madeira, Brown sauce, Tomato sauce	**8** 0.^{2}g	**15** 0.^{3}g	**23** 0.^{5}g	**30** 0.^{6}g
2	Canned Au Jus, Burgundy Wine sauce, Horseradish, Hot sauce, Picante sauce, Salsa	**5** 0g	**10** 0g	**15** 0g	**20** 0g

Gravies, Sauces, & Spreads

	Calories	Fat (g)	Sodium (mg)	Exchanges
Per 2T:				
Aioli Sauce (garlic oil)	195	21	5	4FAT
Alfredo Sauce	75	7	180	1½FAT
Au Jus, canned	5	0	150	FREE
Au Jus, drippings	60	6	100	1FAT
Barbecue	30	0	500	½CHO
Béarnaise	120	12	220	2½FAT
Béchamel	51	5	70	1FAT
Buerre Blanc	154	16	2	3½FAT
Buerre Noir	136	15	148	3FAT
Bolognese, cream-based	50	$3.^5$	45	1FAT
Bolognese, tomato-based	32	$1.^6$	146	¼ST+¼FAT
Bordelaise	22	$1.^5$	150	¼FAT
Brown Sauce	15	$0.^1$	30	FREE
Burgundy Wine Sauce	10	$0.^3$	5	FREE
Butter, unsalted	216	24	4	5FAT
Butter, salted	216	24	246	5FAT
Butter Wine Sauce	140	14	140	3FAT
Caper Sauce	60	5	265	1FAT
Cheese Sauce	60	4	180	1FAT
Chili Cream Sauce	72	8	33	1½FAT
Chili Sauce	35	0	380	½ST
Chutney	55	0	0	½FR+½CHO
Cocktail Sauce	40	0	320	½CHO
Cranberry Sauce	52	0	10	½CHO
Cream Sauce, thick	108	12	40	2½FAT
Cream Sauce, thin	50	4	180	1FAT
Creamy Dijon Sauce	96	8	90	1½FAT
Creamy Dill Sauce	126	13	90	2½FAT
Gravy	40	3	150	½FAT
Hollandaise	135	14	105	3FAT
Honey Mustard Cream Sauce	91	9	30	1½FAT
Horseradish, 1T	6	0	14	FREE
Creamy Horseradish Sauce	110	10	220	2FAT
Hot Sauce, 1t	0	0	20	FREE
Guacamole	55	5	210	1FAT
Ketchup	36	0	360	½CHO
Lemony Dill Sauce	72	7	283	1½FAT
Lemon Butter Sauce	176	19	250	4FAT
Madeira	15	$0.^5$	30	FREE
Margarine	200	23	200	4½FAT
Marinara	25	1	150	½V+¼FAT
Mayonnaise	200	22	160	4½FAT
Meuniére	130	14	510	3FAT
Mornay	64	5	160	1FAT
Mushroom Sauce	40	3	87	½FAT
Mustard, 1T	15	1	190	FREE

Gravies, Sauces, & Spreads (continued)

	Calories	Fat (g)	Sodium (mg)	Exchanges
Per 2T continued:				
Mustard Sauce	43	3	200	½FAT
Newburg	55	5	200	1FAT
Oil, Clarified Butter	240	28	6	3FAT
Orange Sauce	53	0	10	1CHO
Oyster Sauce	55	4	150	1FAT
Pesto	155	15	244	3FAT
Picante Sauce	10	0	220	FREE
Rémoulade Sauce	200	22	210	4½FAT
Salad Dressings, average	160	16	300	½FAT
Salsa	10	0	150	½V
Sour Cream	52	5	12	1FAT
Soy Sauce, 1t	3	0	340	FREE
Soy Sauce, reduced sodium, 1t	3	0	170	FREE
Steak Sauce	30	0	200	FREE
Sweet and Sour Sauce	55	0	70	½CHO
Sweet Pickle Relish	40	0	210	½CHO
Tarragon Sauce	90	8	153	1½FAT
Tartar Sauce	140	16	440	3FAT
Teriyaki Sauce, 1T	15	0	610	FREE
Teriyaki Sauce, reduced sodium, 1T	15	0	320	½CHO
Tomato Coulis	30	2	70	½V+½FAT
Tomato Sauce	14	0.[4]	20	FREE
Velouté	30	2	25	½FAT
Veracruz	42	4	177	½V+½FAT
Whipped Butter	162	18	186	3½FAT
Whipped Margarine	140	14	140	3FAT
White Sauce, thin	36	3	96	½FAT
Worcestershire	22	0	465	FREE

Accompaniments

The previous chapter's recommendation to eat only half of your entrée may bring about a concern of "that's not much of a meal." In the majority of restaurants, the entrée covers the plate while the vegetables and starch (if even offered) appear to be simply plate garnishments.

For better health each of us should strive for eating smaller servings of animal protein along with larger portions of accompaniments (including starchy foods and vegetables). Starchy foods (such as rice, potatoes, bread, and pasta) are low in fat when prepared simply. Vegetables are high in fiber, vitamins, and minerals; the American Cancer Society suggests we eat at least five servings of fruits 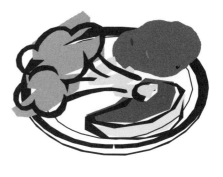 and vegetables each day. When prepared without a lot of butter or oil, vegetables, are also low in calories and fat. Here are some other guidelines for dining lean.

✔ **Split your entrée with a friend and order extra vegetables, starches,** and or a salad. Most restaurants will comply. Ordered this way, the foods fill the plate just as they would have before but the meal is lower in fats and calories and just as filling.

✔ **Ask for steamed vegetables and request no butter or other fats to be added**. Don't be fooled by assuming that the term "steamed" vegetables refers to fat-free vegetables. Most restaurants use the low fat steaming method for cooking vegetables and then add on butter, margarine, oil, or cheese sauce. Some vegetables, however, are prepared ahead of time in bulk and may not be available without butter. In that case, ask the server to drain the vegetables well when serving.

Take a look at what a difference added fat on vegetables makes.

Order the Steamed Vegetables without added Fat:

	Calories	Fat (g)
Steamed asparagus (½ c) with 1t melted butter	60	4
Steamed asparagus (½ c)	25	0
Savings:	**35**	**4**

Order the Broccoli without Cheese Sauce:

	Calories	Fat (g)
Broccoli (½ c) with Cheese Sauce (3T)	115	6
Steamed broccoli (½ c)	25	0
Savings:	**90**	**6**

✔ **Canned vegetables will be higher in sodium than fresh or frozen vegetables.** Canned vegetables contain approximately 300-400 mg sodium per ½ cup cooked portion.

✔ **The addition of french fries or onion rings can easily double the calories** of your meal. Consider asking for a lower calorie substitute, splitting an order with a friend, or requesting that they only put a half order of the fried vegetable on your plate. See the *Burgers & Fast Food* chapter for more details.

✔ **Order your mashed potatoes without gravy or with gravy on the side.** Gravies served by a quick service restaurant are usually prepared from low fat gravy mixes. More upscale restaurants use meat drippings, butter, and/or cream to prepare gravies with far more calories and fat. To be on the safe side, enjoy your mashed potatoes without gravy or have it served on the side so you can use sparingly.

Order the Gravy on the Side:

	Calories	Fat (g)
Mashed Potatoes (½ c) with Gravy (2T)	160	8
Mashed Potatoes (½ c)	120	5
Savings:	**40**	**3**

✔ **Order the baked potato "dry."** Ask for butter, sour cream, and other condiments on the side (to be used wisely or not at all). Other low fat/low calorie toppings include salsa alone or combined with sour cream, mustard, or low fat ranch dressing.

The Baked Potato Difference:

	Calories	Fat (g)
Loaded Baked Potato, 9 oz plus toppings	572	39
Dry Baked Potato, 9 oz	185	0
Savings:	**387**	**39**

Baked Potato Calorimeter: Calories & Fat per serving

	Calories & Fat (g) per serving				
	3 oz	6 oz	9 oz	12 oz	16 oz
Plain	**80**	**160**	**270**	**360**	**470**
	0g	0g	0g	0g	0g
w/ butter only	**116**	**232**	**378**	**522**	**686**
	4g	8g	12g	18g	24g
	(1t)	*(2t)*	*(1T)*	*(1½T)*	*(2T)*
w/sour cream only	**88**	**177**	**296**	**399**	**522**
	1g	2g	3g	4g	5g
	(1t)	*(2t)*	*(1T)*	*(1½T)*	*(2T)*
w/cheese only	**99**	**198**	**327**	**446**	**584**
	2g	4g	5g	8g	10g
	(2t)	*(4t)*	*(2T)*	*(3T)*	*(¼ c)*
w/butter & sour cream	**124**	**249**	**404**	**561**	**738**
	5g	10g	15g	22g	29g
	(1t each)	*(2t each)*	*(1T each)*	*(1½T ea)*	*(2T each)*
w/butter, sour cream & cheese	**143**	**287**	**461**	**647**	**852**
	7g	14g	20g	30g	39g

**All of the potato condiments are in level amounts (shown in italics), not heaping spoonfuls.
Your potato may have more or less.**

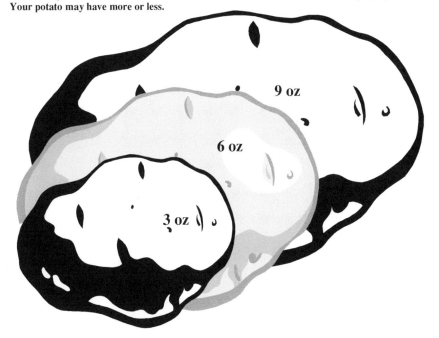

9 oz

6 oz

3 oz

For green salads, coleslaw, and potato salad, please review the *Salads* chapter.

Accompaniments

	Calories	Fat (g)	Sodium (mg)	Exchanges
Sauces:				
Butter, 1t	36	4	40	1FATna
Cheese Sauce, 2T	60	4	180	1FAT
Vegetables (½ c unless noted):				
Avocado, ¼	85	7	5	1½FAT
Artichoke, 1	50	0.[2]	80	2V
Broiled Tomato, ½ w/butter, cheese	80	6	na	1V+1FAT
Creamed Spinach	185	15	550	1V+3FAT
Greens, spinach, *or* cabbage seasoned with bacon or meat	60	4	300	1V+1FAT
Greens, spinach, *or* cabbage sauteed in oil	120	12	150	1V+2½FAT
Grilled Vegetables: eggplant, onions, peppers, squash, tomatoes	135	12	210	1V+2½FAT
Mushrooms, ¼ c sautéed in butter	110	11	125	2FAT
Okra & Tomatoes	40	2	300	1V+½FAT
Onion Rings, 1 ring	82	6	91	½ST+1FAT
Fried Whole Onion	800	64	na	2½ST+1V+13FAT
Ratatouille, ¾ c	75	4	80	1½V+1FAT
Spinach Soufflé	140	9	na	1V+2FAT
Steamed Vegetables w/out added fat: asparagus, broccoli, cabbage, carrots, cauliflower, green beans, greens, okra, spinach, yellow & zucchini squash, tomatoes, turnip, wax beans	25	0.[1]	5	1V
Steamed Vegetables w/melted butter *or* butter sauce: asparagus, broccoli, cabbage, carrots, cauliflower, green beans, greens, okra, spinach, yellow & zucchini squash, tomatoes, turnip, wax beans	60	4	45	1V+1FAT
Steamed Vegetables w/2T cheese sauce: asparagus, broccoli, cauliflower	85	4	185	1V+1FAT
Stewed Tomatoes	55	2	na	1V+½FAT
Vegetables Hollandaise	210	20	na	1V+4FAT
Zucchini Marinara	60	3	310	1V+½FAT
Starchy Vegetables (½ c):				
Corn on the cob, 3", no butter	80	1.[5]	20	1ST
Corn on the cob, 3", w/butter	115	5.[5]	60	1ST+1FAT

Accompaniments (continued)

	Calories	Fat (g)	Sodium (mg)	Exchanges
Potato, Baked, medium 9 oz	270	0	17	3¼ST
1T butter	110	12	123	2½FAT
1T sour cream	26	3	6	½FAT
1T shredded cheese	30	3	45	½MFM
1T crumbled bacon	30	2	80	½FAT
Potato, 9 oz loaded w/ all above	466	20	271	2½ST+½MFM+3½FAT
Potato, Baked, large 16 oz	470	0	30	5½ST
2T butter	215	24	245	5FAT
2T sour cream	52	5	12	1FAT
2T shredded cheese	60	5	90	1MFM
2T crumbled bacon	60	5	160	1FAT
Potato, 16 oz loaded w/ all above	857	39	537	5½ST+1MFM+7FAT
2T Bacon bits	60	2	260	1LM
Twice Baked, 8 oz	380	14	140	2½ST+1HFM+1½FAT
Potatoes, mashed w/butter	120	5	300	1ST+1FAT
Hashbrowns, homefries, puffs	165	10	50	1ST+2FAT
New Potatoes, buttered	120	5	60	1ST+1FAT
Au Gratin	160	9	530	1ST+2FAT
Scalloped Potatoes	140	5	420	1ST+1FAT
French Fries	150	8	80	1ST+1½FAT
Fries covered w/ ¼ c cheese sce	270	16	440	1ST+2FAT
Potato Pancakes, 1-4"	170	10	400	1ST+2FAT
Starchy vegetables (corn, green peas) seasoned w/out butter	70	0.[1]	5	1ST
Starchy vegetables (corn, green peas) seasoned w/butter	105	4	45	1ST
Sweet Potatoes w/butter, marshmallows	200	2	na	2¼ST+½FAT

Starches (½ c):

	Calories	Fat (g)	Sodium (mg)	Exchanges
Beans, Baked or Black beans	120	1	500	1½ST
Boston Baked Beans	170	3	600	1ST+1CHO+½FAT
Refried Beans	250	13	325	1ST+2½FAT
Black eyed Peas w/bacon or meat	135	4	450	1ST+1FAT
Couscous, no butter	170	0	4	2ST
Couscous, w/ butter	205	4	45	2ST+1FAT
Noodles or pasta w/out butter or sauce	80	0	3	1ST
Noodles or pasta, buttered	115	4	40	1ST+1FAT
Spaetzle, German noodle dish	190	5	160	1½ST+1FAT
Polenta, no butter	120	0	180	2ST
Fried Polenta, 2" X 2½" X ½"	90	4	130	1ST+1FAT
Popovers, Herbed, 1	160	7	130	1¼ST+1½FAT
Parmesan, 1	170	8	90	1¼ST+1½FAT
Red Beans w/rice, no meat	160	1	na	2ST
Red Beans w/rice, w/meat	280	10	na	2ST+2FAT

Accompaniments (continued)

	Calories	Fat (g)	Sodium (mg)	Exchanges
Starches (½ c) continued:				
Rice, steamed white	120	0	200	1½ST
Fried Rice	185	6	450	1½ST+1FAT
Rice Pilaf	160	3	520	1½ST+½FAT
Sausage (Dirty) Rice	175	9	500	1½ST+1HFM
Risotto w/butter	170	5	280	1½ST+1FAT
Risotto w/cheese	180	6	na	1½ST+½HFM+1FAT
Stuffing	205	9	650	1ST+2FAT
Condiments (2T):				
Corn Relish	26	0	120	1V
Gravy	40	3	150	½FAT

Desserts

Chapter Contents:

■ Frozen Yogurt, Soft Serve, & Ice Cream
■ Your Favorite Ice Cream & Yogurt Shops
■ Other Desserts

If you can still afford some calories after you have eaten your meal, enjoy some dessert. Below are some general guidelines for selecting desserts within your calorie and dietary fat recommendation.

✔ **Request fresh fruit** "without cream or other topping." Often this is enough to satisfy a sweet tooth.

✔ **Order one dessert and several forks** so everyone at the table can share. Our taste buds are the most sensitive in the first few bites; that's when a sweet and rich dessert offers the most satisfaction. Having just a few bites is also sensible because most desserts have anywhere from 300 to over 1000 calories per restaurant serving.

✔ **Eat the lower calorie part of the dessert and leave the rest**. Do you like the pie filling but don't care for the crust? Fine! Eat just the filling – it's lower in fats and calories than the crust anyway.

✔ **Ask the server for a smaller portion of dessert**. They will still charge you for the whole piece, but you've saved the calories. Remember you can't eat what isn't there.

✔ **Enjoy a small cup of low fat or fat-free frozen yogurt**. It's sweet, satisfying and, other than fruit, one of the lowest calorie desserts.

✓ **Enjoy a cup of flavored tea or coffee** for a satisfying finish to a meal with the benefit of fewer calories than a rich dessert.

Fruit

✓ **Have fresh fruit for dessert**. Even if fruit is not listed on the menu, most restaurants have it available. At fewer than 100 calories per serving, fresh fruit may be the sweet taste you are looking for at the end of the meal. If sugar is added to the fruit, the calories will increase but not significantly.

✓ **Ask for the fruit plain.** What can destroy a perfectly healthy dish of fruit is the heavy cream or excessive whipped topping that is often added to the fruit – or the sugar cookie that is placed on the side. Be specific that you want fresh fruit only – no toppings.

Fruit & Toppings

	Calories	Fat (g)	Sodium (mg)	Exchanges
Fresh Fruit*, ½ c	20-70	0	<10	½-1FR
Fruit packed in sugar or prepared with sugar*, ½ c	75-120	0	<10	1-2FR
Whipping Cream, pressurized, 2T	23	2	4	½FAT
Whipping Cream, pressurized, ¼ c	46	4	8	1FAT
Whipping Cream, whipped, 2T	50	6	6	1FAT
Heavy Cream or Crème Fraiche, 2T	104	11	12	2FAT

*Nutritional information for a wide variety of fruit is listed in the *Breakfast* chapter.

Frozen Yogurt, Soft Serve, & Ice Cream

Many restaurants are serving frozen yogurt as an option to high fat desserts. In addition, freestanding frozen yogurt and ice cream shops sell a variety of frozen yogurt, ice milks, and other frozen desserts.

✓ **Select nonfat or lowfat frozen yogurt instead of packed ice cream**. Frozen yogurt is considerably lower in calories and fat grams than ice cream. Here's a comparison of small portion, just a half cup, without toppings! How much ice cream can you eat?

Choose Yogurt instead of Ice Cream:

	Calories	Fat (g)
Ice Cream, ½ c	250-350	12-24
Non Fat Frozen Yogurt, ½ c	100	0
Savings:	**150-250**	**12-24**

✓ **Order frozen yogurt instead of soft serve**. Frozen yogurt is typically lower than soft serve as well. If restaurants have a self-serve machine and it is not labeled as frozen yogurt, assume that it is soft serve.

Choose Frozen Yogurt for Cups, Cones, & Shakes:			
		Calories	Fat (g)
Soft Serve, ½ c		140	5
Soft Frozen Yogurt, ½ c		100	0
	Savings:	40	5
DQ® Regular Heath Blizzard		820	33
DQ® Regular Heath Breeze		710	18
	Savings:	90	15

✓ **Select lower fat ice cream, sherbet, or sorbet**. Many ice cream shops are offering lower fat ice creams that still taste rich and creamy.

Choose Low Fat Ice Cream:			
		Calories	Fat (g)
Ice Cream, ½ c		250-350	12-24
Friendly's Mocha Fudge Low Fat Ice Cream, ½ c		140	$2.^5$
	Savings:	110-210	$9.^5$-$21.^5$

Choose Sorbet over Sherbet:			
		Calories	Fat (g)
Sherbet, ½ c		135	2
Friendly's Sorbet, ½ c		110-130	0-1.5
	Savings:	5-25	$0.^5$-2

✓ **Order a small portion**. Obviously, the bigger the cup of yogurt or ice cream, the more calories there are. Most people watching calories should order the children's cup, child's cup, or the small size. These usually range between 4-8 fluid ounces of dessert.

Calculating the Calories & Fat Grams in Frozen Yogurt

When restaurants provide nutritional information, be honest about the portion size you were served. Sometimes the portion served is considerably larger than the portion size indicated on the restaurant's nutrition information chart.

> **Quiz:** You are buying soft-serve frozen yogurt. The brochure states that each 4 fluid ounces contains 100 calories. You notice the cup sizes are labeled: Small (5 oz), Medium (8 oz), and Large (12 oz). You select the 8 oz cup. How many calories are in your yogurt?

200 calories, you say? Wrong. It has 300! How?

The brochure stated that the product contains 100 calories per *fluid* ounce. The labeled cup sizes were to demonstrate the *weight* ounces of the yogurt when the cup is filled. *Fluid* ounces and *weight* ounces are not always the same. They *are* the same for water, juice, and milk. In other words, one measuring cup of water, juice, or milk has both 8 *fluid* (volume) ounces and 8 *weight* ounces. That's probably why we assume that fluid ounces and weight ounces are the same for *everything*. They are not the same with everything and they are not the same for frozen yogurt.

When your cup of frozen yogurt is **weighed** (for quality control or for pricing) keep in mind that you can not calculate the calories directly from this number. In the process of making frozen yogurt (and other soft serve products), air is incorporated into the product. Companies refer to this in terms of "percent overrun."

If the company has a 50% overrun (as is most common), simply multiply the weight ounces by 1½. Therefore, a cup of frozen yogurt weighing 4 oz (4 *weight* ounces) will equate to 6 *fluid* ounces. Here's a chart to make calculations easier.

Calories in Frozen Yogurt & Soft Serve* per serving size

Size of Cup or Cone	Calories & fat (g) per 4 fluid oz serving as labeled:							
	40	60	80	100	110	120	140	150
4 oz (6 fl oz)	60	90	120	150	165	180	210	225
	0g	0g	0g	1g	2g	3g	5g	8g
5 oz (7½ fl oz)	75	115	150	190	205	225	265	280
	0g	0g	0g	1g	2g	4g	6g	10g
6 oz (9 fl oz)	90	135	180	225	250	270	315	340
	0g	0g	0g	2g	3g	5g	7g	12g
7 oz (10½ fl oz)	105	160	210	265	290	315	370	395
	0g	0g	0g	2g	3g	6g	8g	14g
8 oz (12 fl oz)	120	180	240	300	330	360	420	450
	0g	0g	0g	2g	4g	6g	9g	16g
9 oz (13½ fl oz)	135	205	270	340	370	405	475	510
	0g	0g	0g	3g	5g	7g	11g	18g
10 oz (15 fl oz)	150	225	300	375	415	450	525	565
	0g	0g	0g	3g	5g	8g	12g	20g

*Assuming 50% overrun. If the liquid ingredients are inadequately frozen, the final product will be very runny. Because there is less air in a runny product, you can fit more yogurt into the cup. More yogurt means even more calories than the chart above demonstrates.

Cone with 4 wt oz (6 fl oz)

✓ **Ask your taste buds**. Per equal portion, frozen yogurt has fewer calories than ice cream. For that reason, some people order an extra large serving of frozen yogurt. Be careful! Ordering a *large* size of frozen yogurt may not be any lower in calories than a *moderate* portion of ice cream. And which would your taste buds prefer today?

Have Discriminating Taste Buds:		
	Calories	Fat (g)
Frozen *Non Fat* Yogurt, 1½ c	300	0
Ice Cream, ½ c	300	18

✓ **Order it served in a cup or small cone.** The small-sized cake or sugar cones have negligible fat and few calories. The large waffle cones are considerably higher in fats and calories. Chocolate, nut dips, and candy sprinkles add even more.

Have a Small Cone:		
	Calories	Fat (g)
Waffle Cone, chocolate covered	300	10
Cake Cone	25	0
Savings:	**275**	**10**

✓ **Sugar free doesn't mean calorie free.** Regular frozen yogurt is typically sweetened with sugar. Sugar-free frozen yogurts and ice creams often use aspartame (such as Nutrasweet®), sorbitol, or fructose. Each sugar-free product has usually a few less calories, but perhaps not as much as you might think.

Sugar Free is not Calorie Free:		
	Calories	Fat (g)
Baskin 31 Robbins® Nonfat Ice Cream, ½ c	100-120	0
Baskin 31 Robbins® No Sugar Added, ½ c	80-100	1-3
Savings:	**20-40**	**1-3g more**

✓ **Watch the sauces and toppings.** Unless you've selected fresh fruit, the toppings will add significantly to the total calories. Most companies use a 2T ladle to spoon on the sauces and toppings. One ladle may be used on the smaller cups, but the larger cups often have 2 or more ladles.

Have It Plain:		
	Calories	Fat (g)
Large Frozen Yogurt Sundae (4T hot fudge sauce, 2T nuts, & ½ c whipped cream)	710	31
Large Cup Frozen Yogurt	270	5
Savings:	**440**	**26**

Cones & Toppings

	Calories	Fat (g)	Sodium (mg)	Exchanges
Cones (1):				
Cake	25	0	35	¼CHO
Sugar	60	0	50	½CHO
Lg. Waffle	120	2	55	1CHO+½FAT
Waffle Cone/Fresh Baked	150	2	5	2CHO+½FAT
Waffle Cone, chocolate covered	300	10	50	3½CHO+2FAT
Waffle Cone, chocolate covered w/nuts	400	19	50	3½CHO+4FAT
Fruit Toppings (2T):				
Fresh strawberries	6	<1	0	FREE _or_ ¼FR
Fresh blueberries	10	<1	1	FREE _or_ ¼FR
Fruit Cocktail, canned in own juice	14	0	1	FREE _or_ ¼FR
Raisins	56	<1	5	1FR
Shredded coconut, dried & sweetened	45	3.^{5}	24	¼CHO+½FAT
Syrups & Toppings (2T):				
Chocolate syrup	90	1	30	1½CHO
Hot Fudge topping	120	5	35	1½CHO+1FAT
No Sugar Added/ Fat-Free Hot Fudge	90	0	96	1½CHO
Butterscotch topping	130	1	110	1½CHO
Caramel topping	120	3	90	1½CHO
Strawberry topping	60	0	5	1CHO
Blueberry or Pineapple topping	70	0	15	1CHO
Walnuts in syrup	130	1	na	1½CHO
Marshmallow creme	90	0	20	1½CHO
Whipped topping	23	1.^{8}	2	½FAT
Grenadine, 1T	60	0	0	1CHO
Candy & Nut Toppings (slightly rounded 2T):				
Chocolate _or_ Yogurt-covered raisins	120	5	30	½FR+1½CHO+1FAT
Sprinkles ("Jimmies")	140	5	0	1¼CHO+1FAT
Cookies, crumbled	135	5	95	1¼CHO+1FAT
Butterfinger, crumbled	130	5	57	1¼CHO+1FAT
Heath bar, crumbled	140	9	106	1CHO+2FAT
Reese's pieces	140	6	47	1¼CHO+1FAT
Plain M&M's®	140	6	15	1¼CHO+1FAT
Peanut M&M's®	150	7	15	1¼CHO+1½FAT
Granola	60	3	30	½CHO+½FAT
Nuts, unsalted	100	9	0	2FAT

Your Favorite Ice Cream & Frozen Yogurt Shops

BASKIN 31 ROBBINS®

	Calories	Fat (g)	Sodium (mg)	Exchanges
Novelties (1):				
Chilly Burgers™:				
Chocolate Chip, Mint Choc. Chip	220	11	100	2CHO+2FAT
Sundae Bars:				
Jamoca Almond Fudge	280	17	60	1½CHO+3½FAT
Peanut Butter Chocolate	340	27	115	1½CHO+5½FAT
Pralines'N Cream	280	17	105	1½CHO+3½FAT
Tiny Toon Adventures™ Ice Cr. Bars:				
Vanilla	140	12	25	½CHO+2½FAT
Blast Bars:				
Cappuccino Blast Bar	100	1	35	1½CHO
Mocha Cappuccino Blast	120	4	35	1½CHO+1FAT
Cones (1):				
Sugar	60	0	50	½CHO
Cake	25	0	35	¼CHO
Lg Waffle	120	1.⁵	55	1CHO+½FAT
Waffle Cone/Fresh Baked	146	2	5	2CHO+½FAT
Reg. Deluxe Ice Cream (1 reg. scoop):				
Banana Strawberry, Peach	240	12	75-70	2CHO+2½FAT
Cherries Jubilee	240	13	75	2CHO+2½FAT
Vanilla	240	14	115	1½CHO+3FAT
Choc. Ribbon, Chunk A Cherry Burn'Love, Rum Raisin	250	13	80-70	2CHO+2½FAT
Jamoca	250	15	85	1½CHO+3FAT
Decorating Vanilla	250	16	85	1½CHO+3FAT
Lemon Custard	260	15	100	2CHO+3FAT
Martian Mint	260	15	140	2CHO+3FAT
Banana Nut	260	17	70	1½CHO+3½FAT
Gold Medal Ribbon	270	13	170	2CHO+2½FAT
Peppermint, Pink Bubble Gum	270	14	75-80	2CHO+3FAT
Strawberry Cheesecake	270	14	130	2CHO+3FAT
Chocolate	270	16	110	2CHO+3FAT
Winter White Chocolate	270	16	90	2CHO+3FAT
Choc. Chip, Mint Choc. Chip	270	18	80-85	1½CHO+3½FAT
Choc. Raspberry Truffle	280	14	95	2CHO+3FAT
Baseball Nut, Jamoca Alm. Fudge, Strawb. Shortck., World Class Choc.	280	16	70-125	2CHO+3FAT
Choco The Irish	280	17	105	2CHO+3½FAT
French Vanilla	280	18	90	1½CHO+3½FAT
Black Walnut, Coconut	280	19	85	1½CHO+4FAT
Chocolate Fudge	290	15	180	2CHO+3FAT

BASKIN 31 ROBBINS® (continued)

	Calories	Fat (g)	Sodium (mg)	Exchanges
Reg. Deluxe Ice Cream (1 reg. scoop) continued:				
English Toffee, Nutty or Nice, Pralines'N Cream	290	16	125-135	2½CHO+3FAT
Caramel Choc. Crunch, Quarterback Crunch	290	17	135-150	2CHO+3½FAT
Triple Chocolate Passion	290	18	110	2CHO+3½FAT
Old Fashioned Peanut Butter	290	20	90	1½CHO+4FAT
Butterfinger	300	15	na	2½CHO+3FAT
Chocoholic's Resolution	300	16	115	2½CHO+3FAT
Choc. Chip Cookie Dough, Chewy Baby Ruth, Rocky Road	300	17	105-125	2CHO+3½FAT
Chunky Heath Bar	300	18	125	2CHO+3½FAT
Cookies'N Cream	300	19	140	2CHO+4FAT
Pistachio-Almond	300	21	80	1½CHO+4FAT
S'Mores	302	13	97	2½CHO+2½FAT
Fudge Brownie, Reeses Peanut Butter	310	19	125-130	2CHO+4FAT
Chocolate Mousse Royale	310	18	105	2CHO+3½FAT
Nutty Coconut	310	21	85	2CHO+4FAT
Chocolate Almond	310	20	100	2CHO+4FAT
Peanut Butter'N Chocolate	330	22	170	2CHO+4½FAT
Ices, Sherbet & Sorbets (1 reg. scoop):				
Daiquiri Ice	130	0	10	1½CHO
Orange Sherbet	160	2	45	2CHO+½FAT
Rainbow Sherbet	160	2	30	2CHO+½FAT
Red Raspberry Sorbet	140	0	25	2CHO
Light/Low Fat (½ c)	100-120	2.^{5}-3	60-75	1½CHO+½FAT
Non-Fat Ice Cream (½ c)	100-120	0	75-105	1½CHO
No Sugar Added (½ c)	80-100	1-2.^{5}	40-70	1CHO+½FAT
Non-Fat Soft Serve (½ c)	120	0	85	1½CHO
Low Fat Frozen Yogurt (½ c)	120	2	70-75	1½CHO
Non-Fat Frozen Yogurt (½ c)				
Vanilla	80	0	80	1CHO
Other Flavors	100-110	0	50-75	1½CHO
Truly Free™ Frozen Yogurt (Fat Free/Reduced Sugar) (½ c)	80-90	0	75-85	1CHO

BASKIN 31 ROBBINS® (continued)

Fountain Drinks:

	Calories	Fat (g)	Sodium (mg)	Exchanges
Blast Drinks, 8 oz (w/out whipped cream):				
Cappy Blast	150	6	55	1½CHO+1FAT
Cappy Non-Fat Blast	90	0	60	1½CHO
Chocolate Blast	240	5	110	3CHO+1FAT
Chocolate Non-Fat Blast	170	0	105	2½CHO
Pina Colada Paradise Blast	190	5	25	2CHO+1FAT
Pina Colada NF Paradise Blast	140	0	35	2CHO
Strawb. Luau Paradise Blast	170	4	40	2CHO+1FAT
Strawb. Luau Non-Fat Paradise Blast	140	0	50	2CHO
Smoothies, 8 oz:				
Blueberry Strawberry	150	0	70	2CHO
Orange Banana	120	0	75	1½CHO
Strawberry Banana	170	0	75	2½CHO
Chocolate Shake, 14 oz	660	31	na	4CHO+1WhMk+4½FAT

For more information, call 1-800-331-0031

CARVEL ICE CREAM BAKERY™

	Calories	Fat (g)	Sodium (mg)	Exchanges
Per 4 fl oz serving:				
Ice Cream, Vanilla	200	10	110	1½CHO+2FAT
Ice Cream, Chocolate	190	10	100	1½CHO+2FAT
No-Fat Ice Cream, Vanilla	120	0	55	1¾CHO
No-Fat Ice Cream, Chocolate	120	0	40	2CHO
Sherbet	140	1	45	2CHO
Specialties:				
Holiday Ice Cream Cake, ¹/₁₅ cake	240	12	100	2CHO+2½FAT
Carvel Ice Cream Cake, 4 oz	270	14	160	2CHO+3FAT
Flying Saucer, Vanilla, 1	240	10	150	2CHO+2FAT
Chocolate, 1	230	9	140	2CHO+2FAT
Vanilla w/Chocolate Covered Sprinkles, 1	340	14	160	3¼CHO+3FAT
Chocolate w/Colored & Chocolate Sprinkles, 1	330	14	150	3¼CHO+3FAT
Low Fat Flying Saucer, Vanilla, 1	180	2.5	140	2½CHO+½FAT
Chocolate, 1	190	2.5	130	2½CHO+½FAT

DAIRY QUEEN®

	Calories	Fat (g)	Sodium (mg)	Exchanges
Cones and Cups:				
DQ® Vanilla Soft Serve, ½ c	140	5	70	1½CHO+1FAT
DQ® Chocolate Soft Serve, ½ c	150	5	75	1½CHO+1FAT
DQ® Nonfat Frozen Yogurt, ½ c	100	0	70	1½CHO
Regular Cup of Yogurt	230	0.5	160	3CHO
Small Vanilla Cone	230	7	115	2½ST+1½FAT
Regular Vanilla Cone	350	10	170	3½CHO+2FAT
Large Vanilla Cone	410	12	200	4CHO+2½FAT
Small Chocolate Cone	240	8	115	2½CHO+1½FAT
Regular Chocolate Cone	360	11	180	3½CHO+2FAT
Regular Yogurt Cone	280	1	170	4CHO
Small Dipped Cone	340	17	130	2½CHO+2½FAT
Regular Dipped Cone	510	25	200	4CHO+5FAT
Queen's Choice® Vanilla Big Scoop®	250	14	100	1½CHO+3FAT
Queen's Choice® Chocolate Big Scoop®	250	14	95	1½CHO+3FAT
DQ® Lemon Freez'r™, ½ c	80	0	10	1CHO
Royal Treats and Sundaes:				
Small Chocolate Sundae	290	7	150	3½CHO+1½FAT
Regular Chocolate Sundae	410	10	210	4CHO+2FAT
Regular Yogurt Strawberry Sundae	300	0.5	180	4CHO
Banana Split	510	11	180	6CHO+2FAT
Peanut Buster® Parfait	730	31	400	6CHO+6FAT
Slushes, Coolers, Malts, & Shakes:				
Small Misty® Slush	220	0	20	3½CHO
Regular Misty® Slush	290	0	30	5CHO
Strawberry Misty® Cooler	190	0	25	3CHO
Small Chocolate Malt	650	16	370	7CHO+3FAT
Regular Chocolate Malt	880	22	500	10CHO+4½FAT
Small Chocolate Shake	560	15	310	6CHO+3FAT
Regular Chocolate Shake	770	20	420	8CHO+4FAT
Bars (1):				
DQ® Sandwich	150	5	115	1½CHO+1FAT
Strawberry Shortcake	430	14	360	4½CHO+3FAT
Chocolate Dilly Bar®	210	13	75	1½CHO+2½FAT
Chocolate Mint Dilly Bar®	190	12	100	1½CHO+2½FAT
Toffee Dilly Bar® w/Heath® Pieces	210	12	100	1½CHO+2½FAT
Fudge Nut Bar™	410	25	250	2½CHO+5FAT
Buster Bar®	450	28	280	2½CHO+5½FAT
Starkiss®	80	0	10	1½CHO

DAIRY QUEEN® (continued)

	Calories	Fat (g)	Sodium (mg)	Exchanges
Bars (1) continued:				
DQ® Caramel & Nut Bar	260	13	90	2CHO+2½FAT
DQ® Fudge Bar	50	0	70	1CHO
DQ® Vanilla Orange Bar	60	0	40	1CHO
Blizzard® and Breeze® (small = 12 oz, Regular = 16 oz):				
Small Butterfinger® Blizzard®	520	18	250	5CHO+3½FAT
Regular Butterfinger® Blizzard®	750	26	360	7CHO+5FAT
Sm. Choc. Sand. Cookie Blizzard®	520	18	380	5CHO+3½FAT
Reg Choc. Sand. Cookie Blizzard®	640	23	500	6CHO+4½FAT
Small Strawberry Blizzard®	400	11	190	4CHO+2FAT
Regular Strawberry Blizzard®	570	16	260	6CHO+3FAT
Small Heath® Blizzard®	560	21	380	5½CHO+4FAT
Regular Heath® Blizzard®	820	33	580	8CHO+6½FAT
Small Choc. Chip Cookie Dough Blizzard®	660	24	440	6½CHO+5FAT
Reg. Choc. Chip Cookie Dough Blizzard®	950	36	660	9½CHO+7FAT
Small Reeses® Peanut Butter Cup Blizzard®	590	24	320	5½CHO+5FAT
Reg. Reeses® Peanut Butter Cup Blizzard®	790	33	430	7CHO+6½FAT
Small Strawberry Breeze®	320	$0.^5$	190	4½CHO
Regular Strawberry Breeze®	460	1	270	6½CHO
Small Heath® Breeze®	470	10	380	5½CHO+2FAT
Regular Heath® Breeze®	710	18	580	8CHO+3½FAT
DQ Treatzza Pizza™ (¹/₈ of Pizza):				
Strawberry-Banana	180	6	140	2CHO+1FAT
Heath®	180	7	160	2CHO+1½FAT
M&M®	190	7	160	2CHO+1½FAT
Peanut Butter Fudge	220	10	200	2CHO+2FAT
DQ® Frozen Cakes (undecorated):				
Log Cake, ¹/₈ cake	280	9	220	3CHO+2FAT
8" Round Cake, ¹/₈ cake	340	12	250	3½CHO+2½FAT
10" Round Cake, ¹/₁₂ cake	360	12	260	3½CHO+2½FAT
Heart Cake, ¹/₁₀ cake	270	9	190	2½CHO+2FAT
Sheet Cake, ¹/₂₀ cake	350	12	270	3½CHO+2½FAT

FRIENDLY®'S

	Calories	Fat (g)	Sodium (mg)	Exchanges
Sorbets (½ c):				
Peach Sorbet	130	1.5	na	na
Chocolate Sorbet	120	0	na	na
Raspberry *or* Lemon Sorbet	110	0	na	na
Low Fat Ice Creams (½ c):				
Butterscotch Ripple Low Fat	150	2.5	na	na
Mocha Fudge Low Fat	140	2.5	na	na
Strawberry Low Fat	120	2	na	na
Chocolate *or* Vanilla Low Fat	120	2.5	na	na
No Fat Frozen Yogurt (½ c):				
Vanilla, Chocolate, Raspberry, Vanilla/Chocolate, *or* Peach No Fat Frozen Yogurt	110	0	na	na
Strawberry *or* Wildberry/Vanilla/ Strawberry No Fat Frozen Yogurt	100	0	na	na

TCBY® FROZEN YOGURT

	Calories	Fat (g)	Sodium (mg)	Exchanges
Soft-Serve (½ c):				
Nonfat Frozen Yogurt	110	0	60	1½CHO
No Sugar Added Nonfat Frozen Yogurt (w/aspartame)	80	0	35	1¼CHO
96% Fat Free Frozen Yogurt	140	3	60	1½CHO
Nonfat & Nondairy Sorbet	100	0	30	1½CHO
Hand-Dipped (½ c):				
Nonfat Ice Cream	120	0	55	1¾CHO
No Sugar Added Lowfat Ice Cream (w/aspartame)	110	2.5	60	1¼CHO
Nonfat Frozen Yogurt	120	0	60	1¾CHO
96% Fat Free Frozen Yogurt	140	3	70	1¾CHO
(Calorie content will vary with flavors)				
Hot Fudge Topping (per scoop):				
Regular	143	7	na	1CHO+1½FAT
Sugar-Free	69	<1	na	1CHO

Other Desserts

Besides frozen yogurt, what other desserts are acceptable on a low fat regime? As mentioned earlier, your best decision would be to order fruit, share a dessert with others, or ask the server to give you just a small portion rather than the usual serving. Here are some additional ideas.

✔ **Choose one of the lower calorie desserts.** Angel food and sponge cake are two cakes which have the least amount of calories per ounce. Reduced fat brownies, cakes, and muffins may also be offered. While these low fat and fat-free baked goods have significantly less fat than their regular counterparts, the calories are still fairly high due to the fact that low fat desserts are often higher in sugar. In addition, even low fat desserts are served in very large portions.

✔ **Skip the piecrust.** Most of the fat and calories in pies, cobblers, and turnovers come from the piecrust. The fruit filling is rather low in calories. So if you like the pie filling more than the crust, don't feel guilty about leaving the crust behind. You'll save more than half the calories. Cobblers are generally lower in calories than pies because they often have just one layer of crust or crumb topping.

✔ **Choose the sugar-free pie.** Because 40% of the pie's calories come from the fat in the piecrust, it's easy to understand why a sugar-free pie does not have significantly fewer calories than regular pie. It still has a piecrust! Notice that all of the savings in calories are coming from carbohydrates, not fat grams.

Choose Pies Made with Equal:		Calories	Fat (g)
Denny's Apple Pie		430	20
Denny's Apple Pie with Equal		370	20
	Savings:	**60**	**0**

✔ **Muffins are very misleading.** Which has less calories and fat: muffins or doughnuts? The muffin? Probably not. It's true that muffins are not fried and may even have fewer calories per ounce than doughnuts. But the muffin may end up having more fat and calories simply because an average doughnut is about 2 - 3 ounces while muffins often weigh more.

Enjoy the Low Fat Muffins:		Calories	Fat (g)
Regular Blueberry Muffin, 4 oz		400	17
Low Fat Blueberry Muffin, 4 oz		320	1
	Savings:	**80**	**16**

Calculating the Calories and Fat in Baked Goods

Shops selling frozen yogurt and low fat ice creams often have nutritional information. Most other desserts do not. So how do you find out the number of calories and grams of fat in the other desserts? It's easy.

You can calculate the calories of *any* desserts as long as you know

❶ the weight of the item and

❷ the calories per ounce as shown on the Desserts Calorimeter below.

The most accurate way to find out the weight of the dessert is to take it home or to the office and weigh it on a postage scale. If that is not an option, estimate the weight by comparing your dessert to the portion sizes depicted throughout this chapter.

Desserts Calorimeter: Calories & fat per serving

Calories Per oz		Calories & Fat (g)				
		1 oz	2 oz	3 oz	4 oz	5 oz
160	Shortbread	160	320	480	640	800
		9g	19g	28g	37g	47g
135	Almond & Choc Almond Biscotti Brownie Cake Doughnuts Chocolate Croissant Chocolate Chip Cookie Macaroons Peanut Butter Brownie *or* Cookie Pound Cake	135 8g	270 15g	405 23g	540 30g	675 38g
125	Cookies: Butter, Oatmeal, Sugar	125 5g	250 10g	375 16g	500 21g	625 26g
120	Plain & Almond Croissant Choc Cream Filled Doughnuts	120 7g	240 13g	360 20g	480 26g	600 33g
110	Cheesecake Coffeecake, Cinn Rolls & Danish Muffins: Chocolate Chip, Lemon Poppy Seed Gingerbread Madeleines Scones Sweet Cheese Croissant Pecan Pie	110 6g	220 11g	330 17g	440 22g	550 28g

Desserts Calorimeter: Calories & fat per serving (continued)

Calories Per oz		Calories & Fat grams (g)				
		1 oz	2 oz	3 oz	4 oz	5 oz
100	Biscotti, plain Fritters, Glazed Fritters Cakes/Cupcakes (plain or frosted) Muffins: fruit or grain Yeast Doughnuts (includ glazed, frosted, crème & jelly filled) Fruit Tarts & Turnovers Pies: Boston Cream, Buttermilk, German Choc, Choc Cream	**100** 4g	**200** 8g	**300** 13g	**400** 17g	**500** 21g
80	Tiraminsu	**80** 5g	**160** 10g	**240** 14g	**360** 19g	**400** 24g
80	Pies: Fruits including Lemon & Lime, Coconut Custard, Mincemeat	**80** 3g	**160** 6g	**240** 10g	**360** 13g	**400** 17g
80	Angel Food Cake Lowfat Muffins Sponge Cake	**80** $0.^3$g	**160** $0.^6$g	**240** $0.^9$g	**320** $1.^2$g	**400** $1.^5$g
60	Pies: Banana Custard, Banana Cream, Custard, Pumpkin	**60** 3g	**120** 6g	**180** 9g	**240** 12g	**300** 15g

Brownie

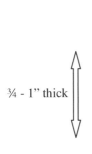

¾ - 1" thick

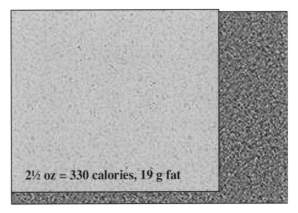

2½ oz = 330 calories, 19 g fat

3½ oz = 475 calories, 28 g fat

Cakes

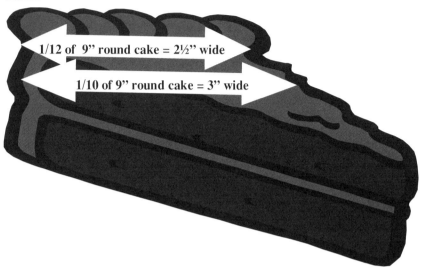

1/12 of 9" round cake = 2½" wide

1/10 of 9" round cake = 3" wide

Cakes, frosted or unfrosted, contain approximately 100 calories per ounce. The amount of ounces per slice vary greatly. Refer to the Cake Calorimeter below or the nutritional information at the end of this chapter for more details.

Cake Calorimeter: Calories & Fat grams per portion

9" Round Cake	Calories & Fat (g)	
	$^1/_{12}$ cake	$^1/_{10}$ cake
Angel Food Cake	**160**	**190**
	0g	0g
Carrot Cake	**521**	**625**
	23g	28g
Chocolate Cake	**575**	**690**
	25g	30g
Italian Rum Custard	**360**	**430**
	20g	24g
Pound Cake	**280**	**340**
	13g	16g
Sponge Cake	**190**	**230**
	3g	4g
Yellow Cake	**540**	**650**
	23g	28g

Cheesecake

3 oz = 330 calories, 23 g fat

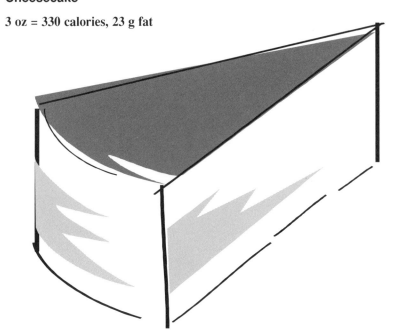

Coffee Cake, Cinnamon Rolls

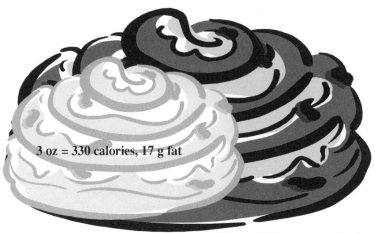

3 oz = 330 calories, 17 g fat

7½ oz = 825 calories, 42 g fat

Cookies

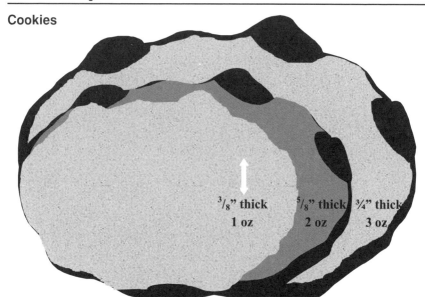

$^3/_8$" thick
1 oz

$^5/_8$" thick
2 oz

$^3/_4$" thick
3 oz

Cookie Calorimeter: Calories & Fat grams per cookie

Cookie	Calories & Fat (g)		
	1 oz	2 oz	3 oz
Peanut Butter, Chocolate Chip, Macadamia Nut, *or* Chocolate Chunk	**135**	**270**	**405**
	8g	15g	23g
Butter, Oatmeal, Oatmeal Raisin, *or* Sugar	**125**	**250**	**375**
	5g	10g	16g

Doughnuts

**2 oz Yeast Raised Doughnut
200 calories, 8 g fat**

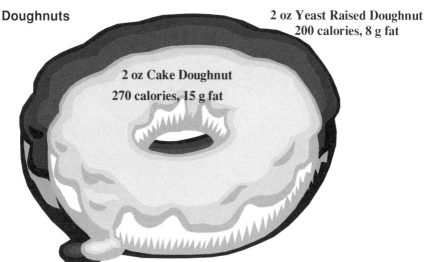

**2 oz Cake Doughnut
270 calories, 15 g fat**

Note that ounce for ounce, the cake doughnuts are smaller and more compact and yet have more calories and fat than yeast raised doughnuts.

Muffins

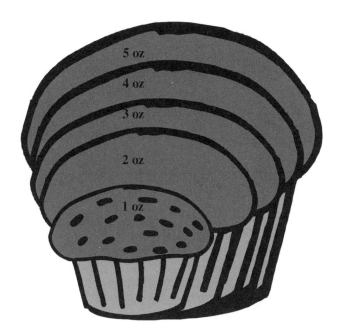

The calories in your muffin vary greatly depending on its size. A 1 oz muffin is very small – almost bite size. The 4 oz muffin is about the size of a baseball; the 5 oz muffin is the size of a softball.

Muffin Calorimeter: Calories & fat grams per muffin

Muffin	Calories & Fat (g)				
	1 oz	2 oz	3 oz	4 oz	5 oz
Chocolate Chip, Lemon Poppy Seed	**110**	**220**	**330**	**440**	**550**
	6g	11g	17g	22g	28g
Fruit or Grain	**110**	**220**	**330**	**440**	**550**
	4g	8g	13g	17g	21g
Fat Free Muffins	**80**	**160**	**180**	**240**	**300**
	$0.^3$g	$0.^6$g	$0.^9$g	$1.^2$g	$1.^5$g

Pies

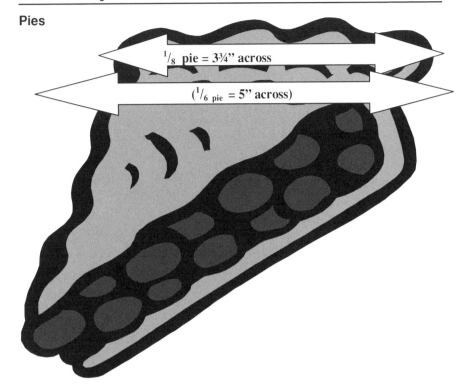

$^1/_8$ pie = 3¾" across

($^1/_6$ pie = 5" across)

Pie Calorimeter: Calories & Fat grams per portion

9" Pie	Calories & Fat (g)	
	$^1/_8$ pie	$^1/_6$ pie
Apple	**270**	**360**
	13g	17g
Banana Cream	**270**	**360**
	12g	16g
Blueberry	**290**	**390**
	13g	17g
Cherry	**350**	**465**
	17g	23g
Chocolate Cream	**290**	**380**
	18g	24g
Coconut Cream	**275**	**365**
	14g	19g
Key Lime	**345**	**460**
	15g	20g
Lemon Meringue	**350**	**465**
	15g	20g
Pecan	**430**	**570**
	24g	32g

Nutritional Information for Other Desserts

Desserts	Calories	Fat (g)	Sodium (mg)	Exchanges
Baklava, 2" X 2"	440	30	na	2CHO+6FAT
Biscotti, 1.[3] oz, 6½" long	112	5	41	1ST+1FAT
Blintz, Cheese, 3" long	80	2	135	¾ST+½LM
Cherry, 3	385	17	na	2ST+1FR+3½FAT
Brownie, 2½ oz, 2"X2¼"X1" high	330	19	100	2CHO+4FAT
3½ oz, 2"X3"X1" high	475	28	150	3CHO+5½FAT
Cakes:				
Angel Food Cake, ¹/₁₂ of tube (2½" slice)	160	0	0	2CHO
Carrot Cake w/cream cheese frosting, ¹/₁₀ of 9" 2 layer	625	28	na	4½CHO+5½FAT
Chiffon Cake, ¹/₁₂ of 10" tube pan	290	12	160	2½CHO+2½FAT
Chocolate w/choc butter cream frosting, ¹/₁₀ of 9" 2 layer	690	30	na	5CHO+6FAT
Devil's Food Cake, ¹/₁₂ of 9" double layer cake	530	19	240	6CHO+4FAT
Fruitcake, ½" X 4" slice	210	7	85	2CHO+1½FAT
Italian Rum Custard Cake, ¹/₁₂	360	20	80	2¼CHO+4FAT
Pound Cake, 1" sl (rectangular pan) or 2½" wide (9" tube)	280	13	130	2CHO+2½FAT
Strawberry Shortcake, 2 ½" biscuit	430	24	240	1ST+1FR+1CHO+5FAT
Sponge Cake, 2½" slice	190	3	160	2CHO+½FAT
Pineapple Upside Down Cake, 3" X 3" X 2" high	360	14	na	1½CHO+1FR+3FAT
Yellow Cake, ¹/₁₂ of 9" cake	540	23	na	4CHO+4½FAT
Cake Icing, chocolate, 2T	140	5	50	1½CHO+1FAT
Vanilla, 2T	150	3	20	2CHO+½FAT
Cheesecake, 3 oz slice, 1½" wide slice from 9" tube, 1½" high	330	23	318	1½CHO+½HFM+4FAT
6 oz slice, 3" wide slice from 9" tube, 1½" high	660	46	636	3CHO+1HFM+7½FAT
Chocolate Mousse, 1c	380	32	na	1CHO+6½FAT
Chocolate Pots de Crème, ²/₃ c	270	21	30	1½CHO+4FAT
Cobblers & Crisps:				
Fruit Cobbler, 1c	330	9	210	1FR+2½CHO+2FAT
Fruit Crisp, 1 c	260	8	100	1FR+2CHO+1½FAT

Desserts (continued)

	Calories	Fat (g)	Sodium (mg)	Exchanges
Cookies (Peanut Butter, Chocolate Chip, Macadamia Nut, Chocolate Chunk):				
1 oz	135	8	100	¾CHO+1½FAT
2 oz	270	15	200	1½CHO+3FAT
3 oz	405	23	300	2¼CHO+4½FAT
Cookies (Butter, Oatmeal Raisin, Sugar):				
1 oz	125	5	100	1CHO+1FAT
2 oz	250	10	200	2CHO+2FAT
3 oz	375	16	300	3CHO+3FAT
Cream Puff, w/out filling	160	11	160	¾ST+2FAT
Cream Puff, w/ filling	300	18	380	1¾CHO+3½FAT
Crème Brûlée, ½ c	405	36	40	1CHO+1MFM+6FAT
Crème Fraische or Heavy Cream, 2T	104	11	12	2FAT
Crepe, 1 w/out filling	135	7	na	1ST+1½FAT
w/ fruit filling, 1	270	11	na	1ST+1¼CHO+2FAT
Crepe Suzette, 3	600	30	na	4CHO+6FAT
Custard, Baked *or* Stirred, ½ c	150	4	70	½CHO+½WhMk+ ½MFM
Doughnut, 2 oz cake	270	15	na	1¾ST+3FAT
2 oz yeast raised	200	8	na	1¾ST+1½FAT
Flan, 1c	220	2	140	3CHO
Funnel Cake, 7" diameter circle, 1" high w/confectioner's sugar	1440	85		9CHO+17FAT
Gelatin, ½ c	80	0	25	1CHO
Marzipan or Almond Paste, 1 oz (1½T)	150	5	70	1½CHO+1FAT
Pies from 9" pan, unless noted (slices from 10" pies are larger & deeper – estimate at least 50% more calories & fat):				
Apple, ⅛	270	13	240	1½ST+1FR+2½FAT
⅙	360	17	320	2ST+1FR+3½FAT
Banana Cream Pie, ⅛	270	12	300	1½ST+1FR+2½FAT
⅙	360	16	400	2ST+1FR+3FAT
Black Bottom Pie, ⅛ of 10"	380	16	na	3CHO+3FAT
⅙ of 10"	506	21	na	4CHO+4FAT
Blueberry Pie, ⅛	290	13	320	1½ST+1FR+2½FAT
⅙	390	17	430	2ST+1FR+3½FAT
Brown Sugar Pie, ⅛ of 10"	590	25	na	4½CHO+5FAT
⅙ of 10"	787	33	na	6CHO+6½FAT

Desserts (continued)

	Calories	Fat (g)	Sodium (mg)	Exchanges
Pies from 9" pan, unless noted (slices from 10" pies are larger & deeper – estimate to contain at least 50% more calories & fat):				
Cherry Pie, $^1/_8$	350	17	410	1½ST+1FR+3½FAT
$^1/_6$	465	23	540	2½ST+1FR+4½FAT
Chocolate Cream Pie, $^1/_8$	290	18	300	1½CHO+3½FAT
$^1/_6$	380	24	395	2CHO+5FAT
Coconut Cream Pie, $^1/_8$	275	14	170	1½CHO+3FAT
$^1/_6$	365	19	220	2½CHO+4FAT
Key Lime Pie, $^1/_6$	460	20	na	3½CHO+4FAT
Lemon Meringue Pie, $^1/_8$	350	15	260	2½CHO+3FAT
$^1/_6$	465	20	345	3½CHO+4FAT
Meringue only for $^1/_8$ pie	45	0	27	½CHO
$^1/_6$ pie	60	0	36	¾CHO
Pecan Pie, $^1/_8$	430	24	230	2½CHO+5FAT
$^1/_6$	570	32	310	3½CHO+6½FAT
Strawberry w/Glaze & whipped topping, $^1/_8$	450	28	na	1½CHO+1FR+5½FAT
Pudding:				
Bread Pudding, ½ c	235	7	290	2CHO+1FAT
Chocolate, ½ c	240	9	110	½WhMk+1½CHO+ 1FAT
Butterscotch, ½ c	200	4	130	½WhMk+1¼CHO+ 1FAT
Vanilla, ½ c	220	8	100	½WhMk+1½CHO+ 1FAT
Rice, ½ c	190	5	50	1ST+1FR+1FAT
Scones, triangular wedge (2"X2"X2¾")	101	5	124	1ST+1FAT
Tiramisu, $^1/_8$ of 9" pan	220	14	na	1CHO+3FAT
Turnover, Fruit	330	15	306	2CHO+½FR+3FAT
Trifle including ½ c pudding, fruit, & 1½ ladyfinger	300	15	60	1ST+1FR+3FAT
Truffles, 1 Chocolate ball	80	7	4	1½FAT
1 Chocolate Nut ball	105	10	4	2FAT
Zabaglione, (Italian frothy egg pudding), ½ c	108	6	10	¾CHO+1FAT

American Style Restaurants & Cafeterias

American Style Restaurants

The general category of "American" restaurants actually encompasses a broad range of restaurants and menu items. American restaurants offer the more popular menu selections from a wide range of ethnic cuisine such as Italian, Mexican, and Chinese along with items normally considered standard American fare such as hamburgers and French fries. Some of the restaurants in this chapter have a diverse menu that they can be considered "eclectic." You are very likely to get food items prepared the way you want, but you will need to be very specific with your requests. Refer to the previous chapters entitled: *Appetizers*, *Beverages*, *Soups*, *Salads*, *Breads & Spreads*, *Entrees & Sauces*, *Accompaniments*, and *Desserts* for more detailed information about how to dine lean in American Style Restaurants.

Cafeterias

Cafeterias are popular places to eat because of their quick service, relatively low cost, and the wide variety of foods available. Whether you get a nutritious, well-balanced meal, however, is often up to you. You might eat less fat simply because the cafeteria portion sizes are usually smaller than in most full-service restaurants. But, unless you are careful, cafeterias can add quite a bit more fat (and subsequently more calories) into your meal than you might think. Here are some ideas to consider when you visit a cafeteria.

✓ **Special order your meal.** Although it appears that you would have to select your food from those displayed, most cafeteria managers say they are willing to cater to your specific nutritional needs. Most are willing to steam vegetables and cook meats without additional fat. Since salad dressing can not be added to tossed salad until close to service, often fresh salad without salad dressing is available if you just ask. You can ask for a roll without the usual butter glaze. Just be prepared though; with special request will come longer waits.

✔ **Talk to the manager.** Ask your local cafeteria manager how they would like to handle special requests. They may allow you to call ahead with your specifications. Some cafeteria managers will ask you to approach the person at the end of the line to make your requests and then get back in line. By the time you advance in the line, your meal will be ready!

✔ **Remove as much fat as you can.** If the cafeteria doesn't permit special requests or you are unwilling to wait, deal with the food yourself. Drain off the excess butter, oil, or salad dressing into an empty dish, trim your meat, and remove the skin from the poultry.

✔ **Take advantage of the small platter special.** Most cafeterias offer a plate that consists of a half portion of meat, two vegetables, and a serving of bread. Choose the meal from the lower fat options including salads with fat-free dressing, fresh fruit, lean protein (beef, ham, baked poultry or fish), vegetables with little added fat, and yeast rolls without the butter glaze.

Your Favorite American Style Restaurants & Cafeterias

BENNIGAN'S®

	Calories	Fat (g)	Sodium (mg)	Exchanges
Health Club Menu Items:				
Health Club™ Chicken Fajitas	783	15	na	5ST+3V+6LM
Health Club™ Chicken Platter	700	9	na	4ST+2V+6LM
Health Club™ Vegetable Lasagna	600	14	na	4ST+3V+3MFM
Health Club™ Club Sandwich	450	10	na	3ST+2V+3LM
Health Club™ Chicken Sandwich	498	8	na	4ST+2V+3LM
Health Club™ Cookie Sundae	807	7	na	2FR+7CHO+1½FAT

BOB EVANS®

Lunch: Salads can be ordered without cheese. Low fat salad dressings include Light Italian and Fat-Free Ranch. The Grilled Chicken Salad includes 3½ oz chicken (cooked wt). Salads are served with fresh baked bread; choose the yeast rolls instead of biscuits.

Order sandwich buns to be grilled *dry* for hamburgers and other grilled sandwiches. The leanest sandwich is the Grilled Chicken Sandwich with BBQ sauce instead of honey mustard.

BOB EVANS® (continued)

Dinner: Leaner dinner entrees, available upon request, include the Grilled Chicken or the Barbecued Chicken. Choose dinner rolls to be served with dinner. The side dishes lowest in fat include Green Beans, Fresh Garden Salad with low calorie salad dressing on the side, Long Grain & Wild Rice, Applesauce, Cottage Cheese, and Baked Potato (with toppings on the side). Also try the Chicken Vegetable Pasta with Light Italian dressing or BBQ sauce instead of the Alfredo sauce. Fruit cup is available for dessert.

BOSTON MARKET

	Calories	Fat (g)	Sodium (mg)	Exchanges
Entrees:				
¼ White Meat Chicken, no skin or wing	160	4	350	4½VLM
¼ White Meat Chicken with skin	330	17	530	6LM
¼ Dark Meat Chicken, no skin	210	10	320	4LM
¼ Dark Meat Chicken with skin	330	22	460	4½MFM
½ Chicken with skin	630	37	960	6LM+4½MFM
Skinless Rotisserie Turkey Breast	170	1	850	5VLM
Ham with Cinnamon Apples	350	13	1750	3MFM+2FR
Meat Loaf & Chunky Tomato Sauce	370	18	1170	4MFM+1½ST
Meat Loaf & Brown Gravy	390	22	1040	1ST+4MFM
Original Chicken Pot Pie	750	34	2380	5ST+3HFM+1V+2FAT
Chunky Chicken Salad	370	27	790	4LM+3FAT
Soups, Salads, and Sandwiches:				
Caesar Salad Entree	520	43	1420	2HFM+3V+5FAT
Caesar Salad without Dressing	240	13	780	2HFM+3V
Chicken Caesar Salad	670	47	1860	1ST+4LM+2HFM+4FAT
Chicken Soup	80	3	470	1V+1LM
Chicken Tortilla Soup	220	11	1410	1ST+1LM+2FAT
Chicken Sandwich w/Cheese & Sauce	750	33	1860	4ST+5LM+3½FAT
Chicken SW, no Sauce or Cheese	430	4.⁵	910	4ST+4VLM
Chicken Salad Sandwich	680	30	1360	4ST+4MFM+2FAT
Turkey SW w/Cheese & Sauce	710	28	1390	4½ST+5MFM
Turkey SW, no Cheese or Sauce	400	3.⁵	1070	4ST+3VLM
Ham Sandwich w/Cheese & Sauce	760	35	1880	4½ST+4MFM+3FAT
Ham SW, no Cheese or Sauce	450	9	1600	4½ST+2MFM
Meat Loaf Sandwich w/Cheese	860	33	2270	6ST+4MFM+2½FAT
Meat Loaf Sandwich, no Cheese	690	21	1610	5ST+3½MFM+½FAT
Ham & Turkey Club Sandwich w/Cheese & Sauce	890	44	2350	5ST+5HFM
Ham & Turkey Club Sandwich, no Cheese or Sauce	430	6	1330	4ST+2½LM

BOSTON MARKET (continued)

	Calories	Fat (g)	Sodium (mg)	Exchanges
Hot Side Dishes:				
Steamed Vegetables, $^2/_3$ c	35	0.^{5}	35	1V
New Potatoes, ¾ c	130	2.^{5}	150	1½ST
Buttered Corn, ¾ c	180	4	170	2ST+1FAT
Zucchini Marinara, ¾ c	80	4	470	2V+1FAT
Mashed Potatoes, $^2/_3$ c	180	8	390	1½ST+1½FAT
Mashed Potatoes & Gravy, ¾ c	200	9	560	1½ST+2FAT
Chicken Gravy, 2Tbs	15	1	170	FREE
Rice Pilaf, $^2/_3$ c	180	5	600	2ST+1FAT
Creamed Spinach, ¾ c	280	21	820	½ST+1V+1HFM+3FAT
Stuffing, ¾ c.	310	12	1140	3ST+2FAT
Butternut Squash, ¾ c	160	6	580	1½ST+1FAT
Macaroni & Cheese, ¾ c	280	10	760	1½ST+1MFM+1FAT
BBQ Baked Beans, ¾ c	330	9	630	3½ST+1LM+1FAT
Hot Cinnamon Apples, ¾ c	250	4.^{5}	45	3½FR+1FAT
Green Bean Casserole, ¾ c	90	4.^{5}	580	2V+1FAT
Cool Side Dishes:				
Fruit Salad, ¾ c	70	0.^{5}	10	1FR
Mediterranean Pasta Salad, ¾ c	170	10	490	1ST+2FAT
Cranberry Relish, ¾ c	370	5	5	5½FR+1FAT
Cole Slaw, ¾ c	280	16	520	2V+1½ST+3FAT
Tortellini Salad, ¾ c	380	24	530	2ST+1MFM+4FAT
Caesar Side Salad, 4 oz	210	17	560	1V+1HFM+2FAT
Baked Goods:				
Corn Bread, 1 loaf	200	6	390	2ST+1FAT
Oatmeal Raisin Cookie	320	13	260	3ST+2½FAT
Chocolate Chip Cookie	340	17	240	3ST+3FAT
Brownie	450	27	190	3ST+5½FAT
Honey Wheat Roll, 1 roll	300	3	560	3½ST+½FAT

Current as of 11/07/97. Please call Boston Market™ Customer Service Department at 1-800-365-7000 for info on new menu items, menu revisions, or specific ingredient info.

CHILI'S®

	Calories	Fat (g)	Sodium (mg)	Exchanges
Guiltless Grill Menu Items (less than 30% of calories from fat):				
GG Veggie Pasta	680	13	na	na
GG Veggie Pasta with Chicken	786	15	na	na
GG Chicken Platter	563	9	na	na
GG Veggie Skewers	474	10	na	na
GG Chicken Sandwich	527	8	na	na
GG Chicken Salad with Dressing	272	5	na	na
Diet By Chocolate Cake w/Yogurt & Fudge Topping	534	3	na	na

COUNTRY KITCHEN®

Right Choice™ Menu Items:	Calories	Fat (g)	Sodium (mg)	Exchanges
Salads (ask for reduced calorie dressing):				
Grilled Chicken Salad	615	23	na	na
Calico Bean Soup & Salad	360	14	na	na
Sandwiches (request fresh fruit instead of fries):				
Grilled Chicken Breast Sandwich	525	21	na	na
French Dip	645	19	na	na
Philly Beef and Cheese	850	27	na	na
Entrees (request a Right Choice™ side dish):				
Beef and Broccoli Stir-Fry	530	18	na	na
Chicken Stir-Fry	420	10	na	na
Oriental Chicken & Fried Rice	465	15	na	na
Herb Chicken with Fresh Tomato Pasta	735	15	na	na
Grilled Chicken Dinner	290	9	na	na
Chicken Stir-Fry Pita (request fresh fruit instead of fries)	385	3	na	na
Side Dish Choices:				
Apple Sauce	90	0	na	na
Glazed Baby Carrots	100	3	na	na
Dinner Salad w/ reduced calorie dressing	170	8	na	na
Baked Potato w/sour cream only	280	6	na	na
Rice Pilaf	70	1	na	na
Cup of Calico Bean Soup	125	4	na	na
Vegetable of the Day	110	6	na	na
Cottage Cheese	105	2	na	na
Children:				
Chicken Strips	500	24	na	na
Kid's Burger	500	24	na	na

DENNY'S®

	Calories	Fat (g)	Sodium (mg)	Exchanges
Fit Fare™ Soups, Sandwiches, & Salads:				
Garden Chicken Delite, w/out dressing	277	5	785	3V+1ST+4VLM
Side Garden Salad, w/out dressing	113	4	147	½ST+1V+1FAT
Fat Free Honey Mustard, 1 oz	38	0	121	½ST
Reduced Calorie Italian, 1 oz	23	1	515	FREE
Vegetable Beef Soup	79	1	820	1ST
Grilled Chicken Sandwich	434	9	1206	4ST+3½VLM

DENNY'S® (continued)

	Calories	Fat (g)	Sodium (mg)	Exchanges
Other Salads (w/out dressing & bread, unless noted):				
Fried Chicken Salad	506	31	1174	3V+1ST+4½MFM+ 1FAT
Oriental Chicken Salad, w/dressing	568	26	1656	3V+2ST+4LM+3FAT
Grilled Chicken Caesar, w/dressing	655	47	1728	1V+1ST+5MFM+4FAT
Buffalo Chicken Salad	615	37	1258	2½ST+4½HFM
Garden Chicken Delite	277	3	785	3V+1ST+4VLM
Side Caesar, w/dressing	338	25	725	1ST+1V+5FAT
Condiments (1 oz unless specified):				
Bleu Cheese Dressing	124	12	405	2FAT
Caesar Dressing	142	15	340	3FAT
French Dressing	106	10	274	2FAT
Reduced Calorie French Dressing	76	5	265	1FAT+½CHO
Fat Free Honey Mustard	38	0	121	½ST
Creamy Italian Dressing	106	10	306	2FAT
Ranch Dressing	101	11	215	2FAT
Reduced Calorie Italian	23	1	515	1FREE
Ranch Dressing	101	11	215	2FAT
Thousand Island Dressing	104	10	208	2FAT
Sour Cream, 1.^{5} oz	91	9	23	2FAT
BBQ Sauce, 1.^{5} oz	47	1	595	1CHO
Horseradish Sauce, 1.^{5} oz	170	20	227	4FAT
Oriental Peanut Dressing	106	8	399	2FAT
Mayonnaise, approx 2T	200	22	159	4½FAT
Other Soups (8 oz):				
Vegetable Beef	79	1	820	1ST
Chicken Noodle	60	2	640	½ST+½FAT
Cream of Potato	222	12	761	1½ST+2FAT
Cream of Broccoli	193	12	818	1ST+2FAT
Cheese	293	23	895	1ST+½HFM+4FAT
Clam Chowder	214	11	903	1½ST+2FAT
Split Pea	146	6	819	1½ST+1FAT
Appetizers (without condiments):				
Sampler	1120	59	3430	7ST+4HFM+5FAT
Buffalo Wings, 12	856	54	5552	13LM+3FAT
Mozzarella Sticks, 8 w/sauce	756	43	5423	3½ST+4HFM+2FAT
Chicken Quesadilla	827	55	1982	3½ST+6½MFM+4FAT
Buffalo Chicken Strips	734	42	1673	3ST+6MFM+2FAT
Chicken Strips, 5	720	33	1666	3½ST+1CHO+5MFM+ 1½FAT
Onion Ring Basket, 7	439	27	1158	3ST+5FAT

DENNY'S® (continued)

	Calories	Fat (g)	Sodium (mg)	Exchanges
Other Sandwiches (you may substitute tomato slices or vegetables *instead* of french fries – *neither* is included in nutritional information):				
French Dip, add horseradish sauce	531	16	1948	3½ST+4½LM
Fried Fish Sandwich	905	56	1778	3ST+3HFM+6FAT
Club Sandwich	718	38	1740	4ST+3HFM+2FAT
Chicken Melt Sandwich	520	29	1170	3ST+2½HFM+2FAT
Super Bird	620	32	1954	3½ST+2½HFM+1FAT
Classic Burger	673	40	1142	3ST+4½MFM+3FAT
Classic Burger w/Cheese	836	53	1595	3ST+6MFM+4½FAT
Charleston Chicken™, add honey mustard or mayo dressing	632	32	1967	3½ST+4HFM
Bacon Cheddar Burger	935	63	na	3ST+7MFM+6FAT
Bacon, Lettuce, & Tomato	634	46	1190	2½ST+1½HFM+7FAT
Patty Melt	695	44	1146	2½ST+4½MFM+3½FAT
Grilled Chicken Sandwich	509	19	1809	3½ST+4VLM
Deluxe Grilled Cheese	482	26	1209	3ST+2½HFM
Delidinger®	852	45	3216	4ST+6HFM+2FAT
Fit Fare™ Entrees (entrée only):				
Grilled Salmon	210	4	103	6VLM
Grilled Chicken Breast	130	4	566	3½VLM
Other Entrees:				
Porterhouse Steak, 14 oz	708	54	713	8MFM+3FAT
T-Bone Steak, 7 oz	530	40	534	6MFM+2FAT
Pork Chop Dinner, 8 oz	386	24	844	5½LM+2FAT
Grilled Alaskan Salmon, 7 oz	296	14	257	6VLM
Battered Cod, 9 oz & tartar sauce	732	47	1335	3ST+3½HFM+4FAT
Chicken Fried Steak, 4 oz	265	17	668	1ST+2HFM
Pot Roast w/gravy, 8 oz	260	11	1085	5½VLM+1FAT
Grilled Chopped Steak, 11 oz	639	44	736	7MFM+2FAT+½ST
Steak & Shrimp, 9 oz	645	42	1143	2ST+4½HFM+1FAT
Shrimp, 8 oz	558	32	1114	3ST+2HMF+3FAT
Roast Turkey & Stuffing, 12 oz	701	27	2346	4ST+5½MFM
Chicken Fried Chicken w/gravy	327	18	993	1ST+3MFM+1FAT
Chicken Strip, 10 oz w/ Honey Mustard Dressing	635	25	1510	3½ST+5MFM
Fit Fare™ Sides:				
Baked Potato, plain	186	0	14	3ST
Rice Pilaf	112	2	328	1½ST
Broccoli in butter sauce	50	2	280	1V+½FAT
Corn in butter sauce	120	4	260	1ST+1FAT
Carrots in honey glaze	80	3	220	½CHO+1V+½FAT
Green Beans with bacon	60	4	390	1V+1FAT
Green Peas in butter sauce	100	2	360	1ST+½FAT

DENNY'S® (continued)

	Calories	Fat (g)	Sodium (mg)	Exchanges
Other Sides:				
French Fries, unsalted, 4 oz	323	14	130	3ST+3FAT
Seasoned Fries, 4 oz	261	12	556	2ST+2½FAT
Onion Rings, 3 oz	264	16	695	2ST+3FAT
Mashed Potatoes, plain, 6 oz	105	1	378	1½ST
Cornbread Stuffing, 2 oz	182	9	405	1ST+2FAT
Hashed Browns, 4 oz	218	14	424	1½ST+2½FAT
Cottage Cheese, 3 oz	72	3	281	1MFM
Applesauce, 3 oz	60	0	13	1FR
Sliced Tomatoes, 3 slices	13	0	6	½V
Brown Gravy, 1 oz	13	0	184	1FREE
Chicken Gravy, 1 oz	14	0.5	139	1FREE
Country Gravy, 1 oz	17	1	93	1FREE
Grilled Mushrooms	14	0	0	1FREE
Dinner Roll	132	2	265	1½ST
Herb Toast	200	11	372	1½ST+2FAT
Pies ($^1/_6$ pie):				
Apple Pie	430	20	390	2ST+1FR+1CHO+4FAT
Apple Pie w/Equal	370	20	360	2ST+1FR+4FAT
Cherry Pie	540	21	430	2ST+1FR+2½CHO+ 4FAT
Chocolate Pecan Pie	790	37	460	2ST+5CHO+7½FAT
Coconut Cream Pie	480	26	440	2ST+2CHO+5FAT
Cheesecake Pie	470	27	280	1ST+2CHO+5½FAT
3 oz Blueberry topping	106	0	15	1FR+½CHO
3 oz Strawberry topping	115	1	12	1FR+½CHO
3 oz Cherry topping	86	0	5	1FR+½CHO
Dutch Apple Pie	440	19	290	2ST+1FR+1CHO+4FAT
French Silk Pie	650	43	220	1ST+3CHO+8½FAT
German Chocolate Pie	580	33	460	1ST+3CHO+6½FAT
Key Lime Pie	600	27	300	1ST+4CHO+5½FAT
Lemon Meringue Pie	460	17	310	1½ST+3CHO+3½FAT
Pecan Pie	600	28	430	2ST+3CHO+5½FAT
Other Desserts:				
Chocolate Cake	370	17	374	1ST+2CHO+3½FAT
Hot Fudge Cake Sundae	687	38	486	2ST+3CHO+7½FAT
Banana Split Sundae	894	43	177	3ST+2½CHO+2FR+ 8½FAT
Double Scoop Sundae w/out toppings	375	27	86	2CHO+5½FAT
Single Scoop Sundae w/out toppings	188	14	43	1CHO+3FAT
Chocolate Shake/Malt	579	27	278	1WhMk+4CHO+4FAT
Vanilla Shake Malt	581	27	236	1WhMk+4CHO+4FAT
Ice Cream Float	280	10	109	3CHO+2FAT

DENNY'S® (continued)

Toppings (2 oz *or* 4 Tbsp):	Calories	Fat (g)	Sodium (mg)	Exchanges
Chocolate Topping	317	25	83	1½CHO+5FAT
Blueberry Topping	71	0	10	1CHO
Cherry Topping	57	0	3	1CHO
Fudge Topping	201	10	96	2CHO+2FAT
Strawberry Topping	77	1	8	1CHO

FURR'S CAFETERIA®

Furr's cafeteria offers an All-You-Can-Eat concept, By-The-Item pricing, or the Delight Plate. The Delight Plate includes a full portion of an entrée with 2 vegetables. The leanest are the Baked Fish (remove bread topping), Roast Beef, and Baked Chicken (remove skin). Portion sizes are about 3 oz cooked. Sugar-free Jello is always available. Light salad dressings are offered; all salad dressings may also be requested *on the side*. Fresh strawberries (without the syrup) are available, just ask.

Salads:	Calories	Fat (g)	Sodium (mg)	Exchanges
Furr's Fruit Salad	120	2	7	1½FR+½FAT
Five Cup Fruit Salad	181	9	57	1½FR+2FAT
German Potato Salad	304	12	762	2½ST+2½FAT
Cauliflower Salad	205	16	670	2V+3FAT
Broccoli & Cauliflower Salad	206	16	672	2V+3FAT
Crunchy Vegetable Salad	144	10	349	2V+2FAT
Sweet Slaw with Nutrasweet	62	4	225	1V+1FAT
Three Bean Salad	145	6	381	1ST+1V+1FAT
Sweet Slaw	141	8	331	1V+½FR+1½FAT
Spanish Slaw	63	3	635	1½V+½FAT
Apple Cabbage Slaw	179	17	126	½V+½FR+3FAT
Carrot Cabbage Slaw	129	10	95	1V+½FR+2FAT
Coleslaw with Sour Cream	64	4	104	1V+1FAT
Colorado Coleslaw	163	13	312	1V+½FR+2½FAT
Country Corn Coleslaw	107	6	320	1V+½ST+1FAT
Cream Slaw w/Raisins Pineapple	153	12	93	1V+½FR+2½FAT
Health Slaw	108	8	68	1½V+1½FAT
Old Fashioned Coleslaw	53	3	450	1V+½FAT
Red Coleslaw	114	11	147	1V+2FAT
Sweet and Sour Slaw	221	10	697	1½V+1½FR+2FAT
Carrot Coconut Pineapple Salad	189	16	133	1V+½FR+3FAT
Carrot and Raisin Salad	127	7	171	1V+½FR+1½FAT
Cauliflower and Olive Salad	171	18	533	½V+3½FAT
Copper Carrot Salad	229	9	448	2V+1½FR+2FAT
Country Style Cucumbers	137	12	559	½V+½FR+2½FAT
Cucumber Salad	42	1	538	1½V
Cucumber in Sour Cream & Mayo	261	25	299	½V+½FR+5FAT
Avocado and Diced Tomato Salad	277	22	653	3V+4½FAT
Carrot Ambrosia	201	8	57	1½V+1½FR+1½FAT

FURR'S CAFETERIA® (continued)

	Calories	Fat (g)	Sodium (mg)	Exchanges
Entrees:				
Mexican Chicken Casserole, 8 oz	517	31	1415	1½ST+4MFM+2FAT
Barbecued Pork Tips, 6 oz pork + 1 c rice	447	19	524	3ST+2MFM+2FAT
Apple Pork Oriental, 6 oz pork + 6 oz rice	550	21	529	3ST+2MFM+1FR+2FAT
Beef and Green Chili Casserole, 8 oz	621	47	1112	1ST+4½HFM+2FAT
Liver and Onions	562	35	576	2ST+3LM+5FAT
Peppery Beef Stir Fry	471	8	597	4ST+2LM+1V+½FAT
Chicken Fried Steak w/ Gravy	626	44	1181	2ST+3HFM+4FAT
Chicken Fry w/Pan Fry Potato	789	51	1387	3½ST+3HFM+5FAT
Side Dishes:				
Lemon Celery Rice Pilaf	241	10	699	2ST+2FAT
Almond Rice Pilaf	232	10	603	2ST+2FAT
Cranberry Orange Relish	232	0	1	4FR
Cranberry Cream	216	7	10	2½FR+1½FAT
Sweet Potato Soufflé	395	17	379	2ST+1½FR+3½FAT
Almond Rice	211	10	445	1½ST+2FAT
Fruited Rice	250	7	39	2ST+1FR+1½FAT
Carrots, Asparagus, Squash	77	3	423	1½V+½FAT
Broccoli w/ Lemon Butter	119	11	377	1V+2FAT
Steamed Broccoli	56	4	283	1V+1FAT
Brussel Sprouts Almondine	111	7	338	1V+1½FAT
Steamed Brussel Sprouts	70	4	284	1V+1FAT
Steamed Cabbage	42	3	315	½V+½FAT
German Boiled Cabbage	90	3	365	2V+½FAT
Scalloped Cabbage	151	9	575	2V+2FAT
Bacon Fried Carrots	106	4	427	2V+1FAT
Braised Carrots and Onion	86	4	354	1½V+1FAT
Carrots and Green Onions	74	2	415	2V+½FAT
Carrots Supreme	121	5	504	2V+1FAT
Glazed Carrots and Celery	128	5	393	1V+1FR+1FAT
Scalloped Corn	272	11	781	2½ST+2FAT
Whole Kernel Corn	152	4	281	2ST+1FAT
Sautéed Mushrooms	148	15	563	1V+3FAT
Green Beans	125	9	820	1V+2FAT
Blackeyed Peas	106	5	468	1MFM+1V
Harlequin Rice	168	4	596	1½ST+1FAT
Seasoned Spinach	63	4	305	1V+½HFM
Breads:				
Jalapeno Cornbread, 3.³ oz	213	9	298	1½ST+2FAT
Cornbread Muffins, 1	176	5	229	1½ST+1FAT
Hard Rolls, 3.⁸ oz	272	5	529	3ST+1FAT
Applesauce Spice Muffins, 1	267	13	76	1ST+1½FR+2½FAT
Brown Sugar Muffins, 1	316	6	245	2ST+2FR+1FAT

FURR'S CAFETERIA® (continued)

	Calories	Fat (g)	Sodium (mg)	Exchanges
Desserts:				
Pumpkin Cake Roll, 1 slice	359	18	273	3ST+3½FAT
Texas Sheet Cake w/Icing	577	28	448	2ST+3FR+5½FAT
Oatmeal Cake, 3"X4"	492	24	297	2ST+2FR+5FAT
Rocky Road Cake	431	20	323	2ST+2FR+4FAT
Lemon Chess Pie	481	21	270	2ST+2½FR+4FAT
Millionaire Pie	427	26	277	1ST+2FR+5FAT
Pecan Pie	584	23	287	2ST+4FR+4½FAT
Pumpkin Pie	333	16	200	2ST+1FR+3FAT
German Chocolate Pie	425	21	446	2ST+1½FR+4FAT
Cool Lime Pie	436	19	278	1ST+3½FR+4FAT
Holiday Billionaire Pie	371	16	286	2ST+1½FR+3FAT
Raspberry Ribbon Pie	359	20	205	2ST+4FAT
Sour Cream Cheese Cake, w/out topping	334	21	204	2ST+4FAT
Butter Chess Pie	486	23	302	2ST+2½FR+4½FAT
Buttermilk Pie	587	36	363	4ST+7FAT
French Pineapple Pie	463	26	383	2ST+1½FR+5FAT
Surprise Pecan Pie	349	18	148	2ST+1FR+3½FAT
Coconut Custard	420	19	257	2ST+1½FR+4FAT
Strawberry Ambrosia	438	25	305	1ST+2½FR+5FAT
No Sugar Added Pies ($^1/_7$ pie):				
Strawberry	194	12	204	1ST+2½FAT
Cherry Cream	338	20	249	1ST+1FR+4FAT
Peach Cream	319	18	260	1ST+1FR+3½FAT
Pineapple Cream	322	18	224	2ST+3½FAT
Banana Cream	312	17	207	1ST+1FR+2½FAT
Strawberry Cream	307	18	224	2ST+3½FAT
Lemon Ice Box	245	16	194	1½ST+3FAT

Two No Sugar Added pies are offered daily and labeled with a sticker. One is a Fruit Pie and the other is a Cream Pie. Both are sweetened with Equal® sweetener.

GOLDEN CORRAL®

Golden Corral has started a "Wise Choice" labeling program in all of their restaurants. This program uses the Wise Choice Owl to label individual products on the buffet that are healthier choices. In some cases the label will state "fat free" or list the fat grams. Golden Corral offers an abundance of fresh vegetables and fruits, fat-free salad dressings, fresh carved meats (including roast turkey, steamed fish and/or baked chicken), fat free and low fat soft serves, and fresh baked bread that all fit into a healthy diet.

HOULIHAN'S®

Entrees:	Calories	Fat (g)	Sodium (mg)	Exchanges
Grilled Chicken Breast	229	6	na	3ST+2LM
Vegetable Stir Fry	355	18	na	2ST+1LM+3FAT
Vegetable Fajitas	275	10	na	1ST+3V+2FAT
Soups:				
Vegetable Soup	117	2	na	1ST+1V+½FAT
Tortilla Soup	205	5	na	2ST+1FAT
Black Bean Soup	240	10	na	1½ST+2LM+1FAT

HOUSTON'S®

No nutritional information is available. The following information is provided to assist in making healthy choices. All weights referred to uncooked portion sizes.

Grilled fish (salmon, swordfish, or halibut) is oiled prior to putting on the grill to prevent sticking to the wood-burning grill. You can request it without the butter baste; fish is still seasoned. Portions are about 9 oz at lunch and 10 oz at dinner. Roasted chicken is a half of a chicken (remove the skin prior to eating). The Barbecue Chicken is a 10 oz boneless breast. You can request it to be grilled without the skin and/or barbecue sauce. The leanest beef portion is the Filet Mignon, a 10 oz portion.

The Traditional Salad can be requested without the chopped egg & bacon and dressing on the side. The Grilled Chicken Salad has 6 oz of grilled chicken. Request both the Honey Lime Vinaigrette and Light Peanut Sauce on the side for your control. Plenty of flavored vinegars (Red Wine, Balsamic, and Apple Cider) or picante sauce are available for a low fat dressing.

The leanest side choices include a 10 oz Baked Potato (request dry), Black Beans with Brown Rice, Couscous, and the Iron Skillet Beans. Fresh Fruit is available in season and can be ordered macerated (softened & tenderized) with balsalmic vinegar and sugar is available for dessert (request without the creme fraise).

HYATT®

Hyatt® Hotels offer "Cuisine Naturelle", items that are lower in calories, but more importantly, represent a balance of necessary nutrients and exceptional flavor. Each dish is created from wholesome foods whose flavors have been enhanced by herbs and the freshness of the product itself. These items are available in Hyatt's Three Meal Restaurants and through Room Service.

MOZZARELLAS AMERICAN CAFE

Several items, with less than 12 grams of fat, are noted on the menu with a heart. These include the following:

Veggie Tator - baked potato topped with fresh roasted vegetables and marinara sauce

Roasted Veggie Pasta - marinara served with roasted fresh vegetables on a bed of spaghetti

Orange Dijon Chicken - 2 skewers of chicken, grilled and brushed with orange dijon sauce, and served on a bed of steamed rice with our vegetable of the day

Sinless Berry Sundae - a dessert made of fat free vanilla ice cream topped w/choice of homemade raspberry strawberry sauce, chocolate sauce, or caramel

Other menu items which can be modified to contain less fat include:

Garden Salad without croutons, cheese, or almonds

Vegetarian Entrée Salad without cheese

Black Bean Vegetarian Burger (request without cheese or mayo)

Roasted Vegetable Sandwich (ask for without cheese and for the bread not to be brushed with oil)

Sierra Grill without cheese or mayo

The Roasted Veggie Pizza can be ordered with less cheese.

Other Tips: The leanest side orders are the Roasted Vegetables and the dry baked potato. Two low calorie dressings are available: Ranch (20 calories/T) and Italian (18 calories/T). Try the low calorie Ranch dressing or Salsa on the baked potato.

OUTBACK® STEAKHOUSE

The leanest entrees are the Chicken Barbie and the Grilled Fish. All weights refer to uncooked weights. Chicken on the Barbie is an 8 oz grilled chicken breast served with barbecue sauce. Grilled Fish, an 11 oz portion, varies daily. Fish choices may be Grouper, Mahi-Mahi, Tuna, Swordfish, or Salmon. The grilled chicken and fish are both brushed with butter prior to flamed broiling, but you may request them without it. Both entrees are served with Fresh Vegetables (request without seasoned butter).

The smallest steak is a 9 oz tenderloin filet; ask for it to be prepared without the clarified butter. Jacket Potato (a Baked Potato) can be served dry or with toppings on the side.

Tangy Tomato Dressing, a non-fat salad dressing, is available upon request. It contains 45 calories per 2T.

PERKINS® FAMILY RESTAURANT

The flexibility and wide variety of wholesome, traditional American foods offered by Perkins allow guests to select food suited to their lifestyles, health needs and taste preferences. Guests interested in products with lower fat and cholesterol may choose from a variety of grilled entrees, including skinless chicken breasts, as well as salads; no fat salad dressings; egg and sugar substitutes; lite syrup; low-fat milk; hot and cold cereals; fresh fruit and low-fat muffins. Because Perkins cooks to order, our guests can and do ask that we adapt our standard recipes to meet special dietary requests.

PICCADILLY CAFETERIA®

Piccadilly Cafeteria is willing to satisfy most special dietary requests. Call ahead to make your request or go to the beginning of the line and ask to speak to the manager. All weights listed below refer to uncooked weights.

Fresh fruits and many salads without dressing are offered. Low fat Ranch salad dressing and fat-free Italian and Ranch salad dressings can be requested. Sugar Free Jello is often available.

The "Dilly Dish" offers a choice of a selected entree, two vegetables, and bread. The leanest Dilly Dish entrees include: Baked Cod, Roast Beef, Quartered Chicken (remove the skin), and Carved Turkey Breast. Each are approximately 4 oz uncooked servings. Another lean entree is the boneless, skinless chicken breast (6 oz) or the baked catfish (6 oz). The leanest steak is the 6 oz choice filet (remove the bacon). The fish is kept on the food line in a sauce that contains mostly chicken broth and is thickened with an oleo/flour roux.

Many vegetables such as broccoli and squash are steamed. The fats are added just before being brought out to the line so you may be able to ask for your portion to be served without fat. Baked potatoes are served dry.

Yeast rolls are 2 oz in weight. Often you can request a roll to be served before it has been brushed with butter. Sugar-free desserts are often served. Lowfat or skim milk is also available.

QUINCYS® FAMILY STEAK HOUSE

Beef:	Calories	Fat (g)	Sodium (mg)	Exchanges
Chopped Steak, 8 oz	499	42	348	4½HFM+1FAT
Country Steak/Gravy, 8 oz	530	25	1161	3HFM+3ST
Filet w/Bacon, 8 oz	340	17	311	7VLM+2FAT
Ribeye Steak, 10 oz	452	29	156	6MFM
Junior Sirloin Steak, 5.5 oz	194	10	199	3½LM
Regular Sirloin Steak, 8 oz	285	16	317	5LM
Large Sirloin Steak, 10 oz	368	20	390	6½LM
Sirloin Tips w/peppers & onions	203	8	793	3½LM+1V
Sirloin Tips w/mushroom gravy	196	7	578	3½LM+1V
T-Bone Steak, 13 oz	521	35	265	7MFM
Cowboy Steak, 14 oz	580	33	1308	8½LM+2FAT

QUINCYS® FAMILY STEAK HOUSE (continued)

	Calories	Fat (g)	Sodium (mg)	Exchanges
Beef continued:				
NY Strip Steak, 10 oz	450	26	156	7½LM+1FAT
Smothered Strip Steak, 10 oz	622	41	239	7½MFM+2V+½FAT
Porterhouse Steak, 17 oz	683	46	346	9MFM
Other Entrees:				
Grilled Chicken, Regular 5 oz	120	2	540	3½VLM
Homestyle Chicken Fillet, 3 oz	217	9	682	1½MFM+1½ST
Grilled Salmon, 7 oz	228	4	112	6½VLM
Southern Breaded Shrimp, 7 oz	546	31	821	3ST+2HFM+2FAT
Steak & Shrimp, 9 oz	677	39	816	6MFM+2ST+2FAT
Roasted Herb Chicken, 14 oz	875	65	1238	10MFM+3FAT
Roasted BBQ Chicken, 14 oz	941	65	1548	10MFM+3FAT+1ST
Breads:				
Banana Nut, 2 oz	165	7	195	1½ST+1½FAT
Biscuit, 2 oz	270	15	610	2ST+3FAT
Cornbread, 2 oz	140	5	340	1½ST+1FAT
Yeast Roll, 2 oz	160	4	285	2ST+1FAT
Side Items:				
BBQ Beans	114	1	604	1½ST
Cinnamon Apples	172	5	149	1FR+1½CHO
Steak Fries	358	19	245	3ST+4FAT
Green Beans	61	4	796	1V+1FAT
Corn	96	1	271	1½ST
Mashed Potatoes	54	6	195	1ST
Baked Potato, plain	115	0	0	1½ST
Broccoli Spears	34	0	50	1V
Broccoli Spears w/cheese sauce	92	5	262	1V+1FAT
Rice Pilaf	119	2	1283	1½CHO
Sandwiches (w/out condiments/mayo):				
Bacon Cheese Burger	663	41	997	5HFM+2ST
⅓ pound Hamburger	565	33	603	4HFM+2ST
Philly Cheese Steak	588	30	1684	4½MFM+2½ST+1FAT
Smothered Steak Sandwich	429	15	846	4LM+2ST+1FAT
Grilled Chicken Sandwich	324	4	1183	4VLM+2½ST
Spicy BBQ Chicken Sandwich	368	5	1608	4VLM+3ST
Salad Dressing (2 T):				
Bleu Cheese	155	16	165	3FAT
French	125	12	500	2½FAT
Honey Mustard	100	6	220	1CHO+1FAT
Italian	135	14	230	3FAT
Light Creamy Italian	65	4	485	½CHO+1FAT
Light French	85	4	285	1CHO+1FAT
Light Italian	20	2	485	½FAT

QUINCYS® FAMILY STEAK HOUSE (continued)

	Calories	Fat (g)	Sodium (mg)	Exchanges
Salad Dressing (2 T) continued:				
Light Thousand Island	65	4	340	½CHO+1FAT
Parmesan Peppercorn	150	14	280	¼CHO+3FAT
Ranch	110	11	195	2FAT
Soups (6 fl oz):				
Chili w/Beans	235	11	920	1½ST+1HFM+½FAT
Clam Chowder	180	9	835	1½ST+2FAT
Cream of Broccoli	170	10	770	1½ST+2FAT
Vegetable Beef	90	2	325	3V+½FAT
Desserts:				
Banana Pudding, 5 oz	240	12	240	1ST+1FR+2½FAT
Brownie Pudding Cake, 4 oz	310	5	395	4½CHO+1FAT
Chocolate Chip Cookie, ½ oz	60	8	35	½CHO+1½FAT
Apple Cobbler, 6 oz	255	8	285	2½CHO+1FR+1½FAT
Cherry Cobbler, 6 oz	410	8	185	2½CHO+1FR+1½FAT
Peach Cobbler, 6 oz	305	8	190	2½CHO+1FR+1½FAT
Frozen Yogurt, 4 oz	135	2	85	2CHO
Caramel Topping, 1 oz	105	1	120	1½CHO
Fudge Topping, 1 oz	105	4	75	1CHO+1FAT
Sugar Cookie, ½ oz	60	3	30	½ST+½FAT

SOUPLANTATION & SWEET TOMATOES

	Calories	Fat (g)	Sodium (mg)	Exchanges - calculated by the author
Fat-Free Signature Prepared Salads (½ c):				
Aunt Doris' Red Pepper Slaw	70	0	480	½CHO+1V
Cucumber Tomato w/chile lime	20	0	20	1V
Marinated Summer Vegetables	80	0	210	3V
Low-Free Signature Prepared Salads (½ c):				
Baja Bean & Cilantro Salad	180	3	190	1ST+1V+½VLM+½FAT
Carrot Raisin Salad	90	3	80	1FR+1V+½FAT
Cowboy Beans Salad	90	2	290	1ST+½FAT
Gemelli Pasta w/chicken in citrus v	130	3	380	1ST+½VLM+½FAT
German Potato Salad	120	3	260	1ST+½FAT
Mandarin Krab Salad	150	3	280	1½FR+½FAT
Mandarin Noodles Salad w/brocc	120	3	380	1ST+1V+½FAT
Mandarin Shells Salad w/almonds	120	3	360	1ST+½FAT
Mediterranean Harvest Salad	120	3	180	1V+½FAT
Moroccan Marinated Vegetables	90	3	230	2V+½FAT
Oriental Ginger Slaw w/krab	70	3	80	1V+½FAT
Southern Dill Potato Salad	120	3	300	1½ST+½FAT
Spicy Southwestern Pasta Salad	130	3	350	1½ST+½FAT
Summer Barley Salad w/blk beans	110	3	280	1ST+½FAT

SOUPLANTATION & SWEET TOMATOES (continued)

	Calories	Fat (g)	Sodium (mg)	Exchanges - calculated by the author
Signature Prepared Salads (½ c):				
Artichoke Rice Salad	160	8	780	1ST+1V+1½FAT
BBQ Potato Salad	160	8	270	1½ST+1½FAT
Carrot Ginger Salad w/herb vinaig.	150	12	40	1V+2½FAT
Chinese Krab Salad	160	8	260	1ST+½VLM+1½FAT
Confetti Pasta w/cheddar & dill	160	9	380	1ST+½HFM+1FAT
Dijon Potato w/garlic dill vinaigr.	140	7	260	1ST+1½FAT
Greek Couscous w/feta cheese	170	9	480	1ST+½HFM+1FAT
Italian White Bean Salad	140	5	480	1ST+1FAT
Jalapeño Potato Salad	140	5	490	1ST+1FAT
Lemon Orzo Salad w/feta & mint	130	5	270	1ST+1FAT
Mazatlan Krab & Pasta Salad	160	9	480	1ST+½VLM+1½FAT
Mediterranean Krab & Rotini Salad	170	10	380	1ST+½VLM+2FAT
Old Fashioned Macaroni w/ham	180	11	360	1ST+2FAT
Pesto Pasta Salad	160	7	320	1ST+1½FAT
Picnic Potato Salad	150	7	320	1ST+1½FAT
Pineapple Coconut Slaw	150	10	190	1FR+2FAT
Poppyseed Coleslaw	120	9	130	2V+2FAT
Roasted Potato Salad with Chipotle Chile Vinaigrette	140	6	250	1ST+1FAT
Spinach Krab Salad	230	12	550	1ST+1V+2½FAT
Thai Noodle Salad w/Peanut Sauce	170	8	310	1ST+1½FAT
Three Bean Marinade Salad	170	6	320	1½ST+1FAT
Tortellini Salad with Basil	170	10	260	1ST+2FAT
Tumbleweed Tortelli Salad	140	9	330	½ST+2FAT
Tuna Tarragon Salad	240	14	480	1½ST+½LM+2½FAT
Turkey Chutney Pasta Salad	230	9	310	1½ST+1LM+1FAT
Zesty Tortellini Salad	190	15	460	1ST+3FAT
Fresh Tossed Salads (1 c):				
Antipasto Salad	140	10	370	1V+½HFM+1FAT
BBQ Chopped Salad	130	9	190	1V+1HFM
California Cobb Salad	180	8	190	1V+1MFM+½FAT
Caribbean Krab Salad	120	7	180	2V+1½FAT
Classic Caesar Salad	190	14	280	2V+3FAT
Country French Salad w/bacon	210	18	420	1V+1HFM+2FAT
Ensalada Azteca	130	9	230	1½V+2FAT
Greek Salad	120	9	320	1V+2FAT
Mandarin Spinach w/carm walnuts	170	11	150	1V+½FR+2FAT
Roasted Vegetables w/feta & olives	140	11	340	1V+2FAT
Roma Tomato, Mozzarella & Basil	120	9	180	1V+½HFM+1FAT
Shrimp & Krab Louis Salad	180	12	340	1V+1LM+1FAT
Sonoma Salad with Artichokes	160	12	640	1V+2½FAT
Spinach & Pasta w/rasp vinaigrette	180	6	620	1ST+1V+1FAT
Traditional Spinach Salad	180	13	360	2V+2½FAT
Won Ton Chicken Salad	150	8	220	½ST+1LM+1FAT

SOUPLANTATION & SWEET TOMATOES (continued)

	Calories	Fat (g)	Sodium (mg)	Exchanges - calculated by the author
Fat-Free Salad Dressings (2T):				
Honey Mustard Dressing	45	0	160	½CHO
Italian Dressing	20	0	340	FREE
Ranch Dressing	50	0	180	½CHO
Low-Fat & Reduced Calorie Salad Dressings (2T):				
Garden Fresh French Tomato	40	1.5	270	½CHO+½FAT
Creamy Cucumber Dressing	80	7	290	1½FAT
Croutons: Parmesan & Garlic Croutons, 10 pieces	40	3	160	½FAT
Salad Dressings (2T):				
Balsamic House Vinaigrete	180	19	190	4FAT
Basil House Vinaigrette	160	17	160	3½FAT
Blue Cheese Dressing	140	14	230	3FAT
Blush Vinaigrette	120	12	320	2½FAT
Honey Ginger Dressing	150	15	200	¼CHO+3FAT
Honey Mustard Dressing	150	13	230	½CHO+2½FAT
Parmesan Pepper Cream Dressing	160	17	330	3½FAT
Ranch House Dressing	130	13	180	2½FAT
Raspberry Vinaigrette	120	13	150	2½FAT
Roasted Garlic Dressing	140	14	300	3FAT
Thousand Island Dressing	110	11	250	2FAT
Zesty Italian Dressing	160	18	280	3½FAT
Low-Fat Soups & Chilies (1 c):				
Chicken Tortilla Soup with Jalapeño Chilies & Tomatoes	100	3	990	1V+1½VLM
Classic Chicken Noodle Soup	160	3	480	1ST+1½LM+½FAT
House Chili	230	3	560	1½ST+1½LM+½FAT
Santa Fe Black Bean Chili	190	3	580	1ST+1VLM+½FAT
Spicy 4-Bean Minestrone	140	3	980	1ST+1V+½FAT
Sweet Tomato Onion Soup	110	3	450	2V+½FAT
Turkey Noodle Soup	170	3	550	1ST+2LM+½FAT
Vegetable Medley Soup	90	1	520	1ST
Soups & Chilies (1 c):				
Albondigas Buenas	190	9	720	1ST+1MFM+1FAT
Arizona Chili	220	8	690	1ST+2MFM
Chesapeake Corn Chowder	310	13	720	2½ST+2½FAT
Chicken Fajitas & Black Bean	280	7	980	1½ST+2½LM
Chicken Jambalaya	160	7	980	1ST+1½LM+1FAT
Chunky Potato Cheese w/Thyme	210	10	480	1ST+1HFM+½FAT
Cream of Broccoli Soup	210	15	960	2V+3FAT
Cream of Chicken Soup	250	15	350	1½ST+1HFM+1½FAT
Cream of Mushroom Soup	290	21	820	½ST+1V+1HFM+2½FAT

SOUPLANTATION & SWEET TOMATOES (continued)

	Calories	Fat (g)	Sodium (mg)	Exchanges - calculated by the author
Soups & Chilies (1 c) continued:				
Green Chile Stew	150	6	980	1V+½ST+1MFM
Irish Potato Leek Soup	260	16	680	1ST+1V+3FAT
Minestrone with Italian Sausage	210	11	890	½ST+1V+1HFM+½FAT
Navy Bean Soup with Ham	340	10	980	1½ST+4LM
New England Clam Chowder	330	20	630	1ST+2LM+3FAT
New Orleans Style Jambalaya	160	8	900	½ST+1V+½MFM+1FAT
Posole	150	6	980	1ST+1FAT
Shrimp Bisque	300	19	880	1ST+1LM+3FAT
Split Pea Soup with Ham	350	10	980	1½ST+4LM
Texas Red Chili	240	8	680	1ST+1V+1HFM
Turkey Vegetable Soup	270	12	990	½ST+1V+2½LM+1FAT
Vegetable Beef Stew	250	14	780	1V+1ST+1MFM+2FAT
Vegetarian Harvest Soup	190	8	990	½ST+2V+1½FAT
Yucatan Chili	280	10	890	1ST+1V+3LM
Hot Tossed Pasta (1 c):				
Bruschetta	260	4	450	2ST+2V+1FAT
Chipotle Chicken w/cilantro	390	16	560	2ST+2½LM+2FAT
Creamy Pesto w/sundried tomatoes	430	21	410	2½ST+1V+1HFM+ 2½FAT
Creamy Bruschetta	360	16	510	2ST+1V+1HFM+1½FAT
Fettucine Alfredo	390	18	580	2½ST+1½HFM+1FAT
Garden Vegetable w/meatballs	270	7	460	2ST+1V+1HFM
Garden Vegetable w/Italian saus.	300	10	540	2ST+1V+1HFM
Italian Vegetable Beef	270	6	470	2ST+1V+1MFM
Jalapeño Salsa	240	4	430	2ST+1V+1MFM
Nutty Mushroom	390	20	410	2ST+1V+1HFM+2½FAT
Smoked Salmon & Dill	360	16	390	2ST+1V+1HFM+1½FAT
Vegetarian Marinara w/basil	260	4	750	2ST+2V+1FAT
Low-Fat Fresh Baked Muffins & Breads (1):				
Apple Cinnamon Bran, Cranberry Orange Bran, *or* Fruit Medley Bran Muffin , 96% fat-free	80	0.5	110	1ST
Buttermilk Corn Bread	140	2	270	1½ST+½FAT
Chile Corn Muffin	140	3	320	1½ST+½FAT
Indian Grain Bread	200	1.5	260	2½ST+½FAT
Sourdough Bread	150	0.5	240	1½ST
Fresh Baked Muffins & Breads (1):				
Apple Raisin, Apricot Nut, Banana Nut, *or* Cherry Nut Muffin	150	7	190	1½ST+1½FAT
Carrot Pineapple Muffin w/Oat Bran	150	6	230	1½ST+1FAT
Choc. Brownie, Choc. Chip, *or* Choc. Chip Mandarin Muffin	170	8	190	1½ST+1½FAT

SOUPLANTATION & SWEET TOMATOES (continued)

	Calories	Fat (g)	Sodium (mg)	Exchanges - calculated by the author
Fresh Baked Muffins & Breads (1) continued:				
Garlic Parmesan Focaccia	100	3	170	1ST+½FAT
Georgia Peach Poppyseed Muffin	150	6	210	1½ST+1FAT
Lemon Muffin	140	4	190	1½ST+1FAT
Mandarin Alm. Muffin w/Oat Bran	140	7	210	1ST+1½FAT
Nutty Peanut Butter Muffin	170	8	210	1½ST+1½FAT
Peanut Butter Choc. Chip Muffin	190	9	230	1½ST+2FAT
Pizza Focaccia	140	6	220	1ST+1FAT
Pumpkin Raisin Muffin	150	6	210	1½ST+1FAT
Roasted Potato Focaccia	150	6	220	1ST+1FAT
Strawberry Buttermilk Muffin	140	6	210	1½ST+1FAT
Tomatillo Focaccia	140	6	270	1ST+1FAT
Wild Maine Blueberry Muffin	140	5	180	1ST+½FR+1FAT
Wild Maine Blueberry Muffin, lg	310	12	380	2ST+1FR+2½FAT
Zucchini Nut Muffin	150	7	190	1½ST+1½FAT
Fat-Free Desserts (½ c unless specified):				
Apple Medley	70	0	5	1CHO
Banana Royale	80	0	5	1CHO
Ghiradelli Choc. Frozen Yogurt	95	0	80	1CHO
Jello, flavored	80	0	40	1CHO
Tropical Fruit Salad	75	0	5	1FR
Low-Fat *or* Reduced Fat Desserts (½ c):				
Chocolate Pudding	140	3	220	1½CHO+½FAT
Nutty Waldorf Salad	80	3	80	1FR+½FAT
Rice Pudding	110	2	50	1ST+½FAT
Tapioca Pudding	140	3	160	1½CHO+½FAT
Vanilla Soft Serve	140	4	70	1½CHO+1FAT
Yogurt Bar Toppings:				
Chocolate Syrup, 2T	70	0	15	1CHO
Candy Sprinkles, 1T	70	2	0	½CHO+½FAT
Granola Topping, 2T	110	4	14	1CHO+1FAT
Desserts:				
Banana Pudding, ½ c	160	4	220	1½CHO+1FAT
Chocolate Chip Cookie, 1 small	70	3	90	½CHO+½FAT
Vanilla Pudding, ½ c	140	4	160	1LfMk+1CHO

WYNDHAM®

Every Wyndham Hotel offers several "Nutritional Cuisine" menu choices that are designed to be lower in calories, fat, and sodium. These are available on every menu including room service. Specific nutrition information is not listed on the menu but is made available upon request.

PART
4

Ethnic Cuisines

Cajun & Creole Restaurants

Chapter Contents:

- ■ Appetizers
- ■ Salads
- ■ Entrees
- ■ Sandwiches
- ■ Accompaniments
- ■ Desserts

Cajun foods are those originating from the Acadian French immigrants living in Louisiana. Creole foods can be broadened to those foods traditionally prepared by a person of European parentage born in the West Indies, Central America, or Gulf States. Most of us think of Cajun and Creole foods as being spicy and flavorful. Here are some general guidelines for dining lean at Cajun/Creole restaurants.

Appetizers

✔ **Avoid the fried appetizers**, share them with a friend, or have them instead of an entrée. More appetizer suggestions and nutritional information can be found in the *Appetizers* chapter.

✔ **Boiled shrimp, boiled crawfish, and oysters on the half shell are low fat** choices. Nutritional information for these choices can be found in the seafood section of the *Entrees & Sauces* chapter.

✔ **Choose the red sauce** for dipping. This selection is much lower in calories than tartar sauce or the butter sauces. Compare the different sauces in the *Entrees & Sauces* chapter.

Salads

✓ **Always order vegetable salads with the dressing on the side**. Or use just vinegar or fresh lemon as a dressing.

✓ **Ask about the salad components**. You may want to omit some of the high fat components such as cheese, olives, and croutons.

✓ **Seafood salads should be ordered "dry."** Unless specified as such, seafood salads come prepared with mayonnaise or other high fat salad dressings.

Entrees

Fish is the most common protein source served in Cajun and Creole restaurants. It is served as an entrée and added to salads, soups, and sauces. Detailed ordering suggestions and nutritional information can be found in the seafood section of the *Entrees & Sauces* chapter. Here are some general recommendations:

✓ **Request that the fish be prepared grilled or broiled**. Fish is also offered fried, stuffed, blackened, or pan broiled. Fried fish has about twice as many calories as grilled or broiled fish. This calorie difference makes a major impact because fish portions are generally about 8-12 oz portions. Stuffed fish are often prepared with additional fat and are best avoided.

✓ **Skip the butter and sauces or ask for them to be served on the side**. Cajun fish is often served with a high fat sauce on top. If you want the taste of the sauce, order it on the side and dip your fork into the sauce with each bite.

Request the Sauces on the Side:		Calories	Fat (g)
6 oz Fish w/Butter & Crab Sauce		390	35
6 oz Fish w/out butter or sauce		180	12
	Savings:	**210**	**23**

✓ **Be sure to ask that the fish be blackened in *very little* oil**. Blackened fish *can be* relatively low in fat although some restaurants add a great deal of oil. Blackened meats and fish can be prepared two different ways. Usually, it is dipped in oil and then in a spice mixture containing the hotter spices such as garlic, cayenne, and white pepper. Some restaurants put oil in the pan or brush on oil and then sprinkle the "meat" with the spices. The "meat" is cooked in a very hot skillet or on the grill so that the outer portion gets crusty and blackened while the inside stays moist and juicy. The meatier fish such as salmon and swordfish hold up best. Blackened chicken is lower in fat than blackened beef.

✔ **Foods prepared with roux contain more fat than it appears**. Roux, a mixture of melted fat and flour, is frequently used for thickening sauces for meats, gravies (etoufeés), and soups such as gumbo. This fat may not be visible but it can increase the calories of a food item much higher than you would guess from appearances.

Entrees	Calories	Fat (g)	Sodium (mg)	Exchanges
Crayfish Étoufeé, 1 c + ¾ c rice	445	21	610	2ST+3LM+2V+2½FAT
Gumbo, seafood & sausage, 2c	460	27	950	2ST+1V+4MFM+ 1½FAT
Jambalaya, chicken & sausage w/rice, 1½ c	360	15	460	1¼ST+2V+2MFM+ 1FAT

Sandwiches

The most common sandwich served in a Cajun restaurant is the Po Boy (or Peaux Boy). This sandwich consists of fried or sautéed fish served in a Hoagie roll (or French bread) with a sauce. The bread is low in fat, but the fish and sauce are not.

✔ **Request a Po Boy sandwich prepared with *broiled or grilled* fish**. Also request the red sauce rather than tartar or remoulade sauce.

Ask for Lower Calorie Sauces:	Calories	Fat (g)
Po Boy: Roll, *Fried* Shrimp+¼c ***Tartar Sauce***	890	54
Po Boy: Roll, *Grilled* Shrimp+¼c ***Cocktail Sauce***	535	11
Savings:	**355**	**43**

✔ **Ask for the dressing on the side**. The dressing is usually a cocktail sauce and tartar sauce mixture; request only cocktail sauce instead and save the difference. Lettuce, tomato, and pickles are also frequently added to Po Boys.

Accompaniments

At Cajun and Creole restaurants, standard accompaniments are red beans & rice, so-called "Dirty" rice (prepared with sausage), and baked potatoes.

✔ **Ask for vegetables to be served without sauce or butter**. Many restaurants offer one vegetable and it is typically prepared steamed.

✔ **Red beans and rice *may* be a low fat choice** depending on the individual recipe used.

✔ **Request plain rice instead of dirty rice**. Dirty rice is not low fat or low cholesterol because it is prepared with a variety of meats including chicken liver, gizzards, sausage, and pork.

✔ **Baked potatoes are often very large but can be prepared dry**. Keep in mind that a 1 pound baked potato contains 400 calories.

Dessert

✔ **Fresh fruit is the leanest choice for dessert**. It is often available even if it's not mentioned on the menu.

Chinese Restaurants

Chapter Contents:

- Appetizers & Soups
- Accompaniments
- Entrees
- Estimating the Calories & Fat in your Stir Fry
- Nutritional Information for Chinese Foods

Chinese cooking combines many of the American foods that we are familiar with such as mushrooms, broccoli, chicken, shrimp, and rice with some not so common foods such as water chestnuts, bok choy, bamboo shoots, and soy sauce. The most common cooking method involves stir-frying with fat or oil. Individual meats and vegetables are cut up, oftentimes precooked, and then further cooked at high temperatures in the wok with oil.

Traditional Chinese cooking is considered healthy because small portions of meat are often combined with large amounts of low fat vegetables and rice or noodles. Unfortunately, many Chinese restaurants in this country use larger portions of meat than in traditional recipes. In addition, more oil is added than absolutely necessary when stir-frying. Fortunately, most dishes are made-to-order so you can ask the cook to prepare your dish according to your dietary specifications.

There are four main regions of China; each region has its own unique cuisine. Dishes are typically served with rice as is common in southern China; northern China is better known for their wheat products such as noodles.

- Cantonese style has its origins in southern China. The flavors are mild and subtle. Foods are often steamed or stir-fried and served with rice. Dim Sum brunches come to us from the Cantonese region. Here dim sum, or dumplings stuffed with meat or fish are served steamed or deep-fried.

■ Beijing/Peking in northern China is noted for the sweet and sour sauces, plum, or hoisin sauces.

■ Szechwan and Hunan cooking is from western China. This style is noted by the hot and spicy food flavored with chilies, garlic, and hot red peppers. This style of food tends to be higher in fat than the others.

■ Shanghai, in Eastern China, uses a combination of soy sauces, wine, and sugar. Braising of foods, with these ingredients, is often referred to as "red" cooking.

The following are some recommendations for dining lean that apply in any Chinese restaurant:

✔ **Avoid fried foods** indicated by the words "fried" or "crispy." The frying process alone may double the calories of any meat or vegetable. Check out the nutritional details in the Entrees & Sauces chapter.

✔ **Order "off the menu" rather than selecting the buffet.** Foods featured on the buffet table are prepared with more oil to prevent sticking and drying out. Check out the shine – it's coming from the fat. If you can afford the extra time, order off the menu.

✔ **Use chopsticks.** If you are inexperienced with using chopsticks, you will find it difficult to eat quickly. Eating slowly allows time for your stomach to signal when you're full.

Appetizers & Soups

✔ **Order steamed dumplings** instead of fried egg rolls.

✔ **Select non-fried foods.** Use caution at Dim Sum lunches; most of the items are fried.

✔ **Fill up on soup**. Most soups, although very high in sodium, are low in fat and calories. Select the Won Ton, Egg Drop (higher in cholesterol because of the egg), Hot & Sour, or Velvet Corn.

Accompaniments

✔ **Request steamed rice or plain noodles rather than fried rice or fried noodles**. Even though steamed rice may not be listed on the menu or offered on the buffet, you can always request steamed rice or plain noodles at no additional charge.

✔ **Enjoy boiled noodles rather than the fried noodles**. The boiled noodles are close to the composition of American wheat noodles.

Entrees

✓ **Avoid restaurants that serve their food** *too fast.* For speed in serving, some restaurants will cut up the meat and poultry in advance and deep-fry them until the inside is cooked but the meat is not browned on the outside. When you order your meal, the individual orders are then stir-fried in the wok with even more oil. It is often difficult to determine whether the meat has been fried prior to being stir-fried because the color of the meat is the same. Be sure to ask how the meat is prepared.

✓ **Order dishes that contain more vegetables than meat.** Beef, poultry, and seafood contain in the range of 120-520 calories per cup. Most vegetables have only about 50 or less! Since most dishes are made to order, you can always request more vegetables than meat. Or ask them to add vegetables to a typical meat-only dish. All of this helps you to lower the total calories and fat grams in the dish.

✓ **Avoid sweet and sour entrees.** Sweet and sour chicken, beef, and shrimp are typically all deep fat fried before the sugar-laden sauce is added.

✓ **"House Specialties" should be avoided**, as a rule. These higher priced items are usually dishes consisting of large portions of meat and little or no vegetables. In addition, these selections are usually high in both fat and calories.

✓ **Avoid dishes with nuts.** Just a handful of nuts, or about ¼ c, will add an extra 200 calories and 20 grams of fat. Your dish could actually have even more nuts! Water chestnuts (at just 20 calories per ¼ c) are a great crunchy, low calorie alternative to nuts.

✓ **Ask that your dish to be prepared with as "little oil as possible" in any stir-fried dish.** Usually 1-2 tablespoons of oil (and sometimes lard) is used to stir-fry an entree. That's 120-240 calories worth of fat. Some restaurants use as much as 4 T!

✓ **Order steamed foods with sauce on the side.** Some restaurant goers are choosing to order their food steamed (cooking it over water or chicken broth. Please consider that steamed foods will taste bland without the zing of traditional Chinese flavors. As a remedy, mix the steamed foods with rice and Plum sauce. Or request a sauce to be made of only thickened broth - and no oil.

✓ **Order fewer meals than the number of people at your table**. It is common practice in Chinese restaurants to share your meal with others at your table. Consider ordering just three meals for a table of four.

✓ **Order Chop Suey instead of Chow Mein.** Chop Suey and Chow Mein are essentially the same mixture of meat and vegetables. Chow Mein is topped with fried noodles, Chop Suey is not.

✓ **Select tofu instead of meat.** Tofu is a soft cheese made from soybeans. It is high in protein and moderate in both calories and fat. Although tofu has little flavor by itself, it soaks up the flavor of the foods in which it was cooked. Avoid dishes prepared with fried tofu.

✓ **Ask for foods prepared without MSG** (Monosodium Glutamate, a flavor enhancer) **if you are sensitive to it's effects.** Some people are sensitive to the MSG and report hot flashes, sweating, and headaches shortly after eating foods prepared with MSG. To reduce the symptoms, simply request that your food be prepared *without MSG*. Other components within the ingredients may still contain MSG, such as the chicken broth, which is used for making a sauce.

✓ **Most Chinese sauces are low in fat, but high in sugar and/or sodium.** If you are not restricting your sodium and sugar intake, these sauces are probably healthier for flavoring your meals than using oil.

■ **Black Bean Sauce** - a thick brown sauce commonly used in Cantonese cooking. It is made of fermented soy beans, wheat flour, and salt.

■ **Hoisin** - a thick sauce that is both sweet and spicy. It is made from soybeans, sugar, garlic, chili, and vinegar.

■ **Oyster sauce** - rich, thick sauce made from oysters and soy sauce. It is frequently used in Cantonese cooking.

■ **Plum sauce** - amber-colored, thick sauce made from plums, apricots, hot peppers, vinegar, and sugar. It has a spicy sweet-and-sour flavor.

■ **Sweet and Sour Sauce** - thick sauce made from sugar, vinegar, and soy sauce.

Estimating the Calories & Fat in Your Stir Fry

Every Chinese restaurant prepares their stir-fry dishes slightly different so it is difficult to list the *exact* calories per serving. On the average, a stir-fried dish contains approximately 2 cups of food. If we assume that each stir-fried dish contains 1 tablespoon (when you request "very little oil") or 2 tablespoons (for most Chinese meals) of oil we can estimate the calories and fat grams:

Chinese Food Calorimeter: Calories & fat (g) per serving

Calories & Fat (g) when stir-fried in 1T oil:				
2c Vegetables	1½c Vegetables ½c Beef *or* Pork	1c Vegetables 1c Beef *or* Pork	½c Vegetables 1½c Beef *or* Pork	2c Beef
220	**335**	**450**	**565**	**680**
14g	22g	30g	38g	44g
	1½c Vegetables ½c Chicken	1c Vegetables 1c Chicken	½c Vegetables 1½c Chicken	2c Chicken
	295	**370**	**445**	**520**
	18g	22g	26g	30g
	1½c Vegetables ½c Seafood *or* Chicken Breast	1c Vegetables 1c Seafood *or* Chicken Breast	½c Vegetables 1½c Seafood *or* Chicken Breast	2c Seafood *or* Chicken Breast
	265	**210**	**355**	**400**
	17g	20g	23g	26g

Calories & Fat (g) when stir-fried in 2T oil:				
2c Vegetables	1½c Vegetables ½c Beef *or* Pork	1c Vegetables 1c Beef *or* Pork	½c Vegetables 1½c Beef *or* Pork	2c Beef
440	**455**	**570**	**685**	**800**
28g	36g	44g	52g	58g
	1½c Vegetables ½c Chicken	1c Vegetables 1c Chicken	½c Vegetables 1½c Chicken	2c Chicken
	415	**490**	**565**	**640**
	32g	36g	40g	44g
	1½c Vegetables ½c Seafood *or* Chicken Breast	1c Vegetables 1c Seafood *or* Chicken Breast	½c Vegetables 1½c Seafood *or* Chicken Breast	2c Seafood *or* Chicken Breast
	385	**330**	**475**	**520**
	31g	34g	37g	40g

Some Chinese restaurants use as much as 4 tablespoons of oil per serving. Since each tablespoon of oil contains 120 calories and 14 grams of fat, the calories may be higher.

Nutritional Information for Chinese Foods

Chinese Foods

	Calories	Fat (g)	Sodium (mg)	Exchanges
Appetizers:				
Egg Foo Yong, 2 – 1oz patties	220	16	na	1½MFM+1V+2FAT
Egg Roll, 1- 4" pork & shrimp fried	300	19	490	¾ST+1LM+1V+3½FAT
Fried Beef or Pork Dumplings, 6	490	27	na	2½ST+1½HFM+3FAT
Fried Chicken Wing, 1	90	7	na	1HFM
Fried Pork & Shrimp Wonton, 1	45	2	100	¼ST+½FAT
Fried Won Ton, 4	340	25	na	1ST+1HFM+3½FAT
Shrimp Balls, 1	172	16	1462	1HFM+1½FAT
Shrimp Toast, 2 small pieces	250	24	220	½ST+1HFM+3FAT
Spareribs, 3 oz	339	26	80	3HFM+½FAT
Steamed Vegetable Dumplings, 6	230	5	na	2ST+1V+1FAT
Soups (1c):				
Chinese Noodle	210	9	1010	1½ST+2FAT
Egg Drop	50	3	1239	½MFM
Hot and Sour	75	2	920	½ST+½FAT
Velvet Corn	165	5	1230	1½ST+1FAT
Won Ton w/ 4 won tons	180	8	1701	1ST+1HFM
Beef & Pork Entrees (1 c unless noted):				
Beef *or* Pork w/asparagus, broccoli, cabbage, *or* green peppers	360	28	na	3MFM+1V+2½FAT
Beef *or* Pork w/cabbage *or* bok choy	395	30	na	3MFM+1V+3FAT
Cashew Beef	580	49	na	4MFM+6FAT
Chop Suey, Beef *or* Pork	220	12	na	1MFM+3V+1½FAT
Chow Mein, Beef *or* Pork	345	17	na	1MFM+1ST+3V+2½FAT
Mongolian Beef w/green onions & rice noodles	375	24	na	2MFM+1ST+3FAT
Oriental Noodles w/beef *or* pork & sauce	385	25	na	1ST+2MFM+3FAT
Pepper Steak, 4 oz	340	21	na	4MFM
Pork in Hoisin Sauce	450	30	na	4MFM+1CHO+2FAT
Shredded Pork w/Garlic or Peking Sauce	390	18	na	4MFM+2½FAT
Stir-fried Beef w/peppers, onions, mushrooms, & snow peas	315	24	na	2MFM+2V+3FAT
Stir-fried Beef *or* Pork w/vegetables	315	24	na	2MFM+2V+3FAT
Szechuan Beef *or* Pork	400	28	na	4MFM+2FAT
Sweet & Sour Beef *or* Pork	525	35	na	4MFM+1CHO+3FAT
Twice Cooked Pork	420	29	na	4MFM+2FAT

Chinese Foods (continued)

	Calories	Fat (g)	Sodium (mg)	Exchanges
Chicken Entrees (1 c unless noted):				
Almond *or* Cashew Chicken	495	40	na	4MFM+4FAT
Chicken & Snow Peas	200	17	na	2LM+1V+2FAT
Chicken Chop Suey	180	9	na	1VLM+3V+1½FAT
Chicken Chow Mein	305	14	na	1VLM+1ST+3V+2½FAT
Chicken Teriyaki, 1 quarter	335	16	na	4MFM+½CHO
Kung Pao Chicken	520	45	na	4MFM+5FAT
Lemon Chicken	720	44	na	4MFM+1CHO+5FAT
Moo Goo Gai Pan	190	9	na	2VLM+2V+1½FAT
Noodles w/chicken & vegetables in Szechuan sauce	290	17	na	1ST+1LM+1V+3FAT
Stir-fried Chicken w/vegetables	175	17	na	2LM+1V+2FAT
Sweet & Sour Chicken	490	30	na	4MFM+1CHO+2FAT
Fish & Shellfish (1 c unless noted):				
Chinese Fried Shrimp, 6 oz	540	30	na	6MFM+1ST
Shrimp Chop Suey	180	10	na	1LM+3V+1½FAT
Shrimp Chow Mein	305	15	na	1LM+1ST+3V+2½FAT
Shrimp w/cashews	460	38	na	4MFM+3½FAT
Shrimp w/Snow Peas	165	17	na	2VLM+1V+2½FAT
Sweet & Sour Shrimp	475	28	na	4MFM+1CHO+1½FAT
Szechuan noodles w/Chinese cabbage, snow peas & scallops	280	16	na	1ST+1LM+1V+2½FAT
Vegetable (½ c):				
Bok Choy, oriental style	55	4	na	1V+1FAT
Chop Suey, vegetable	44	3	na	1V+½FAT
Snow Pea, Mushroom, & Bamboo	40	3	na	1V+½FAT
Snow Peas & Water Chestnuts	40	3	na	1V+½FAT
Stir-Fried Broccoli	70	5	na	1V+1FAT
Stir-Fried String Beans	70	5	na	1V+1FAT
Szechuan noodles w/Chinese cabbage & snow peas	195	11	na	1ST+1V+2FAT
Szechuan-Style Eggplant	135	11	na	1V+2FAT
Tofu, ½ c pieces raw firm	185	11	17	2½MFM
Tofu, ½ c pieces fried	275	22	17	2½MFM+2FAT
Water Chestnuts	50	0	6	1V
Rice & Noodles:				
Steamed Rice, 1 c	240	0	400	3ST
Fried Rice, 1 c	370	12	900	3ST+2½FAT
Crispy Chow Mein Noodles, ½ c	250	11	440	2ST+2FAT
Oriental Noodles, ½ c	95	1	na	1ST

Chinese Foods (continued)

	Calories	Fat (g)	Sodium (mg)	Exchanges
Sauces & Oils (2T unless noted):				
Chinese BBQ Sauce	45	0	570	¾CHO
Mustard Sauce	60	6	na	1FAT
Oil, vegetable 1T	120	13	0	2½FAT
Plum or Duck Sauce	60	4	170	½CHO+1FAT
Sesame Oil, 1T	120	13	0	2½FAT
Sesame Soy Dip, 1T	30	2	na	½FAT
Soy Sauce, 1t	3	0	340	FREE
Soy Sauce, reduced sodium, 1t	3	0	170	FREE
Sweet and Sour Sauce	55	0	70	1CHO
Teriyaki Sauce, 1T	15	0	610	FREE
Teriyaki Sauce, reduced sodium, 1T	15	0	320	FREE
Worcestershire Sauce, 1T	10	0	235	FREE
Beverage:				
Tea, 1 c	0	0	0	FREE
Desserts:				
Fortune Cookie, 1	30	0	na	½CHO
Lychee, fruit/syrup, ½ c	60	0	na	1FR

Indian Restaurants

Chapter Contents:

- Appetizers & Soups
- Entrees
- Breads
- Accompaniments

Indian restaurants use some of the same ingredients as the Middle Eastern countries including rice, yogurt, onions, tomatoes, eggplant, legumes, and lamb. But Indian food more closely resembles the cuisine from Thailand because of the commonality of spices and curries. Spices used in Indian cooking includes: cardamon, cinnamon, clove, coriander, cumin, fennel, mint, saffron, and tumeric.

The many religions practiced in this country play a role in what is served in the particular regions of India. Many Buddhists practice vegetarianism. Moslems avoid pork and pork products while Hindus do not eat beef.

South Indian cuisine is hotter than foods from the northern part of India. Chilies, peppers, and hot pickles are more common. Rice, seafood, and chutney are served frequently. The Northern region's food is milder and uses more wheat products. Restaurants in the United States serve food from all over India.

Sesame oil and coconut oil are the fats commonly used in Indian cuisine. While sesame oil is an unsaturated fat, coconut oil is a highly saturated (unhealthy) fat. Ask which fat is being used before you make your selection.

Curries are often made with very high fat coconut milk but can also be prepared without. Yogurt is used in most recipes; typically whole milk is the norm, but low fat is becoming more popular.

Appetizers & Soups

✔ **Choose these lower fat starters to your meal:**

■ **Allu Chat** – appetizer of diced potatoes, chopped tomatoes, cucumber, and little or no oil

■ **Dahl Rasam** – pepper soup with lentils

■ **Mulligatawny** – lentil & vegetable soup

■ **Vegetable Salad** – usually dressing is on the side

✔ **Limit the amount of these fried appetizers:**

■ **Samosa** – vegetable turnover, stuffed & fried

■ **Papadum** – fried, crispy, thin lentil wafers served with dipping sauces

■ **Cheese** *or* **Chicken Pakoras** – deep fried, homemade cheese or chicken

Entrees

✔ **Ask for the meats to be sautéed in very little oil** or ghee (clarified butter).

✔ **Request curries to be prepared without coconut milk or cream.** Curry sauce is prepared by first sautéing onions in oil; yogurt and spices are then added. The addition of coconut milk or cream can be left off, if requested.

✔ **Split an entrée with a friend.** The tandori chicken is usually an 8 oz portion.

✔ **Plain rice comes with most entrees.**

✔ **Choose these lower fat entrees:**

■ **Aloo Chole** – chick peas cooked with tomatoes and potatoes

■ **Chicken** *or* **Shrimp Tandoori** – chicken or shrimp marinated in spices & yogurt and roasted in a tandoor (clay oven)

■ **Chicken** *or* **Fish Tikka** – roasted in an oven with mild spices

■ **Chicken, Fish,** *or* **Beef Vandaloo** – cooked with potatoes and hot spices

■ **Chicken** *or* **Fish Masala** – cooked with spices and a thick curry sauce made of yogurt

■ **Kebobs** – chunks of meat (preferably chicken) and vegetables cooked on a skewer. Request without the butter for basting.

■ **Shrimp** *or* **Lamb Bhuna** – cooked with onions and tomatoes

■ **Chicken** *or* **Lamb Saag** – cooked with spinach in a spicy curry sauce. Ask for without coconut milk or cream

- ■ **Vegetable Curry** – ask for it without coconut milk or cream
- ■ **Paneer** – homemade "cottage cheese." Ask for the high fat sauces to be served on the side.

✓**Limit these higher fat entrees:**

- ■ **Chicken Kandhari** – cooked with cream sauce and cashews
- ■ **Shrimp Mali** - cooked with cream and coconut
- ■ **Beef or Vegetable Korma** – curry cooked with cream

Breads

✓ **Ask for these low fat breads:**

- ■ **Chapati** – thin, dry whole wheat bread
- ■ **Nan** – leavened baked bread
- ■ **Tandori roti** – unleavened bread similar to pita bread

✓**Limit these higher fat breads:**

- ■ **Poori** – light, puffed bread
- ■ **Paratha** – fried bread, may be stuffed with potatoes or meats

Accompaniments

✓ **Select these low fat accompaniments:**

- ■ **Biryani** – rice dish that contains chicken, shrimp, or beef, along with vegetables and dried fruit
- ■ **Chutney** – usually mango or onion chutney
- ■ **Dahi** – plain, unflavored yogurt
- ■ **Pullao** – basmati rice, an aromatic long grain rice. Pullao is low fat when cooked plain; the fat content increases when cooked along with meat, nuts, paneer, or vegetables such as peas.
- ■ **Raita** –yogurt with grated cucumbers, onions, and spices

✓ **Limit these higher fat accompaniments:**

- ■ **Dahl** – lentil-based, spicy sauce

Italian Restaurants

Chapter Contents:

- Appetizers, Antipasto, & Salads
- Pasta
- Meats & Cheese
- Sauces
- Nutritional Information for Italian Foods
- Your Favorite Italian Restaurants

When we think of Italian foods, the foods that often come to mind are pizza and pasta. For more information on how to order a leaner pizza refer to the *Pizza* chapter.

A moderate portion of pasta, by itself, is low in fat and relatively low in calories. Additions such as sauce, cheese, meats, and oil determine if a meal remains low fat.

Olive oil is one of the most common staples in Italian cooking. It is often considered a healthy fat because it contains no cholesterol and is high in monounsaturated fats. Keep in mind that, like other oils, it still has 120 calories per tablespoon. To eat lean, avoid excessive amounts of meat, cheese, fried foods or those foods that have liberal amounts of oil added.

Appetizers, Antipasto, & Salads

✓ **Consider squid, mussels, or clams in a herb wine sauce.** Stay away from fried appetizers such as fried eggplant and fried cheese.

✔ **Inquire as to what comes with appetizers of Carpaccio or Prosciutto ham**. These thin slices of beef, fish, or ham are very high in fat but are often served in small portions. Refer to the *Entrees & Sauces* chapter for nutritional information. If these offerings are a must, enjoy them instead of a meat entrée and ask for the Carpaccio or Prosciutto to be served with vegetables or fruit such as melon. Often drizzled with olive oil or served with mayonnaise, this plate is lower in fat if eaten plain or with lemon juice.

✔ **Minestrone and Bean Soups are often prepared low fat** and are a good way to fill up prior to a meal.

Low Fat Soups can Fill You Up:		
	Calories	Fat (g)
Minestrone Soup, 8 oz	95	3
Bean Soup, 8 oz	180	6

✔ **Request Bruschetta to be prepared with very little oil.** This oil-ladened toast is best enjoyed in small quantities. The same advice is appropriate when restaurants offer you bread with a dish of oil for dipping - use little or no oil and keep your bread portion minimal.

Bruschetta can be Modified:		
	Calories	Fat (g)
1 oz Bread + 1T oil	198	15
1 oz Bread + 1t oil	118	6
Savings:	80	9

✔ **Order a vegetable salad with balsamic vinegar** or with the salad dressing on the side. Caesar salad is best avoided because of its high fat ingredients including eggs, Parmesan cheese, and Italian dressing.

✔ **Watch the high fat additions of olives, pine nuts, cheese, and oil**. Whenever possible, ask for your meal to be prepared without these ingredients or in limited amounts.

These Foods can Quickly Add Calories to Your Meal:		
	Calories	Fat (g)
Parmesan or Romano Cheese, 2T	46	3
Olive Oil, 1T	120	14
Pine Nuts, 1 oz *or* small handful	161	17
Olives, 6 super Colossal ripe	78	7

✔ Nutritional information on a variety of Appetizers, Soups, and Salads can be found in their respective chapters.

Pasta

✓ **Pasta noodles, made of mostly flour and water, are very low in fat**. Freshly prepared pasta noodles may have eggs as an added ingredient. This will add about 50 mg of cholesterol per cup and a few grams of fat. Some restaurants offer dried pastas, made without egg, for patrons who are closely monitoring their cholesterol.

✓ **Each half cup portion of pasta has only 100 calories** but serving sizes are often 2 cups. Frequently, appetizer portions can be ordered instead of a large entree portion; or you can request a doggie bag. This is what a half cup portion of spaghetti looks like.

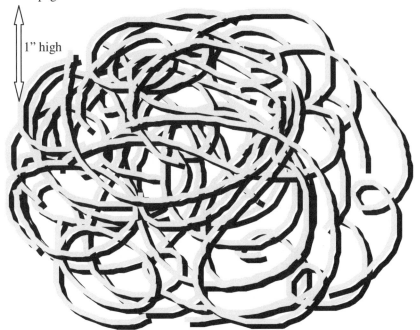

1" high

½ c plain pasta = 100 calories, ½ g fat

✓ **Here's a description of the most common pastas:**

■ **Straight (thinnest to widest):** Capellini (Angel hair), Vermicelli, Spaghetti, Linguine, Fettuccine, Lasagna

■ **Tubular:** Mostaccioli, Penne, Rigatoni, Ziti, Cannelloni (stuffed), Manicotti (stuffed)

■ **Other Shapes:** Capellitti (little hats), Farfalle (bowties), Fusilli (long pasta which is spiral shaped), Gnocchi (little dumplings), Ravioli (stuffed & usually square), Rotelle (corkscrew spirals), Shells

Meats & Cheese

✓ **Chicken, seafood, and veal are the leanest "meats" as long as they are not fried**. Pancetta (Italian bacon) and sausage are best avoided due to their high fat content.

✓ **Request for the meat to be steamed or grilled** instead of sautéed or fried even if the menu suggests otherwise. Nutritional information for a variety of meats can be found in the *Entrees & Sauces* chapter.

✓ **Choose "pasta with meat" rather than an entrée serving of meat**. In addition, choose a low fat sauce such as a tomato sauce.

Choose "Pasta with Meat" rather than a Meat Entree:	Calories	Fat (g)
8 oz Beef Entrée + 1 c pasta w/tomato sauce	1090	71
2 c Pasta w/ 2 oz beef in tomato sauce	780	30
Savings:	**310**	**41**

But don't Blow it with a High Fat Sauce:	Calories	Fat (g)
2 c Pasta w/ 2 oz beef in Alfredo sauce	1380	91
2 c Pasta w/ 2 oz beef in tomato sauce	780	30
Savings:	**600**	**61**

✓ **Also, ask that "no oil" be added to the preparation of the "meats"**; wine or broth can often be substituted. Request that the skin be removed from the poultry dishes.

✓ **Avoid dishes with excessive cheese.** Instead of pasta stuffed with cheese, choose pasta with a sprinkling of cheese.

Avoid Pasta Stuffed with Cheese:	Calories	Fat (g)
Manicotti, 2 stuffed	695	42
1½ c Pasta Primavera w/3T grated cheese	360	10
Savings:	**335**	**32**

✓ **Partially skimmed cheeses are not as low fat as you might think**. Occasionally, you may find dishes prepared with partially skimmed cheeses; while lower in fat, they are not fat-free.

Partially skimmed cheeses are lower in fat:	Calories	Fat (g)
Ricotta Cheese, ½ c	215	16
Ricotta Cheese, part skim, ½ c	170	10
Savings:	**45**	**6**

✔ **Avoid Parmigiana meals**. Parmigiana refers to food that is floured, fried, and topped with a marinara sauce and cheese. These dishes are very high in fat whether made from chicken, veal, or eggplant. Instead, you can request the meat to be *grilled* and topped with a marinara sauce and cheese. Or consider ordering an appetizer (or luncheon) portion of your favorite parmigiana instead of the entrée portion. This option is often available even if it is not suggested on the menu.

Sauces

✔ **Ask for a lower calorie/fat sauce.** Even if the menu states a particular sauce you can always substitute a healthier sauce.

✔ **If you want the higher fat sauce, ask them to put on less or request the sauce to be served on the side.**

✔ **Order Pasta Primavera (pasta with vegetables) prepared with a tomato sauce or *very little* oil** instead of the typical butter or Alfredo sauce.

✔ **When ordering a side order of pasta, consider asking for no sauce to be added**. Use the sauce from the meat entrée to mix with the pasta instead.

✔ **Know your sauces:**

    ■ **Alfredo Sauce** - a very high fat cream sauce prepared with butter, heavy cream and parmesan cheese.

    ■ **Bolognese Sauce** - a cream or tomato-based sauce with a variety of meats, vegetables, and wine added.

    ■ **Carbonara Sauce** - made with butter, eggs, bacon, sausage, parmesan cheese, and cream.

    ■ **Meat Sauce** - a tomato sauce with added ground beef or sausage. Calories and fat grams are dependent upon the amount of meat added; sausage is higher in calories and fat than ground beef.

    ■ **Pesto Sauce** - a very high fat sauce prepared from fresh basil, pine nuts, parmesan cheese, and oil. If you want a dish prepared with pesto – request that it be prepared with "just a little."

    ■ **Red Clam Sauce** - consists of oil, tomatoes, and clams.

    ■ **Tomato Sauces** (such as marinara, spicy marinara, and pomodori) are typically the lowest fat sauces. Caution: creamy tomato sauce is much higher in fat and calories.

    ■ **White Clam Sauce** (Vongole) - made of butter, oil, white wine and clams.

✔ **Hold the oil.** Upscale Italian restaurants offer dishes of pasta combined with a variety of meat, chicken, seafood, and/or vegetables. These combinations are generally mixed with a sauce or simply with flavored oil. Ask for a tomato sauce or *very little* oil. Many restaurants will use broth instead of oil to add moisture and flavor with the addition of very few calories.

Consider the Difference:

	Calories	Fat (g)
2 c Pasta combined w/shrimp, prosciutto, peas, & tomatoes, in a cream sauce	1470	87
Above prepared with a tomato sauce instead	850	22
Savings:	**620**	**65**

Pasta Calorimeter: Calories & fat per serving

	Calories & Fat (g)			
	½ c	1 c	1 ½ c	2 c
Plain Pasta	**100**	**200**	**300**	**400**
	$0.^5$g	1g	2g	2g
w/ Tomato sauce (½ c sauce/1 c pasta)	**145**	**290**	**435**	**580**
	3g	6g	9g	12g
w/ Red Clam sauce (½ c sauce/1 c pasta)	**160**	**320**	**480**	**640**
	5g	9g	14g	18g
w/ Bolognese sauce (½ c sauce/1 c pasta)	**165**	**330**	**495**	**660**
	4g	7g	11g	14g
w/ White Clam sauce (½ c sauce/1 c pasta)	**190**	**380**	**570**	**760**
	5g	10g	15g	20g
w/ meat sauce ($^2/_3$ c sauce/1 c pasta)	**235**	**475**	**710**	**945**
	9g	18g	27g	36g
w/ Pesto sauce (5 T sauce/1 c pasta)	**248**	**495**	**743**	**990**
	14g	28g	42g	56g
w/ Creamy Tomato Sauce (¾ c sauce/1 c pasta)	**260**	**515**	**775**	**1030**
	14g	27g	41g	54g
w/Alfredo sauce ($^2/_3$ c sauce/1 c pasta)	**300**	**600**	**900**	**1200**
	20g	39g	58g	77g
w/ Carbonara sauce ($^2/_3$ c sauce/1 c pasta)	**320**	**640**	**965**	**1280**
	20g	39g	58g	77g

Nutritional information is based upon sauces added according to average amounts indicated in parentheses. Your portion sizes may vary.

Nutritional Information for Italian Foods

Italian Food	Calories	Fat (g)	Sodium (mg)	Exchanges
Entrees:				
Cannelloni Florentine (4 noodles stuffed w/veal, spinach, beef)	450	27	na	2ST+2MFM+3FAT
Chicken Cacciatore (6 *oz w/out skin*), w/sauce	585	23	na	2ST+6LM+2V+1FAT
Chicken Parmesan, 6 oz w/sauce	675	43	na	1ST+6LM+2V+5FAT
Chicken Saltimbocca (5 oz chicken + 1 oz prosciutto)	747	52	585	6LM+7FAT
Chicken Scaloppini, 6 oz	582	34	250	6LM+3FAT
w/ 3T Lemon Butter Sauce	845	63	625	6LM+9FAT
Chicken Tetrazzini, 1 c	425	21	na	2ST+1V+2MFM+2FAT
Eggplant Parmesan, 3" X 4"	310	22	1180	1ST+1V+1HFM+3FAT
Fettuccine Alfredo, 1½ c	360	15	370	3ST+3FAT
Lasagna, traditional, 3"X3" square	340	16	1020	1½ST+1V+2HFM
Lasagna with meat & cream sauce, 3" X 4" square	685	45	538	1½ST+3HFM+4FAT
Manicotti, 2 stuffed	695	42	1835	2ST+5HFM
Ravioli, Cheese, 1 c	340	10	220	2½ST+1HFM+½FAT
w/red sauce	430	15	490	2½ST+1HFM+1V+2FAT
w/Alfredo sauce	740	48	1180	4ST+2½HFM+4½FAT
Ravioli, Beef or Chicken, 1 c	280	9	350	2½ST+1HFM
w/red sauce	370	14	620	2½ST+1HFM+1V+1FAT
w/Alfredo sauce	680	47	1310	3½ST+2½HFM+5½FAT
Tortellini, meat & cheese, 1 c	450	11	560	3½ST+1½HFM
w/red sauce	540	16	830	3½ST+1½HFM+1V+1FAT
w/Alfredo sauce	840	48	1520	5ST+3HFM+5FAT
Veal Scaloppini, 6 oz cooked	700	50	300	6MFM+4FAT
w/ 3T Lemon Butter Sauce	964	79	675	6MFM+10FAT
Veal Saltimbocca, 5 oz veal + 1 oz prosciutto	650	42	600	6MFM+2½FAT
Sauces for Entrees (2T):				
Butter Wine Sauce	140	14	140	3FAT
Cream Sauce, thin	50	4	180	1FAT
Cream Sauce, thick	108	12	50	2½FAT
Lemon Butter Sauce	175	19	250	4FAT
Meuneire Sauce	130	14	510	3FAT
Tomato Sauce	23	1	190	1V
Pasta:				
Pasta, no sauce or oil, ½ c	100	0.5	2	1¼ST
Pasta, no sauce or oil, 1 c	200	1	4	2½ST

Italian Food (continued)

Pasta continued:	Calories	Fat (g)	Sodium (mg)	Exchanges
Pasta Primavera, 1 c pasta + vegetables in very light oil	290	5	50	2½ST+2V+1FAT
Pasta Primavera, 1 c pasta + vegetables in tomato sauce	300	6	270	2½ST+3V+1FAT
Pasta Primavera, 1 c pasta + vegetables in Alfredo sauce	700	43	1080	2½ST+2V+1FAT
Pasta Puttanesca, 1 c pasta + sauce	388	16	910	2½ST+2V+3FAT

Accompaniments:

Gnocchi Dumplings, 2 small	80	1	na	1ST
Meatballs, 1 @ 2" diameter	80	6	na	1MFM
Polenta, 2½ X 4" piece	120	0	180	2ST
Fried Polenta, 2" X 2½" X ½"	90	4	130	1ST+1FAT
Polenta Pasticciata, w/sauce	375	23	470	2ST+4½FAT
Prosciutto, Italian ham, 1 oz	80	6	na	1MFM
Risotto w/ butter, ½ c	170	5	280	1½ST+1FAT
Roasted Potatoes, ½ c	155	7	na	1ST+1½FAT

Cheeses:

Ricotta Cheese, ½ c	215	16	104	2HFM
Ricotta Cheese, part skim, ½ c	170	10	155	2MFM
Parmesan or Romano Cheese, 1T	23	1.^{5}	93	¼HFM
Mozzarella, 1 oz	90	7	106	1HFM
Part skim, 1 oz	72	4.^{5}	132	1MFM
Feta Cheese, 1 oz	75	6	316	1MFM
Cream Cheese, 1 oz (2T)	100	10	84	2FAT
Light, 1 oz (2T)	62	4.^{7}	160	1FAT

Sauces (½ c):

Alfredo Sauce	300	28	720	1ST+1HFM+4FAT
Bolognese Sauce, cream-based	200	14	180	1½MFM+1V+1½FAT
Bolognese Sauce, tomato-based	130	6	585	1MFM+2V
Carbonara Sauce	330	28	770	2HFM+2½FAT
Creamy Tomato Sauce	210	17	313	1HFM+1V+2FAT
Marinara Sauce	85	4	750	1V+1FAT
Meat Sauce (little meat)	160	10	290	1V+½HFM+1½FAT
Meat Sauce (chunky w/meat)	250	16	300	1V+1HFM+2FAT
Pesto Sauce	600	60	880	1HFM+10FAT
Pomodoro (Tomato Sauce)	90	5	270	2V+1FAT
Puttanesca (tomatoes & anchovies)	126	10	605	2V+2FAT
Red Clam Sauce	110	8	240	1V+½MFM+1FAT
Spinach, Mushrooms, & Cream	190	19	160	1V+4FAT
White Clam Sauce	180	9	510	¼ST+1HFM+1FAT

Desserts:

Stuffed Cannoli, 1, 4"	315	19	70	2CHO+4FAT
Pirouline, 3 thin rolled cookies	150	7	25	1½CHO+1½FAT
Fruit Sorbet, ½ c	120	0	0	2CHO

Your Favorite Italian Restaurants

FAZOLI'S®

	Calories	Fat (g)	Sodium (mg)	Exchanges
Spaghetti:				
Spaghetti w/Tomato Sauce	343	7	175	na
Spaghetti w/Meat Sauce	372	8	161	na
Spaghetti w/Meat Balls	582	25	864	na
Large Spaghetti w/Tomato Sauce	509	10	244	na
Large Spaghetti w/Meat Sauce	553	12	223	na
Large Spaghetti w/Meat Balls	829	34	1163	na
Specialty Items:				
Ravioli w/Tomato Sauce	332	15	714	na
Ravioli w/Meat Sauce	361	16	700	na
Fettuccine Alfredo	400	13	711	na
Large Fettuccine Alfredo	596	20	1048	na
Broccoli Fettuccine	424	13	731	na
Large Broccoli Fettuccine	619	20	1068	na
Chicken Parmesan	481	14	368	na
Baked Ziti	331	13	347	na
Lasagna	533	24	1148	na
Broccoli Lasagna	571	27	1443	na
Meat Ball Sub	650	30	1534	na
Sampler Platter	607	20	904	na
Shrimp Pasta	552	19	1121	na
Soup, Salad, Bread:				
Breadstick	131	4	330	na
Breadstick, dry	99	$0.^{8}$	204	na
Minestrone Soup	90	1	1038	na
Bean & Pasta Soup	174	7	1079	na
Italian Chef Salad	391	30	1307	na
Pasta Salad	397	20	1030	na
Garden Salad	28	$0.^{3}$	17	na
House Italian Dressing, 1 oz	138	30	224	na
Reduced Calorie Ital Dressing, 1 oz	69	4	112	na
Honey French Dressing, 1 oz	160	14	230	na
Thousand Island Dressing, 1 oz	140	14	230	na
Ranch Dressing, 1 oz	180	20	250	na
Pizza:				
Cheese Pizza, double slice	360	11	622	na
Pepperoni Pizza, double slice	430	17	908	na
Combination Pizza, double slice	484	21	1042	na

FAZOLI'S® (continued)

Desserts:	Calories	Fat (g)	Sodium (mg)	Exchanges
Lemon Ice, 12 oz	142	0	9	na
Cheesecake, plain	270	21	208	na
Choc Chocolate Chip Cheesecake	298	22	201	na
Strawberry Topping, 1 oz	40	0	1	na

OLIVE GARDEN®

Lunch Entrees:	Calories	Fat (g)	Sodium (mg)	Exchanges
Capellini Pomodoro	360	9	540	na
Capellini Primavera	260	5	560	na
Capellini Primavera w/Chicken	420	8	640	na
Chicken Giardino	360	9	900	na
Linguine Alla Marinara	310	6	105	na
Penne Fra Diavolo	300	5	640	na
Shrimp Primavera	410	8	840	na
Dinner Entrees:				
Capellini Pomodoro	610	16	940	na
Capellini Primavera	400	7	950	na
Capellini Primavera w/Chicken	560	10	1030	na
Chicken Giardino	550	11	1000	na
Grilled Chicken Marsala	590	9	1110	na
Linguine Alla Marinara	500	9	160	na
Penne Fra Diavolo	420	7	940	na
Shrimp Primavera	740	15	1630	na
Soup:				
Minestrone, 6 fl oz bowl	80	1	450	na
Dessert:				
Apple Carmellina	560	2	190	na

Note: Recipes and their respective nutritional information are subject to change.
Other tips: You may request alternative food preparation or serving instructions including cheese topping omitted, sauce served on the side, or lunch portions at dinner.

SPAGHETTI WAREHOUSE®

	Calories	Fat (g)	Sodium (mg)	Exchanges
Lunch:				
Minestrone Soup	77	2	1040	½ST+1V+½FAT
Grilled Chicken Marinara	527	8	395	3½ST+4VLM+2V+ ½FAT
Spaghetti with Marinara Sauce #12	438	5	404	4½ST+2V+1FAT
Seafood Marinara	384	5	398	3½ST+1LM+1½V+ ½FAT
Spaghetti with Tomato Sauce	425	5	490	4½ST+1V+1FAT
Spicy Marinara Sauce Spaghetti	282	4	280	2½ST+1V+1FAT
Vegetable Primavera	337	4	344	3ST+3V+1FAT
Dinner:				
Minestrone Soup, Cup	57	1	772	¼ST+1V
Minestrone Soup, Bowl	111	2	1495	½ST+1½V+½FAT
Grilled Chicken Marinara	637	10	550	4½ST+4VLM+2V+ 1FAT
Spaghetti with Marinara Sauce #12	515	6	390	5½ST+2V+1FAT
Seafood Marinara	520	7	605	4½ST+1½LM+2V+ 1½FAT
Spaghetti with Tomato Sauce	526	6	653	5½ST+2V+1FAT
Spicy Marinara Sauce Spaghetti	330	6	407	3ST+2V+1FAT
Vegetable Primavera	608	8	662	5½ST+4½V+1½FAT
Grilled Halibut	878	15	778	5½+6LM+3V
Grilled Marinated Chicken Breast	912	17	826	5½ST+5LM+4½V+ ½FAT

Other tips: Sourdough bread is served with a blend of low-fat margarine, garlic, and romano cheese. Plain margarine is available upon request. Order all salad dressings on the side; Lite Italian dressing is available.

Mexican Restaurants

Chapter Contents:

If you like hot, spicy foods, Mexican restaurants may top your list of favorite ethnic cuisines. Common foods served in Mexican restaurants include beans, rice, tortillas as well as tomatoes, onions, salsa, and jalapeño peppers. Most people think that Mexican restaurants are definitely off the list when watching their fat intake. However, there are lean choices available.

Appetizers

✔ **Ask for baked chips**. Few restaurants serve baked chips when you are seated, but may prepare them upon request.

Ask for Baked Chips:		Calories	Fat (g)
Restaurant Style Tortilla Chips, 20		460	20
Baked Tortilla Chips, 20		240	2.5
	Savings:	220	17.5

✔ **Move the fried chips**. Count out the chips you have allotted yourself and then ask the server to remove the rest. Or move the chips out of your reach.

✔ **Ask for regular corn tortillas**. Some patrons ask for regular corn tortillas for dipping into the salsa. Try it! There's no crunch but plenty of flavor.

✔ **Enjoy the salsa.** Salsa and pico de gallo are made with little or no fat added and can be used freely.

✔ **Share the nachos with everyone.** Don't make nachos your meal. Instead, have just a few. Chips are high in fats and calories; so are all the nacho toppings.

Nachos are High Calorie – Even Just Six:	Calories	Fat (g)
Tortilla Chips, 6 large	130	6
Cheese, 2T	120	10
Refried Beans, ¼ c	125	7
Guacamole, 2T	55	3
Sour Cream, 2T	50	5
TOTAL:	**480**	**31**

✔ **Enjoy ceviche as an entrée.** Ceviche is fish "cooked" with lemons or limes and onions and jalapeno – not with heat. It's low fat and low calorie.

Soups

✔ **Ask about the tortilla soup.** Tortilla soup is often prepared from a simple low fat vegetable soup. The added bacon, cheese, avocado, and strips of fried tortilla is what contributes most of the calories and fat; some or all of these components can often be omitted.

Tortilla Soup:	Calories	Fat (g)
Vegetables in a broth	70	2
Cheese, 1T	60	5
Chicken, ½ oz	30	1
Avocado, 1/8	40	4
Tortilla Strips	40	2
TOTAL:	**240**	**14**

✔ **Have Black Bean soup.** This is often prepared with less fat than pinto beans.

✔ **Enjoy chili (made with beans)** rather than chili con carne (beans with meat). Ask what toppings are added such as sour cream and cheese; you can ask for them to be omitted.

Salads

✓ **Ask about the components of the salad.** While lettuce and tomato are low in fat, most other additions are not. Ask yourself what components (such as cheese, sour cream, or avocado) you can do without.

✓ **Select the chicken fajita salad** over the beef fajita salad. These are both healthier options than the taco salad, which is prepared with ground beef.

✓ **Use the picante sauce or pico de gallo for a low calorie and spicy dressing.** If you want to tone down the spiciness, try mixing sour cream and picante sauce for a dressing with less than 20 calories per tablespoon.

✓ **Don't eat the shell**. Taco salads and fajita salads are often served in a fried flour tortilla shell. It's tempting to nibble away at the shell. Request that the salad be served on a plate for a savings of hundreds of calories.

Don't Eat the Fried Shell:	Calories	Fat (g)
Taco Salad	930	69
Taco Salad without the Shell	510	39
Savings:	**420**	**30**

Entrees

✓ **Order ala carte**. Instead of ordering a complete meal, order only the items that you want. Chicken fajitas or chicken tacos al carbon can be ordered individually in most restaurants as a lean entrée. Both selections will have 1-2 oz of meat in each. Lettuce, tomatoes, and onions can be requested to accompany this order.

✓ **Ask for high calorie components to be left off the plate** – especially if you are likely to eat them just because they are there, rather than because you like them. The higher calorie accompaniments include refried beans, Mexican rice, guacamole, sour cream, and cheese. The side orders of lettuce, tomato, onion, salsa, and pico de gallo are acceptable.

Eat it Plain:	Calories	Fat (g)
Beef Fajita: 2-6½" flour tortillas, 3 oz meat, ¼ avocado, 2T sour cream & 2T shredded cheese	600	36
Beef Fajita: 2-6½" flour tortillas, 3 oz meat, shredded, lettuce, tomato, onion	415	19
Savings:	**185**	**17**

✓ **Trim the meat.** This extra step will save at least 20 calories an ounce or more than 100 calories in a typical serving.

✓ **Choose menu items prepared with soft tortillas rather than crispy.** Crispy tortillas have been fried and are, therefore, higher in fat and calories than the plain corn or flour tortilla. Commonly served entrees with fried tortillas include the chimichanga, chalupa, crispy taco, and crispy burrito.

✓ **Ask that the fajitas be prepared with very little oil.** The fajita dinner is usually served with sautéed (with oil) green peppers and onions. The meat is then brushed with oil before serving to give it more shine.

✓ **Request these lower calorie entrees.** When prepared with chicken, fish or shrimp these will be leaner than with beef or cheese.

  ■ **Fajitas** – marinated and grilled beef, chicken, or shrimp.

  ■ **Tacos al carbon** *or* **Soft Taco**– Chicken or beef fajita strips wrapped in a flour tortilla.

  ■ **Soft Burritos** – Non-fried large flour tortilla wrapped around chicken or beef fajitas.

  ■ **Chicken Enchiladas**, corn tortillas dipped in hot oil, filled with chicken, and then rolled. Baked with a red or green tomato-based enchilada sauce. These can be requested without the cheese sauce topping.

  ■ **Camarones de Hacha** – shrimp sautéed in red or green tomato sauce.

  ■ **Arroz con Pollo** – boneless chicken breast served with Mexican rice.

✓ **Limit the higher calorie entrees:**

  ■ **Chalupas** *or* **Tostadas** - flat, fried corn tortilla topped with beans, meat, and/or cheese.

  ■ **Chimichanga or Fried Burrito -** flour tortilla filled with beef, chicken, cheese and/or beans and then deep fried. This is often covered with a picante or cheese sauce.

  ■ **Beef or Cheese Enchiladas -** corn tortillas dipped in hot oil and then rolled with cheese, or beef. These are generally served with a red or green tomato-based enchilada sauce.

  ■ **Flauta con crema** – crisp tortillas stuffed with beef or chicken and covered with a cream sauce.

  ■ **Chicken or Beef Mole** – chicken or beef cooked with mole, a high fat, high calorie sauce.

  ■ **Tacos -** fried corn tortilla filled with shredded chicken, beef, beans, and/or cheese.

  ■ **Tamale** – corn husks spread with maize and covered with shredded beef, chicken, or pork. These are rolled up and cooked.

Accompaniments

✓ **Choose corn tortillas over flour tortillas**. Tortillas are great tasting when they are freshly made. While many restaurants make their own flour tortillas, few restaurants prepare corn tortillas fresh. If you think you don't like the taste of corn tortillas, find a restaurant that makes their own. You just might like them better than the higher calorie flour tortillas.

Corn Tortillas are lower in Fat & Calories:		
	Calories	Fat (g)
Flour Tortilla	110	3
Corn Tortilla	70	0.5
Savings:	**40**	**2.5**

✓ **Decide how many tortillas fit into your calorie and fat budget**. Plan ahead and you won't blow it!

✓ **Be selective with the accompaniments**. Many of us eat chips, rice, beans, *and* tortillas. This can add up to a very high fat and high caloric meal. Which of these accompaniments do you really enjoy and which do you eat simply because they are there?

✓ **Ask for cooked pinto or black beans instead of refried beans**. You may see the cooked beans listed on the menu as bean soup, Beans ala charra, or borracho beans. These are usually prepared with bacon or other fat. For that reason, it is best to eat the beans and leave the broth and added fat in the bowl. Every restaurant prepares their refried beans differently. They can be prepared with little fat or quite a bit of fat. You can't tell the difference by simply looking at it. Since most restaurants use lard, it is best to avoid the refried beans.

Dessert

✓ **Flan is a healthier choice than sopappillas.** Flan, a baked custard made with egg and whole milk, is usually served in a small portion. Sopapillas, fried flour dough sprinkled with sugar and cinnamon, is best shared with friends.

Nutritional Information for Mexican Foods

Mexican Foods				
	Calories	Fat (g)	Sodium (mg)	Exchanges
Appetizers:				
Tortilla Chip, 1 large	23	1	15	¼ST
5 Tortilla Chips	125	5.^{8}	65	1ST+1FAT
5 Baked Chips	75	1	65	1ST
Tortilla Chip, 1 regular size	18	0.^{8}	8	¼ST
5 Tortilla Chips	90	4	40	¾ST+1FAT
5 Baked Chips	60	0.^{6}	40	¾ST
Nacho w/Cheese only, 1 chip	42	2.^{5}	35	¼ST+¼HFM+½FAT
w/Bean & Cheese, 1 chip	80	5	105	¼ST+¼HFM+½FAT
w/Bean, Meat & Cheese, 1 chip	115	8	200	¼ST+½HFM+1FAT
Ceviche, 4 oz	150	5	na	4VLM
Soups (1c):				
Tortilla Soup	240	14	840	1V+¾ST+½HFM+2FAT
Gazpacho Soup	90	2	475	2V+½FAT
Black Bean Soup	180	4	1000	1½ST+1VLM+½FAT
Chili (beans only)	180	6	860	1½ST+1VLM+1FAT
Chili con Carne	310	13	1080	2ST+2MFM+½FAT
Salads w/ 2 oz meat (w/out fried bowl _or_ dressing):				
Taco Salad, w/chili meat	510	39	na	2V+3HFM+3FAT
Chicken Taco Salad	400	29	850	2V+2MFM+1HFM+ 2½FAT
Chicken Fajita Salad	350	22	na	2V+2LM+1HFM+2FAT
Beef Fajita Salad	440	31	na	2V+2MFM+1HFM+ 3FAT
Fried Taco Shell Bowl	420	30	250	2ST+6FAT

To estimate tortilla size, note this book is 5½" wide by 8½" high.

Corn Tortillas:				
Corn Tortilla, 5" diameter	50	0.5	30	¾ST
Tostada Chip, crispy, 4½" diameter	50	1	50	½ST
Taco Shell, crispy, small	50	2	70	½ST+½FAT
Taco Shell, crispy, large	100	6	130	1ST+1FAT
Flour Tortillas:				
Flour Tortilla, 6½" diameter	100	3	200	1ST+½FAT
Flour Tortilla, 8"	150	5	350	1½ST+1FAT
Flour Tortilla, 10"	250	8	450	2ST+1½FAT
Fried Flour Tortilla, 8"	220	11	350	1½ST+2FAT
Fried Flour Tortilla, 10"	325	16	450	2ST+3FAT
Rice & Beans (½ c):				
Mexican Rice	150	4	550	1½ST+1FAT
Refried Beans	250	13	325	1ST+2½FAT

Mexican Foods (continued)

	Calories	Fat (g)	Sodium (mg)	Exchanges
Rice & Beans (½ c) continued:				
Beans, cooked whole, drained	120	3	350	1ST+½FAT
Black Beans, whole	120	2	250	1ST+½FAT
Toppings:				
Avocado, ¼	78	8	5	1½FAT
Avocado, ⅛ slice	40	4	3	1FAT
Avocado + Salsa Verde, 2T	35	3	180	½V+½FAT
Cheddar Cheese, ¼ c	120	10	176	2MFM
Cheddar Cheese, 2T not packed	57	5	88	1MFM
Enchilada Sauce (red or green), 2T	15	$0.^8$	130	FREE
Cheese Sauce (Queso), 2T	100	8	580	½HFM+1FAT
Guacamole, ¼ c	110	10	420	2FAT
Hot Sauce, 1t	0	0	20	FREE
Jalapeño, 1	20	0	3	FREE
Mole Sauce, 2T	200	13	480	1CHO+2½FAT
Olives, ea	5	0	30	FREE
Picante Sauce, 2T	10	0	220	FREE
Pico de Gallo, 2T	15	1	150	FREE
Salsa Verde (Green Sauce), 2T	10	0	150	FREE
Salsa, 2T	10	0	150	½V
Sour Cream, 2 T	52	5	12	1FAT

To estimate meat portions, note that 3 oz meat is the size of a deck of cards.

	Calories	Fat (g)	Sodium (mg)	Exchanges
Lean Meats (1 oz):				
Chicken Fajita Meat, white	35	2	250	1VLM
Chicken Fajita Meat, dark	55	$3.^5$	250	1VLM
Chicken Breast, marinated & grilled	35	2	150	1VLM
Shrimp, marinated & grilled (3)	35	1	200	1VLM
Medium Fat Meats (1 oz):				
Beef Fajita Meat, trimmed	70	$4.^3$	250	1MFM
High Fat Meats (1 oz):				
Beef Fajita Meat, untrimmed	90	7	250	1HFM
Beef Taco Meat, about ¼ c	90	7	275	1HFM
Cheddar or Jack Cheese, ¼ c loosely packed	110	9	175	1HFM
Chorizo (Mexican sausage)	105	10	250	1HFM

Mexican Foods (continued)

	Calories	Fat (g)	Sodium (mg)	Exchanges
Entrees:				
Arroz Con Pollo, 2 c	405	14	1600	2½ST+1V+2LM+ 1½FAT
Soft Burritos: Bean & Cheese, 6½"	300	12	850	2ST+1HFM+1FAT
Bean & Beef Burritos, 1	280	10	820	2ST+1HFM+½FAT
Chicken Burritos, 1	260	7	730	2ST+1MFM+1FAT
Chicken Enchiladas, 2	260	11	1110	1½ST+3LM+1FAT
Cheese Enchiladas, 2	480	32	900	1½ST+3HFM+1FAT
Beef Fajita – 1½ oz trimmed meat in a 6½" flour tortilla	205	9	575	1ST+1½MFM+½FAT
Beef Fajita – 2 oz trimmed meat in a 8" flour tortilla	290	14	850	1½ST+2MFM+1FAT
Chicken Fajita – 1½ oz white meat in a 6½" flour tortilla	160	6	575	1ST+1½VLM+½FAT
Chicken Fajita – 2 oz white meat in a 8" flour tortilla	220	9	850	1½ST+2MFM+1FAT
Shrimp Fajita – 5 marinated shrimp in a 6½" flour tortilla	160	5	500	1ST+1½VLM+½FAT
Shrimp Fajita – 7 marinated shrimp in a 8" flour tortilla	220	7	750	1½ST+2VLM+1FAT
Quesadilla, 6½"	430	24	760	2ST+2HFM+1FAT
Chicken Quesadilla, 6½"	465	26	1010	2ST+2HFM+1LM+ 1FAT
Quesadilla, 10"	960	52	1620	4ST+4HFM+3FAT
Chicken Quesadilla, 10"	1030	56	2120	4ST+4HFM+2LM+ 3FAT
Taco w/beef & cheese, 2 small	395	27	870	1ST+3HFM+½FAT
Tamales, 4	350	17	500	2ST+1HFM+2FAT
Taquito filled w/shredded beef, 5	350	12	460	2½ST+1HFM+1FAT
Bean & Cheese Tostada, 3 @ 4½"	465	23	630	1ST+3HFM+1FAT
Desserts:				
Flan, ½ c w/caramel topping	290	8	110	1VLM+3CHO+1½FAT
Soppapilla, 1 piece	95	5	50	½ST+½CHO+1FAT
Honey, 1T	64	0	0	1CHO
Fruit Filled Chimichanga fried w/ caramel topping	660	29	600	1½ST+2FR+3CHO+ 6FAT

Your Favorite Restaurants

CHI-CHI'S®

	Calories	Fat (g)	Sodium (mg)	Exchanges
Low Fat Chicken Soft Taco (two grilled soft tacos, served with Spanish rice, Mexi-Veggies, and Salsa)	692	7.[4]	1379	5ST+3V+4LM
Low Fat Chicken Enchiladas (two soft flour tortillas filled with chicken, served with Spanish rice and Mexi-Veggies)	688	18.[6]	2325	5ST+3V+2LM+2½FAT

EL CHICO®

	Calories	Fat (g)	Sodium (mg)	Exchanges
Tablano Chicken Salad	na	6	na	na
Santa Fe Chicken Burrito	na	8	na	na
Light Chicken Fajitas	na	10	na	na

Other tips: The Tortilla Soup can be requested without avocado and cheese for fewer calories and fat. Frijoles Rancheros (vegetarian beans) are available a la carte or instead of the usual refried beans.

The leanest salads are the Chicken Fajita Salad and Toblano Chicken Salad. The Chicken Fajita Salad includes 5 oz (raw weight) chicken and 1 oz of cheddar cheese. Request corn or flour tortillas instead of the fried flour tortilla wedges. Ask for corn or flour tortillas on the side instead of the fried flour tortilla shell. Request guacamole on the side and salsa for a low calorie dressing. A Light Ranch Dressing is also available.

EL POLLO LOCO®

	Calories	Fat (g)	Sodium (mg)	Exchanges
Chicken:				
Breast, 3 oz±	160	6	390	3½LM
Leg, 1¾ oz±	90	5	150	1½LM
Thigh, 2 oz±	180	12	230	2MFM
Wing, 1½ oz±	110	6	220	1½LM
± edible portion				
Tortillas:				
Flour Tortilla, 1 oz each	90	3	224	1ST+½FAT
Corn Tortilla, 1 oz each	70	1	35	1ST
Side Dishes:				
Cole Slaw, 5 oz	160	12	269	2V+2½FAT
Corn-on-Cob, 5½"	146	2	18	2ST

EL POLLO LOCO® (continued)

	Calories	Fat (g)	Sodium (mg)	Exchanges
Side Dishes continued:				
French Fries, 4.[4] oz	323	14	330	3ST+3FAT
Pinto Beans, 6 oz	185	4	744	1ST+1MFM
Potato Salad, 6 oz	256	14	527	2ST+3FAT
Smokey Black Beans, 5 oz	255	13	609	2ST+2FAT
Spanish Rice, 4 oz	130	3	397	1½ST
Side Buffet (selected restaurants):				
Broccoli Slaw	203	17	365	3V+3FAT
Crispy Green Beans	41	2	667	1V+½FAT
Cucumber Salad	34	0	11	1V
Fiesta Corn	152	6	397	1½ST+1FAT
Cornbread Stuffing	281	12	832	2½ST+2FAT
Gravy	14	0	139	FREE
Honey Glazed Carrots	104	6	403	½CHO+1V+1FAT
Lime Parfait	125	3	107	2CHO
Macaroni & Cheese	238	12	919	1ST+1MFM+2FAT
Mashed Potatoes	97	1	369	1½ST
Rainbow Pasta Salad	157	1	533	2ST
Southwest Cole Slaw	178	13	267	½ST+1V+3FAT
Sliced Apples	146	0	139	1CHO+1FR
Burritos:				
BRC	482	15	1250	4½ST+1MFM+1FAT
Classic Chicken	556	22	1499	4ST+3MFM
Grilled Steak	705	32	1689	4ST+4MFM+2FAT
Loco Grande	632	26	1649	4½ST+3½MFM+1FAT
Smokey Black Bean	566	22	1337	4½ST+1MFM+3FAT
Spicy Hot Chicken	559	22	1503	4ST+3MFM
Whole Wheat Chicken	592	26	1199	4ST+2½MFM+2FAT
Specialties:				
Veggie Bowl	388	7	1165	4ST+1½V+1FAT
Steak Bowl	616	26	1743	4ST+4LM+2FAT
Chicken Soft Taco	224	12	585	1ST+2MFM
Flame-Broiled Chicken Salad	167	5	765	3VLM+2V
Garden Salad	29	0	20	1V
Light Italian Dressing, 2 oz	25	1	990	FREE
Ranch Dressing, 2 oz	350	39	500	8FAT
1000 Island Dressing, 2 oz	270	27	460	6FAT
Bleu Cheese Dressing, 2 oz	300	32	590	6FAT
Pollo Bowl	504	13	2068	4ST+4LM+1V
Taco al Carbon – Chicken	265	12	223	2ST+1HFM
Taco al Carbon – Steak	394	22	473	2ST+2HFM
Taquito	370	17	690	3ST+1MFM+2FAT

EL POLLO LOCO® (continued)

	Calories	Fat (g)	Sodium (mg)	Exchanges
Specialties continued:				
Tostado Salad - Chicken, no shell, no sour cream	332	14	1280	2ST+4½VLM
Tostado Salad - Steak, no shell, no sour cream	525	31	1206	2ST+5MFM
Shell	440	27	610	3ST+5FAT
Condiments:				
Guacamole, 1.⁷⁵ oz	52	3	280	1V+½FAT
Jalapeño Hot Sauce, 1 pkt	5	0	110	FREE
Light Sour Cream, 1 oz	45	3	25	1FAT
Salsa, 1 oz, House	6	0	96	FREE
Verde	6	0	90	FREE
Picante	5	0	66	FREE
Chipotle	8	0	156	FREE
Pico de Gallo	11	1	131	FREE
Desserts:				
Churro, 1¼ oz	149	8	160	1ST+1½FAT
Flan	220	2	140	3CHO
Foster's Freeze	38	1	na	na

EL TORITO

	Calories	Fat (g)	Sodium (mg)	Exchanges
Lite Specialties:				
Sonoro Burrito	625	20	1598	na
Vegetable Fajitas	505	7	1265	na
Chicken Fajitas Lite with 3 Flour Tortillas	550	7	1233	na
Chicken Quesadilla Lite	530	19	800	na

TACO BELL®

	Calories	Fat (g)	Sodium (mg)	Exchanges
Tacos & Tostadas:				
Taco	170	10	280	½ST+1MFM+1FAT
Soft Taco	210	10	530	1ST+1MFM+1FAT
Taco Supreme®	220	13	290	1ST+1MFM+1½FAT
Soft Taco Supreme®	260	14	540	1½ST+1MFM+1½FAT
DOUBLE DECKER™ Taco	340	15	700	2ST+1MFM+2½FAT
DOUBLE DECKER™ Taco Supreme®	390	18	710	2ST+1MFM+3½FAT
Steak Soft Taco	200	7	500	1ST+1MFM+1FAT
BLT Soft Taco	340	23	610	1ST+1MFM+4FAT

TACO BELL® (continued)

	Calories	Fat (g)	Sodium (mg)	Exchanges
Tacos & Tostadas continued:				
Kid's Soft Taco Roll-Up	290	16	790	1½ST+1MFM+2FAT
Chicken Soft Taco	250	11	380	1½ST+1MFM+1FAT
Kid's Chicken Soft Taco	240	11	320	1½ST+1MFM+1FAT
Burritos:				
Bean Burrito	380	12	1140	3ST+1MFM+1½FAT
Burrito Supreme®	440	18	1220	3ST+1MFM+3FAT
Big BEEF Burrito Supreme®	520	23	1450	3ST+2MFM+3FAT
7-Layer Burrito	540	24	1310	4ST+1MFM+3FAT
Chili Cheese Burrito	330	13	880	2ST+1MFM+2FAT
Chicken Club Burrito	540	31	1290	2½ST+2MFM+4FAT
Bacon Cheeseburger Burrito	560	30	1360	2½ST+3MFM+3FAT
Specialties:				
Tostada	300	14	700	2ST+1MFM+1½FAT
Mexican Pizza	570	36	1050	2½ST+2MFM+5FAT
BIG BEEF MexiMelt®	300	16	860	1ST+2MFM+1½FAT
Taco Salad with Salsa	840	52	1670	3ST+2V+3MFM+7FAT
Taco Salad w/Salsa, w/out Shell	420	21	1420	1ST+2V+3MFM+1FAT
Cheese Quesadilla	370	20	730	2ST+2MFM+1FAT
Chicken Quesadilla	420	22	1020	2ST+3MFM+1FAT
Border Wraps™:				
Steak Fajita Wrap™	460	21	1130	3ST+2MFM+1½FAT
Chicken Fajita Wrap™	460	21	1220	3ST+2MFM+1½FAT
Veggie Fajita Wrap™	420	19	920	3ST+1V+1MFM+ 1½FAT
Steak Fajita Wrap™ Supreme	510	25	1140	3ST+2MFM+2½FAT
Chicken Fajita Wrap™ Supreme	500	25	1230	3ST+2MFM+2½FAT
Veggie Fajita Wrap™ Supreme	460	23	930	3ST+1V+1MFM+ 2½FAT
Nachos and Sides:				
Nachos	310	18	540	2ST+3FAT
BIG BEEF Nachos Supreme™	430	24	720	2½ST+1MFM+3½FAT
Nachos BellGrande®	740	39	1200	5ST+1MFM+6FAT
Pintos'N Cheese	190	8	690	1ST+1MFM+½FAT
Mexican Rice	190	10	510	1½ST+1½FAT
Cinnamon Twists	140	6	190	1ST+1FAT
Sauces and Condiments:				
Green Sauce	5	0	150	FREE
Guacamole	35	3	140	1FAT
Hot Taco Sauce	0	0	85	FREE
Mild Taco Sauce	0	0	75	FREE

TACO BELL® (continued)

	Calories	Fat (g)	Sodium (mg)	Exchanges
Sauces and Condiments continued:				
Nacho Cheese Sauce	120	10	470	½ST+2FAT
Picante Sauce	0	0	110	FREE
Pico de Gallo	5	0	65	FREE
Red Sauce	10	0	260	FREE
Salsa	25	0	490	1V
Cheddar Cheese	30	2	45	½FAT
Pepper Jack Cheese	25	2	105	½FAT
Sour Cream	40	4	10	1FAT
Drinks:				
Lipton® Brisk Iced Tea, sweetened	140	0	60	1¾CHO
Orange Juice	80	0	0	1½FR

TACO JOHN'S

	Calories	Fat (g)	Sodium (mg)	Exchanges
Burritos:				
Bean Burrito	387	11	866	3ST+ 1LM+1½ FAT
Beef Burrito	449	20	863	3ST+2MFM+2FAT
Combination Burrito	418	16	865	3ST+1½MFM+1½FAT
Meat & Potato Burrito	503	24	1341	3ST+1MFM+4FAT
Ranch Burrito	447	23	804	3ST+1MFM+3½FAT
Super Burrito	465	19	922	3ST+1½MFM+2FAT
Fajitas:				
Chicken Fajita Burrito	370	12	1536	3ST+1½LM+1½FAT
Chicken Fajita Salad in Bowl, no dressing	557	33	1541	3ST+2LM+5FAT
Chicken Fajita Softshell	200	7	903	1½ST+1LM+1FAT
Kid's Meals:				
Kid's Meal, with Crispy Taco	579	34	789	3ST+1MFM+6FAT
Kid's Meal, with Softshell Taco	617	33	1037	4ST+1MFM+5½FAT
Platter:				
Chimichanga Platter	979	38	2341	8ST+2HFM+4FAT
Double Enchilada Platter	967	42	1921	7ST+3HFM+3½FAT
Sampler Platter	1406	61	2875	10ST+5HFM+4FAT
Smothered Burrito Platter	1031	40	2351	8ST+2HFM+5FAT
Special Features:				
Mexi Rolls® with Nacho Cheese	863	48	1392	4½ST+2½HFM+5½FAT
Potato Olés Bravo®	579	38	1550	3ST+1HFM+6FAT
Sierra Chicken Fillet Sandwich	534	29	1406	2½ST+3MFM+3FAT
Super Nachos	919	56	1484	4½ST+1½HFM+9FAT
Taco Salad in Bowl, no dressing	584	38	766	2½ST+2HFM+3FAT

TACO JOHN'S (continued)

	Calories	Fat (g)	Sodium (mg)	Exchanges
Tacos:				
Crispy Tacos	182	11	272	½ST+1HFM+½FAT
Softshell Tacos	230	10	520	1½ST+1HFM+½FAT
Taco Bravo®	346	14	677	2½ST+1HFM+1FAT
Taco Burger	280	12	576	1½ST+1½HFM
Side Orders & Extras:				
Beans, "refried"	357	9	1032	3ST+1VLM+1½FAT
Chili	350	21	865	1ST+2½VLM+3½FAT
Mexican Rice	567	18	1293	2½ST+3½FAT
Nachos	333	21	611	1½ST+½HFM+3½FAT
Nacho Cheese	120	10	600	1HFM+½FAT
Potato Olés®	363	23	964	2ST+4½FAT
Potato Olés® Large	484	30	1285	3ST+6FAT
Potato Olés®, with Nacho Cheese	483	33	1564	2½ST+6½FAT
Sour Cream	60	5	15	1FAT
Desserts:				
Churro	147	8	160	1ST+1½FAT
Apple Flauta	84	1	72	1ST
Cherry Flauta	143	4	110	1½ST+1FAT
Cream Cheese Flauta	181	8	135	1½ST+1½FAT
Choco Taco	320	17	100	1½CHO+3½FAT
Italian Ice	80	0	5	1CHO

Middle Eastern Restaurants

Chapter Contents:

■ Appetizers & Salads
■ Entrees
■ Accompaniments
■ Desserts
■ Nutritional Information for Middle Eastern Foods

Middle Eastern cuisine includes foods which are native to Greece, Syria, Lebanon, Iran, Iraq, Turkey, Armenia, and surrounding areas. Some of the staples common to this region include eggplant, olives, olive oil, wheat, rice, legumes, yogurt, dates, figs, and lamb. Plain yogurt, a frequent ingredient in sauces and salads, is most commonly homemade with whole milk. Tahini or sesame seed butter (made of crushed sesame seeds, lemon juice, and spices) is a high fat ingredient added to a variety of dishes. Rice is served with most meats.

Frequently used spices are parsley, mint, cilantro, and oregano. The common Indian spices such as cinnamon, coriander, cumin, and ginger are also used. Middle Eastern food is generally healthy food with a few exceptions. Below are some general guidelines for dining lean in Middle Eastern restaurants.

✔ **Avoid fried foods** such as falafel.

✔ **Request "no oil" to be added on top of the dishes.** You may not be able to avoid the olive oil that is frequently used in the preparation of Middle Eastern dishes. But, you can always ask for "no oil to be added" on top of the dishes prior to serving.

✔ **Request tomato sauce rather than lemon & butter sauce or cream sauce.**

Appetizers & Salads

✓ **Choose these lower fat starters to your meal:**

■ **Avgolemono soup** - traditional Greek soup made with chicken broth, rice, vegetables, lemon, and eggs. Enjoy this high fat soup only if lower fat vegetarian (rather than meat) dishes are chosen for the rest of the meal.

■ **Falafel** - fried patty consisting of mashed fava beans and chick peas.

■ **Fried Calamari** - fried squid

■ **Fish Roe Dip**

■ **Kasseri Casserole** - fried Kasseri cheese served with lemon & butter sauce

■ **Spanikopita** - spinach & feta cheese pie layered with phyllo dough

■ **Taramolsalata** - caviar blended with olive oil and lemon juice. Served with pita bread.

✓ **Limit these higher fat appetizers and salads:**

■ **Avgolemono soup** - traditional Greek soup made with chicken broth, rice, vegetables, lemon, and eggs. Enjoy this high fat soup only if lower fat vegetarian (rather than meat) dishes are chosen for the rest of the meal.

■ **Falafel** - fried patty consisting of mashed fava beans and chick peas.

■ **Fried Calamari** - fried squid

■ **Fish Roe Dip**

■ **Kasseri Casserole** - fried Kasseri cheese served with lemon & butter sauce

■ **Spanikopita** - spinach & feta cheese pie layered with phyllo dough

■ **Taramolsalata** - caviar blended with olive oil and lemon juice. Served with pita bread.

Entrees

✓ **Choose chicken rather than beef or lamb** (such as a chicken pita sandwich rather than gyros made with beef and lamb)

✓ **Meat dishes rather than casseroles.** Casseroles are typically prepared with ground meat and have added sauces.

✓ **Ask for the sauces on the side** including the commonly served tzateki sauce. Casseroles are made in advance and, therefore, sauces can't be substituted. Tomato sauces are leaner than the cream sauces.

✓ **Choose these lower fat entrees:**

- **Chicken in pita bread**

- **Dolma** - boiled stuffed grape leaves (green leaves of a grape vine stuffed with a rice, meat, and spice mixture).

- **Lah Me June** - Armenian pizza topped with ground meat, tomatoes, and spices

- **Kafta** - grilled ground beef with spices

- **Kibbeh** - cracked wheat, meat, sautéed onions, and pine nuts

- **Sheik el Mahski** - baked eggplant stuffed with ground lamb, pine nuts, onions, spices, and tomato sauce

- **Shish Kebobs -** chunks of meat and vegetables cooked on a skewer. Chicken kabobs would be the meat leanest choice. Request without the butter for basting.

- **Souvlaki** - marinated and grilled fish or chicken. Often served with tzateki sauce

✓ **Limit these higher fat entrees:**

- **Falafel** - fried patty consisting of mashed fava beans and chick peas

- **Gyros -** beef and lamb cut thin and stuffed into a pita pocket or other bread. Ask for the tzateki dressing, a spicy yogurt-based sauce, to be served on the side.

- **Moussaka** - a casserole of layered eggplant, lamb, and cheese topped with a white sauce

- **Spanikopita** - spinach and feta cheese pie made with phyllo dough

- **Pasticchio** - baked macaroni with ground beef and eggs, topped with a creamy sauce

■ **Fried Kalamari** - squid

■ **Omelets** - 3 eggs combined with feta cheese, sausage and/or other meat

■ **Loukanika** - sausage

Accompaniments

✔ **Choose these low fat accompaniments:**

■ **Pita bread -** a flat round bread with a hollow center that is low in fat. It is eaten as an accompaniment to a meat or stuffed as a sandwich. Be aware, pita bread is sometimes served buttered and grilled; this would be much higher in fat.

■ **Couscous** - cooked cracked wheat

■ **Steamed rice**

■ **Rice pilaf** - a cooked rice dish made with sautéed vegetables and seasoned with butter and saffron. Although higher in fat than steamed rice, it is still relatively lean.

■ **Steamed vegetables**

Desserts

✔ **Choose fresh fruit or rice pudding** (rizogalo).

✔ **Share baklava.** This sweet, rich dessert is made up of layers of phyllo dough, butter, honey, and nuts. If you must order it, share your dessert with others.

Nutritional Information for Middle Eastern Foods

Middle Eastern Foods				
	Calories	Fat (g)	Sodium (mg)	Exchanges
Appetizers & Salads:				
Falafel Patties, 3 oz fried	155	10	na	1ST+2FAT
Fattoush, 1½ c w/out dressing	95	1	na	2V+½ST
1T dressing	85	9	145	2FAT
Greek Salad - 1 c of lettuce only	25	0	5	1V
+3 Kalamata olives	39	3	435	¾FAT
+1 oz feta cheese	75	6	315	1MFM
+2T lemon/herb dressing	170	18	290	3½FAT
Greek Salad w/olives, cheese, & dressing	309	27	1045	1V+1MFM+4½FAT
Hummus, ¼ c	100	5	300	1ST+1FAT
Humus, ¼ c+1T oil	220	18	300	1ST+3½FAT
Lentil Soup, 8 oz	190	5	1300	1½ST+1VLM+1FAT

Middle Eastern Foods (continued)

	Calories	Fat (g)	Sodium (mg)	Exchanges
Appetizers & Salads continued:				
Pine Nuts, 1 oz or ¼ c	161	17	20	1LM+3½FAT
Stuffed Eggplant, 1 slice	270	23	na	1V+1MFM+3½FAT
Tabouli Salad, ½ c	140	6	na	1ST+½V+1FAT
Tahini (sesame butter), 1T	90	8	17	1½FAT
Yogurt & Cucumber Salad, ½ c	110	7	na	1V+¼WhMk+1FAT
Entrees:				
Dolmades, 3	220	9	na	1V+1ST+1MFM+1FAT
2 T lemon & egg sauce	175	19	250	4FAT
Moussaka, 4" X 4"	420	24	730	½ST+2V+3MFM+2FAT
Gyro, 4 oz beef & lamb on pita bread w/out sauce	505	21	na	2½ST+4MFM
Tzatziki sauce, 2T	45	3.^{5}	na	½FAT
Gyro, 4 oz beef & lamb on pita bread w/4T tzatziki sauce	595	28	na	2½ST+4MFM+1FAT
Chicken on Pita, 4 oz chicken breast on pita bread	310	3	na	2½ST+4VLM
w/f1 oz feta cheese & 1T olive oil	505	22	na	2½ST+4VLM+4FAT
Greek-style Lamb w/orzo, 4 oz lamb +2 oz orzo	505	25	na	4MFM+2ST+1FAT
Shish Kebab, 1 skewer w/2 oz beef & vegetables basted	240	14	na	2MFM+1V+1FAT
Shish Kebab, 1 skewer w/2 oz chicken & vegetables basted	190	11	na	2LM+1V+1FAT
Lamb & artichoke w/lemon sauce	310	11	na	
Baked Chicken Quarter, Greek Style w/potatoes, onions, lemon sauce	550	35	na	3MFM+1½ST+1V+ 4FAT
Sheik el Mahshi, 1 c	175	10	na	1MFM+2V+1FAT
Kibbeh, 1 c	225	10	na	1ST+1MFM+1V+1FAT
Accompaniments:				
Rice, plain, ½ c	120	0	4	1½ST
Rice Pilaf, ½ c	160	4	520	1½ST+¼V+1FAT
Couscous, plain, ½ c	170	0	4	2ST
Couscous, buttered, ½ c	210	5	na	2ST+1FAT
Pita Bread, 6½" round diameter	190	1.^{5}	510	2½ST
Hummus, 2T	50	2.^{5}	150	½ST
Desserts:				
Yogurt, plain whole, ¼ c	35	2	30	¼WhMk
Baklava, 2" X 2"	440	30	na	2CHO+6FAT

Index

To schedule Dr. Joanne Lichten to speak to
your company, group, or association
call 1-888-431-LEAN

Topics include:

How to Stay Healthy & Fit on the Road

Dining Lean

Keeping Your Energy Up All Day Long

There's No Such Thing as Willpower: Getting from "I know it" to "I do it"

Stress Solutions for Busy People

Swimming in a Sea of Priorities: How to Get Your Life in Balance

Order Form

For credit card orders
or to inquire about quantity discounts
call 1-888-431-LEAN

_____ copies of Dining Lean @ $16.95 each _____

If shipping to Texas add 6¼% ($1.06 ea)_____

Shipping cost $4/book_____

Total _____

Name:_____

Address:_____

City:_____ State:_____ Zip:_____

Send check or money order to:
Nutrifit Publishing
PO Box 690452
Houston, TX 77269-0452

To schedule Dr. Joanne Lichten to speak to
your company, group, or association
call 1-888-431-LEAN

Topics include:

How to Stay Healthy & Fit on the Road

Dining Lean

Keeping Your Energy Up All Day Long

**There's No Such Thing as Willpower: Getting
from "I know it" to "I do it"**

Stress Solutions for Busy People

**Swimming in a Sea of Priorities: How to Get
Your Life in Balance**

Order Form

**For credit card orders
or to inquire about quantity discounts
call 1-888-431-LEAN**

_____ copies of Dining Lean @ $16.95 each _____

If shipping to Texas add 6¼% ($1.06 ea)_____

Shipping cost $4/book_____

Total _____

Name:_____

Address:_____

City:_____ State:_____ Zip:_____

Send check or money order to:
Nutrifit Publishing
PO Box 690452
Houston, TX 77269-0452